D1429307

Visual Diagnosis and Treatment in
Pediatrics

Third Edition

Editor-in-Chief
Esther K. Chung, MD, MPH
Professor
Department of Pediatrics
Sidney Kimmel Medical College of Thomas Jefferson University
Jefferson Pediatrics/Nemours-Philadelphia
Philadelphia, Pennsylvania
Alfred I. duPont Hospital for Children
Wilmington, Delaware

Associate Editors
Lee R. Atkinson-McEvoy, MD
Clinical Professor of Pediatrics
Director of UCSF Pediatric Primary Care Clinic
Associate Chief General Pediatrics
Associate Residency Program Director
Department of Pediatrics
University of California, San Francisco School of Medicine
San Francisco, California

Naline L. Lai, MD
Primary Care Attending Physician
The Children's Hospital of Philadelphia Care Network-Newtown
Newtown, Pennsylvania
Department of Pediatrics
St. Mary Medical Center
Langhorne, Pennsylvania
Department of Pediatrics
Doylestown Hospital
Doylestown, Pennsylvania

Michelle Terry, MD
Clinical Professor of Pediatrics
University of Washington School of Medicine
Seattle, Washington

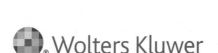

. Wolters Kluwer

Philadelphia • Baltimore • New York • London
Buenos Aires • Hong Kong • Sydney • Tokyo

Acquisitions Editor: Jamie M. Elfrank
Product Development Editor: Ashley Fischer
Editorial Assistant: Brian Convery
Production Project Manager: Alicia Jackson
Design Coordinator: Elaine Kasmer
Manufacturing Coordinator: Beth Welsh
Marketing Manager: Stephanie Kindlick
Prepress Vendor: S4Carlisle Publishing Services

Third edition

Copyright © 2015 Wolters Kluwer Health

© 2010 by Lippincott Williams & Wilkins, a Wolters Kluwer business
© 2006 by Lippincott Williams & Wilkins

9   8   7   6   5   4   3   2   1

Printed in China

Library of Congress Cataloging-in-Publication Data

Visual diagnosis and treatment in pediatrics / editor in chief, Esther K. Chung ; associate editors, Lee R. Atkinson-McEvoy, Naline Lai, Michelle Terry. — Third edition.
    p. ; cm.
  Includes bibliographical references and index.
  ISBN 978-1-4511-9118-9 (alk. paper)
  I. Chung, Esther K., editor.   II. Atkinson-McEvoy, Lee R., editor.   III. Lai, Naline, editor.   IV. Terry, Michelle, editor.
  [DNLM: 1. Pediatrics—Handbooks.   2. Child.   3. Diagnosis, Differential—Handbooks.   4. Medical History Taking—Handbooks.   5. Physical Examination—Handbooks. WS 39]
  RJ50
  618.92'0075—dc23

2014028963

LWW.com

We dedicate this book to:

*My parents, Dr. Okhyung Kang and the late Dr. Ed Baik Chung;
my husband, Dennis; and my daughters, Marissa and Emma*
—Esther

*My parents, Patrick and Beverly Atkinson; my husband Michael; and
my children Amara, Mason, and Noah*
—Lee

My advisors and family, in particular my children Emily, Abigail, and Michael
—Naline

*My mother, Mercedes Riley Terry, and for all of the lessons in and
out of the library*
—Michelle

Photo Credits

Bethlehem Abebe-Wolpaw, MD
HS Assistant Clinical Professor
Department of Pediatrics
University of California
San Francisco, California

Joyce A. Adams, MD, FAAP, FSAM
Clinical Professor of Pediatrics
Division of General Academic Pediatrics
and Adolescent Medicine
University of California-San Diego
San Diego, California

Benjamin Alouf, MD
Medical Director
Aetna Northeast Regional Care
Management
Bluebell, Pennsylvania

Lee R. Atkinson-McEvoy, MD
Clinical Professor of Pediatrics
Director of UCSF Pediatric
Primary Care Clinic
Associate Chief General Pediatrics
Associate Residency Program Director
Department of Pediatrics
University of California, San Francisco
School of Medicine
San Francisco, California

M. Douglas Baker, MD
Director of Pediatric Emergency
Medicine
Vice Chairman for Community
Outreach
Visiting Professor of Pediatrics
Johns Hopkins Children's Center
Baltimore, Maryland

Douglas A. Barnes, MD
Chief of Staff, Pediatric
Orthopaedic Surgery
Shriners Hospitals for Children
Houston, Texas

Roy Benaroch, MD
Adjunct Assistant Professor
Pediatrics
Emory University
Atlanta, Georgia

Dean John Bonsall, MD, MS, FACS
Associate Professor
Department of Ophthalmology
University of Cincinnati
Associate Professor
Division of Pediatric Ophthalmology
Cincinnati Children's Hospital
Cincinnati, Ohio

Julie A. Boom, MD
Associate Professor
Department of Pediatrics
Baylor College of Medicine
Director
Infant and Childhood Immunization
Center for Vaccine Awareness and
Research
Attending Physician
Residents' Primary Care Group Clinic
Texas Children's Hospital
Houston, Texas

Mary L. Brandt, MD
Baylor College of Medicine
Houston, Texas

Brooke Burkey, MD
Instructor of Surgery and Pediatrics
Drexel University College
of Medicine
Attending Plastic Surgeon
Section of Plastic Surgery
St. Christopher's Hospital for Children
Philadelphia, Pennsylvania

Gerardo Cabrera-Meza, MD
Baylor College of Medicine
Houston, Texas

Esther K. Chung, MD, MPH
Professor
Department of Pediatrics
Sidney Kimmel Medical College
of Thomas Jefferson University
Jefferson Pediatrics/
Nemours-Philadelphia
Philadelphia, Pennsylvania
Alfred I. duPont Hospital
for Children
Wilmington, Delaware

Sophia M. Chung, MD
Professor
Department of Ophthalmology
St. Louis University School of Medicine
St. Louis, Missouri

Jayme L. Coffman, MD
Medical Director, CARE Team
Cook Children's Medical Center
Fort Worth, Texas

Steven P. Cook, MD
Medical Director
Division of Otolaryngology,
Department of Surgery
Alfred I. duPont Hospital
for Children
Wilmington, Delaware

Kathleen Cronan, MD
Associate Professor
Department of Pediatrics
Sidney Kimmel Medical Center
Philadelphia, Pennsylvania
Attending Physician
Department of Pediatrics
Division of Pediatric Emergency
Medicine
Nemours/Alfred I. duPont Hospital
for Children
Wilmington, Delaware

Theodore P. Croll, DDS
Private Practice
Doylestown Pediatric
Dentistry, P.C.
Doylestown, Pennsylvania

Carrie Ann R. Cusack, MD
Associate Professor
Department of Dermatology
Drexel University College
of Medicine
Philadelphia, Pennsylvania

George A. Datto, III, MD
Instructor
Department of Pediatrics
Sidney Kimmel Medical Center
of Thomas Jefferson University
Philadelphia, Pennsylvania
Pediatrician
Department of Pediatrics
Alfred I. duPont Hospital for Children
Wilmington, Delaware

Wellington Davis, MD
Assistant Professor of Pediatrics
and Surgery
Drexel University College of Medicine
Philadelphia, Pennsylvania

Allan R. De Jong, MD
Clinical Professor
Department of Pediatrics
Sidney Kimmel Medical Center
Thomas Jefferson University
Philadelphia, Pennsylvania
Medical Director, Children at Risk
Evaluation (CARE) Program
Department of Pediatrics
Nemours/Alfred I. duPont Hospital for
Children
Wilmington, Delaware

Christopher D. Derby, MD
Cardiothoracic Surgeon
Nemours Cardiac Center
Alfred I. duPont Hospital for Children
Wilmington, Delaware

Ellen S. Deutsch, MD
ENT-Otolaryngologist, Ped
Otolaryngology (ENT)
St. Christopher's Hospital for Children
Wilmington, Delaware

Michael C. DiStefano, MD
Assistant Professor of Pediatrics
University of Colorado-Denver
Children's Hospital Colorado-Anschutz
Medical Campus
Denver, Colorado

Jan Edwin Drutz, MD
Professor of Pediatrics
Department of Pediatrics
Baylor College of Medicine
Director of the Continuity Clinic
Teaching Program
Department of Pediatrics
Texas Children's Hospital
Houston, Texas

T. Ernesto Figueroa, MD
Clinical Associate Professor
Department of Urology
Thomas Jefferson University
Philadelphia, Pennsylvania
Chief, Division of Pediatric Urology
Alfred I. duPont Hospital for Children
Wilmington, Delaware

Christine Finck, MD
Section of General Surgery
St. Christopher's Hospital for Children
Philadelphia, Pennsylvania

Darren M. Fiore, MD
Assistant Clinical Professor
Division of Pediatric Hospital Medicine
Department of Pediatrics
University of California, San Francisco
Benioff Children's Hospital
San Francisco, California

Susan A. Fisher-Owens, MD, MPH
Associate Professor
Department of Pediatrics
University of California
San Francisco, California

Brian J. Forbes, MD, PhD
Attending Surgeon
Associate Professor of Ophthalmology,
Perelman School of Medicine at the
University of Pennsylvania
The Children's Hospital of Philadelphia
Philadelphia, Pennsylvania

Lourdes Forster, MD, FAAP
Assistant Professor of Clinical
Pediatrics
Department of Pediatrics
University of Miami, Miller School of
Medicine
Miami, Florida

Martin Fried, MD
Pediatric Gastroenterologist
Jersey Shore University Medical
Center
Ocean, New Jersey
Neptune, New Jersey

Ilona J. Frieden, MD
Professor of Clinical Dermatology
Departments of Dermatology and
Pediatrics
University of California
San Francisco, California

Jeff Friedman, MD

John A. Germiller, MD, PhD
Attending Surgeon
Director of Clinical Research
Assistant Professor of
Otorhinolaryngology: Head and Neck
Surgery, Perelman School of Medicine
at the University of Pennsylvania
Philadelphia, Pennsylvania

Amy E. Gilliam, MD
Dermatologist
Department of Dermatology
Palo Alto Medical Foundation
Freemont, California

Scott M. Goldstein, MD
Oculoplastic and Aesthetic Surgeon
Wills Eye Hospital
Philadelphia, Pennsylvania

Vani V. Gopalareddy, MD
Division of Gastroenterology
Levine Children's Hospital
Carolinas Medical Center
Charlotte, North Carolina

Bettina M. Gyr, MD
Assistant Professor, Orthopaedics
Childress Institute
Wake Forest Baptist Health-Brenner's
Children's Hospital
Winston-Salem, North Carolina

Steven D. Handler, MD, MBE
Associate Director
Professor, Otorhinolaryngology-Head
and Neck Surgery
Perelman School of Medicine at the
University of Pennsylvania
The Children's Hospital
of Philadelphia
Philadelphia, Pennsylvania

Fernando L. Heinen, MD
Deutsches Hospital of Buenos
Aires
Buenos Aires, Argentina

Lior Heller, MD
Associate Professor
Baylor College of Medicine
Department of Surgery,
Plastic Surgery
Texas Children's Hospital
Houston, Texas

Martin J. Herman, MD
Associate Professor of Orthopedic
Surgery and Pediatrics
Drexel University College of Medicine
Attending Orthopedic Surgeon
St. Christopher's Hospital for Children
Philadelphia, Pennsylvania

Alejandro Hoberman, MD
Professor of Pediatrics
University of Pittsburgh School
of Medicine
Chief, Division of General Academic
Pediatrics
Children's Hospital of Pittsburgh
Pittsburgh, Pennsylvania

Larry H. Hollier, Jr., MD, FACS
Chief of Plastic Surgery
Baylor College of Medicine
Chief of Pediatric Plastic Surgery
Texas Children's Hospital
Houston, Texas

David A. Horvath, MD
Plastic Surgeon
Horvath Plastic and Cosmetic
Surgery Center
Abington, Pennsylvania

Glenn Isaacson, MD, FACS, FAAP
Professor, Otolaryngology-Head and
Neck Surgery
Assistant Professor, Pediatrics
Director, Pediatric Otolaryngology
Temple University-School of Medicine
Philadelphia, Pennsylvania

Jason R. Kaplan, DDS, MS
Kaplan Orthodontics
Dunwoody, Georgia

Douglas A. Katz, MD
Assistant Professor of Pediatrics-Surgery
Thomas Jefferson University Hospital
Philadelphia, Pennsylvania
duPont Hospital for Children
Wilmington, Delaware
Division of Pediatric General Surgery,
Department of Surgery
St. Christopher's Hospital for Children
Philadelphia, Pennsylvania

Hans B. Kersten, MD
Associate Professor of Pediatrics
Department of Pediatrics
Drexel University College of Medicine
Attending Physician
Department of General Pediatrics
St. Christopher's Hospital for Children
Philadelphia, Pennsylvania

Aida Z. Khanum, MD
Pediatrician
Houston Area Community Services
Houston, Texas

Shirley P. Klein, MD, FAAP
Pediatrician
Medical Group of Christiana Care
Wilmington Hospital Health Center
Wilmington, Delaware

Jean Labbé, MD
Professor of Pediatrics
Université Laval
Québec, Canada

Naline L. Lai, MD
Primary Care Attending Physician
The Children's Hospital of Philadelphia
Care Network-Newtown
Newtown, Pennsylvania
Department of Pediatrics
St. Mary Medical Center
Langhorne, Pennsylvania
Department of Pediatrics
Doylestown Hospital
Doylestown, Pennsylvania

Kevin P. Lally, MD, MS, FACS
A.G. McNeese, Chair in Pediatric
Surgery
Richard Andrassy Distinguished
Professor
Professor and Chairman
Department of Pediatric Surgery
University of Texas Medical Sciences
Center at Houston
Houston, Texas

Michael Lemper, DMD
Pediatric Dentist
Children's Dental Health
Chadds Ford, Pennsylvania
Lancaster County Pediatric Dentistry
Willow Street, Pennsylvania

Moise L. Levy, MD
Dermatology Specialist
Specially for Children Group
Dell Children's Medical Center of
Central Texas
Austin, Texas

John Loiselle, MD
Pediatric Emergency Medicine
Physician
Alfred I. duPont Hospital for Children
Wilmington, Delaware

Joseph Lopreiato, MD, MPH, FAAP
Dean for Simulation Education
Uniformed Services University of Health
Sciences
Bethesda, Maryland

Steven Manders, MD
Director of Pediatric Dermatology
Professor of Dermatology and Pediatric
Dermatology
Department of Dermatology
Dermatologist
Cooper University Healthcare
Camden, New Jersey
Virtua Marlton
Marlton, New Jersey

Gary Marshall, MD
Division Chief, Pediatric Infectious
Diseases
Department of
Pediatrics, Infectious Diseases
University Louisville School of Medicine
Louisville, Kentucky

Paul S. Matz, MD
Pediatrican
Advocare Haddon Pediatric Group
Haddon Heights, New Jersey

James W. McManaway, III, MD
Ophthalmologist
Hershey Pediatric Ophthalmology
Associates
Hershey, Pennsylvania

Denise W. Metry, MD
Associate Professor
Section of Pediatric Dermatology
and Pediatrics
Baylor College of Medicine
Houston, Texas

Monte D. Mills, MD, MS
Professor of Clinical Ophthalmology
Perelman School of Medicine at the
University of Pennsylvania
Chief, Division of Ophthalmology
The Children's Hopsital of Philadelphia
Philadelphia, Pennsylvania

Leonard B. Nelson, MD
Associate Professor of Ophthalmology
and Pediatrics
Ophthalmology
Sidney Kimmel Medical Center
Thomas Jefferson University
Philadelphia, Pennsylvania
Director
Wills Eye Strabismus Center
Wills Eye Institute
Philadelphia, Pennsylvania

Tony Olsen, MD
Senior Consultant
Department of Pediatrics
Naestved Hospital
Naestved, Denmark

Barry Oppenheim, MD
Pediatric Ophthalmologist
Bucks County Eye Group
Wrightstown, Pennsylvania

Eden Palmer
Medical Photographer
Vascular Anomalies Clinic
Seattle Children's Hospital

Jonathan Perkins, DO
Professor of Pediatric
Otolaryngology-Head & Neck Surgery
Director of Vascular Anomalies Program
Seattle Children's Hospital

William Phillips, MD
Baylor College of Medicine
Houston, Texas

Joseph Piatt, MD
Section of Neurosurgery
St. Christopher's Hospital for Children
Philadelphia, Pennsylvania

Hanah Raverby, MD
Temple University School of Medicine
Center for Urban and Bioethics and
Humanities
Philadelphia, Pennsylvania

Kenneth Rosenbaum, MD
Medical Genetics Doctor
Children's National Medical Center
Children's Hospital
Washington, DC

Amy Ross, MD
Dermatologist
Palm Harbor Dermatology
Palm Harbor, Florida

Denise A. Salerno, MD, FAAP
Professor of Clinical Pediatrics
Pediatrics Clerkship Director
Department of Pediatrics
Temple University School of Medicine
Philadelphia, Pennsylvania

Steven M. Selbst, MD
Professor
Department of Pediatrics
Sidney Kimmel Medical Center
Philadelphia, Pennsylvania
Vice-Chair for Education, Residency
Program Director
Department of Pediatrics
Nemours/Alfred I. duPont Hospital
for Children
Wilmington, Delaware

Philip T. Siu, MD
Instructor
Thomas Jefferson University Hospital
Associate Medical Director
Greater Philadelphia Health Action
Clinical Director
Chinatown Medical Services
Philadelphia, Pennsylvania

Peter Sol, MD
Deceased

Parul Patel Soni, MD, MPH
Assistant Professor of Pediatrics
Department of Pediatrics
Feinberg School of Medicine/
Northwestern University
Attending Physician
Emergency
Ann and Robert H. Laurie
Children's Hospital of Chicago
Chicago, Illinois

Julia L. Stevens, MD
Department of Opthalmology
University of Kentucky Chandler
Medical Center
Ophthalmologist
Central Baptist Eyes
Lexington, Kentucky

Valarie Stricklen, MD, FAAP
Pediatrician
The University of Toledo Medical Center
Toledo, Ohio

Sidney Sussman, MD
Pediatrican
Cooper University Hospital
Camden, New Jersey

Daniel R. Taylor, DO
Associate Professor
Department of Pediatrics
Drexel University College of Medicine
Philadelphia, Pennsylvania
General Pediatrician
General Pediatrics
St. Christopher's Hospital for Children
Philadelphia, Pennsylvania

Tom D. Thacher, MD
Department of Family Medicine
Mayo Clinic
Rochester, Minnesota

E. Douglas Thompson, Jr., MD
Assistant Professor
Department of Pediatrics
Drexel University College of Medicine
Chief of the Section of Hospital
Medicine
Department of Pediatrics
St. Christopher's Hospital for Children
Philadelphia, Pennsylvania

Sujata R. Tipnis, MD, FAAP, MPH
Pediatrician
Palo Alto Medical Foundation -
Fremont Center
Fremont, California

David Tunkel, MD
Director of Pediatric Otolaryngology
Professor of Otolaryngology-Head and
Neck Surgery
Johns Hopkins University School of
Medicine
Balitmore, Maryland

Scott VanDuzer, MD
Pediatric Plastic Surgeon
Philadelphia, Pennsylvania

Mark A. Ward, MD
Associate Professor of Pediatrics
Director of Pediatric Residency Program
Department of Pediatrics
Baylor College of Medicine
Houston, Texas

Evan J. Weiner, MD, FAAP
Assistant Professor of Pediatrics and
Emergency Medicine
Drexel University College of Medicine
Attending Physician
Department of Emergency Medicine
St. Christopher's Hospital for Children
Philadelphia, Pennsylvania

D'Juanna White-Satcher, MD, MPH
Assistant Professor
Academic General Pediatrics
Baylor College of Medicine
Staff
Residents Primary Care Group
Texas Children's Hospital
Houston, Texas

Michael J. Wilsey, Jr., MD, FAAP
Associate Program Director
Pediatric Residency Training Program
University of South Florida College of
Medicine
Tampa, Florida

Jeoffrey K. Wolens, MD
Staff Physician
Department of General Medicine
Texas Children's Hospital
Houston, Texas

Risa L. Yavorsky, MD
Resident Pediatrician
Pediatrics
Icahn School of Medicine at Mount
Sinai
New York, New York
Resident Physician
Pediatrics
The Mount Sinai Hospital
New York, New York

Lisa E. De Ybarrondo, MD
Assistant Professor
Department of Pediatrics
University of Texas Health Center
LBJ Pediatric Clinic Director
Department of Pediatrics
Lyndon B. Johnson General Hospital
Houston, Texas

Terri L. Young, MD
Professor of Ophthalmology
and Pediatrics
Duke University Medical Center
Duke University Hospital
Duke University Eye Center
Durham, North Carolina

Andrea L. Zaenglein, MD
Professor of Dermatology and Pediatric
Dermatology
Penn State Hershey Dermatology
Hershey, Pennsylvania

Robert L. Zarr, MD, MPH, FAAP
Pediatrician
Unity Health Care, Inc.
Washington, DC

Seth Zwillenberg, MD
Chairman of the Division of
Otolaryngology
Albert Einstein Medical Center
St. Christopher's Hospital for Children
Philadelphia, Pennsylvania

Contributors

Bethlehem Abebe-Wolpaw, MD
HS Assistant Clinical Professor
Department of Pediatrics
University of California
San Francisco, California

Michael Amirian, MD
Department of Urology
Thomas Jefferson University
Philadelphia, Pennsylvania

Lee R. Atkinson-McEvoy, MD
Clinical Professor of Pediatrics
Director of UCSF Pediatric Primary
Care Clinic
Associate Chief General Pediatrics
Associate Residency Program Director
Department of Pediatrics
University of California, San Francisco
School of Medicine
San Francisco, California

Eliza Hayes Bakken, MD
Assistant Clinical Professor
Department of Pediatrics
University of California San Francisco
Primary Care Coordinator
Children's Health Center
Department of Pediatrics
San Francisco General Hospital
San Francisco, California

Barbara W. Bayldon, MD
Assistant Professor
Feinberg School of Medicine
Northwestern University
Head
Section of Primary Care, General
Academic Pediatrics
Department of Pediatrics
Children's Memorial Hospital
Chicago, Illinois

Roy Benaroch, MD
Adjunct Assistant Professor
Pediatrics
Emory University
Atlanta, Georgia

Darshita P. Bhatia, MD
Clinical Instructor
Department of Pediatrics
Drexel University College of Medicine
Chief Resident
Department of Pediatrics
St. Christopher's Hospital for Children
Philadelphia, Pennsylvania

David J. Breland, MD, MPH
Assistant Professor of Pediatrics
Pediatrics
University of Washington School of
Medicine
Attending
Adolescent Medicine
Seattle Children's Hospital
Seattle, Washington

Esther K. Chung, MD, MPH
Professor
Department of Pediatrics
Sidney Kimmel Medical College
of Thomas Jefferson University
Jefferson Pediatrics/
Nemours-Philadelphia
Philadelphia, Pennsylvania
Alfred I. duPont Hospital for Children
Wilmington, Delaware

Kathleen Cronan, MD
Associate Professor
Department of Pediatrics
Sidney Kimmel Medical Center
Philadelphia, Pennsylvania
Attending Physician
Department of Pediatrics
Division of Pediatric Emergency
Medicine
Nemours/Alfred I. duPont Hospital for
Children
Wilmington, Delaware

Allan R. De Jong, MD
Clinical Professor
Department of Pediatrics
Sidney Kimmel Medical Center of
Thomas Jefferson University
Philadelphia, Pennsylvania
Medical Director, Children at Risk
Evaluation (CARE) Program
Department of Pediatrics
Nemours/Alfred I. duPont Hospital for
Children
Wilmington, Delaware

Lisa E. De Ybarrondo, MD
Assistant Professor
Department of Pediatrics
University of Texas Health Center
LBJ Pediatric Clinic Director
Department of Pediatrics
Lyndon B. Johnson General Hospital
Houston, Texas

Colette R. Desrochers, MD
Clinical Professor of Pediatrics
Department of Pediatrics
University of Pennsylvania
School of Medicine
Attending Physician
General Pediatrics Primary Care
Children's Hospital of Philadelphia
Philadelphia, Pennsylvania

Blair J. Dickinson, MD, MS
Assistant Professor
Pediatrics
Drexel University College of Medicine
Philadelphia, Pennsylvania
Attending Physician Hospital Medicine
Associate Resident/Program Director
Pediatrics
St. Christopher's Hospital for Children
Philadelphia, Pennsylvania

Yolanda N. Evans, MD, MPH
Associate Professor
Department of Pediatrics
University of Washington
Associate Professor
Department of Pediatrics
Division of Adolescent Medicine
Seattle Children's Hospital
Seattle, Washington

T. Ernesto Figueroa, MD
Clinical Associate Professor
Department of Urology
Thomas Jefferson University
Philadelphia, Pennsylvania
Chief, Division of Pediatric Urology
Department of Surgery
Alfred I. duPont Hospital for Children
Wilmington, Delaware

Darren M. Fiore, MD
Assistant Clinical Professor
Division of Pediatric Hospital Medicine
Department of Pediatrics
University of California, San Francisco
Benioff Children's Hospital
San Francisco, California

Lourdes Forster, MD, FAAP
Assistant Professor of Clinical Pediatrics
Department of Pediatrics
University of Miami, Miller School of
Medicine
Miami, Florida

Anand Gourishankar, MD
Assistant Professor
Pediatrics
University of Texas Medical School
of Houston
Attending Physician
Pediatrics
Children's Memorial Hermann Hospital
Houston, Texas

William R. Graessle, MD
Associate Professor
Department of Pediatrics
Cooper Medical School of Rowan
University
Director of Pediatric Medical Education
Department of Pediatrics
Cooper University Hospital
Camden, New Jersey

Larry H. Hollier, Jr., MD, FACS
Chief of Plastic Surgery
Baylor College of Medicine
Chief of Pediatric Plastic Surgery
Texas Children's Hospital
Houston, Texas

Shonul Agarwal Jain, MD
Assistant Professor
Department of Pediatrics
University of California, San Francisco
Medical Director, Children's Health
Center
Department of Pediatrics
San Francisco General Hospital

Sunitha V. Kaiser, MD
Assistant Professor
Pediatrics
University of California, San Francisco
San Francisco, California

Shareen F. Kelly, MD
Assistant Professor
Department of General Pediatrics
Drexel College of Medicine
Attending Physician
Ambulatory Pediatrics
St. Christopher's Hospital for Children
Philadelphia, Pennsylvania

Hans B. Kersten, MD
Associate Professor of Pediatrics
Department of Pediatrics
Drexel University College of Medicine
Attending Physician
Department of Pediatrics
St. Christopher's Hospital for Children
Philadelphia, Pennsylvania

David Y. Khechoyan, MD
Baylor College of Medicine
Texas Children's Hospital
Houston, Texas

Abena B. Knight, MD
Clinical Assistant Professor
Department of Pediatrics
University of Washington School of
Medicine
Pediatric and Surgical Hospitalist
Division of Hospital Medicine
Seattle Children's Hospital
Seattle, Washington

Naline L. Lai, MD
Primary Care Attending Physician
The Children's Hospital of Philadelphia
Care Network-Newtown
Newtown, Pennsylvania
Department of Pediatrics
St. Mary Medical Center
Langhorne, Pennsylvania
Department of Pediatrics
Doylestown Hospital
Doylestown, Pennsylvania

Ilse A. Larson, MD
Assistant Professor
Department of Pediatrics
Oregon Health & Science University
Portland, Oregon

Tomitra Latimer, MD
Attending, Division of Academic
General Pediatrics, *Ann & Robert H.*
Lurie Children's Hospital of Chicago
Assistant Clinical Professor of Pediatrics,
Northwestern University Feinberg
School of Medicine
Attending, *Ann & Robert H. Lurie*
Children's Pediatrics-Uptown
Primary Care
Chicago, Illinois

Ellen Laves, MD
Assistant Clinical Professor
Department of Pediatrics
University of California, San Francisco
Pediatrician
Department of Pediatrics
San Francisco General Hospital
San Francisco, California

Kelly R. Leite, DO
Associate Professor
Department of Pediatrics
Penn State College of Medicine
Attending Physician
Department of Pediatrics
Penn State Hershey Children's Hospital
Hershey, Pennsylvania

LaTanya J. Love, MD
Assistant Professor
Pediatrics and Internal Medicine
The University of Texas Health Science
Center
Staff Physician
Pediatrics
Children's Memorial Hermann Hospital
Houston, Texas

Elizabeth C. Maxwell, MD
Fellow
Division of Gastroenterology,
Hepatology, and Nutrition
Department of Pediatrics
Children's Hospital of Philadelphia
Philadelphia, Pennsylvania

Liana K. McCabe, MD
Pediatrician
Virginia Mason University Village
Medical Center
Seattle, Washington

Leora N. Mogilner, MD
Assistant Professor
Department of Pediatrics
Mount Sinai School of Medicine
New York, NY
Director, Advocacy and Community
Block
Department of Pediatrics
Kravis Children's Hospital
at Mount Sinai
New York, New York

Laura. A. Monson, MD
Assistant Professor
Division of Plastic Surgery
Baylor College of Medicine
Houston, Texas

Colette C. Mull, MD
Clinical Associate Professor of
Pediatrics
Division of Emergency Medicine
Thomas Jefferson University
Faculty
Division of Emergency Medicine
Nemours/Alfred I. duPont Hospital for
Children
Wilmington, Delaware

Alison Nair, MD
Fellow, Pediatric Critical Care
Department of Pediatrics
University of California, San Francisco
School of Medicine
San Francisco, California

Leonard B. Nelson, MD
Associate Professor of Ophthalmology
and Pediatrics
Ophthalmology
Sidney Kimmel Medical Center
Thomas Jefferson University
Philadelphia, Pennsylvania
Director
Wills Eye Strabismus Center
Wills Eye Institute
Philadelphia, Pennsylvania

Kimberly A. Neutze, DO
Pediatric Ophthalmology Fellow
Division of Ophthalmology
Nemours/Alfred I. duPont Hospital for
Children
Wilmington, Delaware

Julieana Nichols, MD, MPH
Baylor College of Medicine
Texas Children's Hospital
Houston, Texas

Julie S. O'Brien, MD
Assistant Clinical Professor
Department of Pediatrics
University of California, San Francisco
School of Medicine
UCSF Benioff Children's Hospital
San Francisco, California

Christopher O'Hara, MD
Assistant Professor of Pediatrics
Department of Pediatrics
Penn State University College of
Medicine
Pediatric Hospital, Division of Pediatric
Hospital Medicine
Pediatrics
Penn State Hershey Children's Hospital
Hershey, Pennsylvania

Kenya Maria Parks, MD, MS, FAAP
Assistant Professor
Community and General Pediatrics
The University of Texas Health Science
Center at Houston
Houston, Texas

Charles A. Pohl, MD
Professor
Department of Pediatrics
Sidney Kimmel Medical Center
Department of Pediatrics
Thomas Jefferson University/Nemours
Philadelphia, Pennsylvania

Amy Elizabeth Renwick, MD, FAAP
Assistant Professor
Department of Pediatrics
Sidney Kimmel Medical College at
Thomas Jefferson University
Philadelphia, Pennsylvania
Attending Physician
Department of General Pediatrics
Alfred I. duPont Hospital for Children
Wilmington, Delaware

Brent D. Rogers, MD
Fellow, Pediatric Emergency Medicine
Division of Emergency Medicine
Nemours/Alfred I. duPont Hospital for
Children
Wilmington, Delaware

Holly M. Romero, MD
Clinical Assistant Professor
Pediatrics
University of Washington
Hospitalist
Pediatrics
Seattle Children's Hospital
Seattle, Washington

Denise A. Salerno, MD, FAAP
Professor of Clinical Pediatrics
Pediatrics Clerkship Director
Department of Pediatrics
Temple University School of Medicine
Philadelphia, Pennsylvania

Jonathon H. Salvin, MD
Assistant Professor
Departments of Pediatrics and
Ophthalmology
Sidney Kimmel Medical Center
Philadelphia, Pennsylvania
Division of Ophthalmology
Nemours/Alfred I. DuPont Hospital for
Children
Wilmington, Delaware

Benjamin W. Sanders, MD, MSPH
Assistant Professor
Department of Pediatrics
Drexel University College of Medicine
Attending Physician
Section of General Pediatrics
St. Christopher's Hospital for Children
Philadelphia, Pennsylvania

Lee M. Sanders, MD, MPH
Associate Professor
Department of Pediatrics
Stanford University
Attending Physician
Department of Pediatrics
Lucile Packard Children's Hospital
Stanford, California

Mark Jason Sanders, MD
Assistant Professor
Department of Pediatrics
University of Texas Health
Children's Memorial Hospital
Houston, Texas

Andrew Saunders, MD
Assistant Clinical Professor
Department of Pediatrics
University of California, San Francisco
School of Medicine
San Francisco, California

Steven M. Selbst, MD
Professor
Department of Pediatrics
Sidney Kimmel Medical Center
Philadelphia, Pennsylvania
Vice-Chair for Education, Residency
Program Director
Department of Pediatrics
Nemours/Alfred I. duPont Hospital for
Children
Wilmington, Delaware

Beth A. Shortridge, MD, PhD
Clinical Assistant Professor
Department of Pediatrics
Sidney Kimmel Medical Center
Thomas Jefferson University
Philadelphia, Pennsylvania
Attending Pediatric Hospitalist
Department of Pediatrics
Bryn Mawr Hospital
Nemours/Alfred I. duPont Hospital for
Children
Bryn Mawr, Pennsylvania

Laura E. Smals-Murphy, MD
Associate Professor of Pediatrics
Department of Pediatrics
Pennsylvania State University College of
Medicine
Vice Chair of Education
Department of Pediatrics
Penn State Hershey Children's Hospital
Hershey, Pennsylvania

Parul Patel Soni, MD, MPH
Assistant Professor of Pediatrics
Department of Pediatrics
Feinberg School of Medicine/
Northwestern University
Attending Physician
Emergency
Ann and Robert H. Laurie Children's
Hospital of Chicago
Chicago, Illinois

Nancy D. Spector, MD
Professor
Department of Pediatrics
Drexel University College of Medicine
Associate Chair of Education and
Faculty
Department of Pediatrics
St. Christopher's Hospital for Children
Philadelphia, Pennsylvania

Christopher C. Stewart, MD
Associate Professor
Department of Pediatrics
University of California, San Francisco
San Francisco, California

Kathryn T. Stroup, MD
Assistant Professor
Department of Pediatrics
Drexel University College of Medicine
Attending Pediatrician
Section of General Pediatrics
St. Christopher's Hospital for Children
Philadelphia, Pennsylvania

Rebecca G. Taxier, MD
Clinical Assistant Professor
Department of Pediatrics
University of Washington
Medical Hospitalist
Hospital Medicine
Seattle Children's Hospital
Seattle, Washington

Daniel R. Taylor, DO
Associate Professor
Department of Pediatrics
Drexel University College of Medicine
Philadelphia, Pennsylvania
General Pediatrician
General Pediatrics
St. Christopher's Hospital for Children
Philadelphia, Pennsylvania

Michelle Terry, MD
Clinical Professor of Pediatrics
University of Washington School of
Medicine
Seattle, Washington

E. Douglas Thompson, Jr., MD
Assistant Professor
Department of Pediatrics
Drexel University College of Medicine
Chief of the Section of Hospital
Medicine
Department of Pediatrics
St. Christopher's Hospital for Children
Philadelphia, Pennsylvania

Kristina Toncray
Clinical Instructor
Department of Pediatrics
Drexel University College of Medicine
Chief Resident
Pediatrics
St. Christopher's Hospital for Children
Philadelphia, Pennsylvania

Renee M. Turchi, MD, MPH, FAAP
Associate Professor
Community Health & Prevention
Drexel University School of Public
Health
Medical Director
Department of Pediatrics
Center for Children with Special Health
Needs
St. Christopher's Hospital for Children
Philadelphia, Pennsylvania

Evan J. Weiner, MD, FAAP
Assistant Professor of Pediatrics and
Emergency Medicine
Drexel University College of Medicine
Attending Physician
Department of Emergency Medicine
St. Christopher's Hospital for Children
Philadelphia, Pennsylvania

D'Juanna White-Satcher, MD, MPH
Assistant Professor
Academic General Pediatrics
Baylor College of Medicine
Staff
Residents Primary Care Group
Texas Children's Hospital
Houston, Texas

Lauren Wilson, MD
Assistant Professor
Department of Pediatrics
University of Washington
Hospitalist
Department of Pediatrics
Seattle Children's Hospital
Seattle, Washington

Risa L. Yavorsky, MD
Resident Pediatrician
Pediatrics
Icahn School of Medicine at Mount
Sinai
Resident Physician
Pediatrics
The Mount Sinai Hospital
New York, New York

Foreword

Perhaps the expression that a picture is worth a thousand words evolved from an exhausted word counter who reached the number of one thousand right before lunch and quit counting in favor of his ham sandwich. The concept certainly continues that a good picture is worth a great deal of discourse and offers a great deal of information, possibly like Mark Twain's dog who, when sitting on a hornet, gained a great deal of information in a very short time. And so here is the third edition of Dr. Chung's *Visual Diagnosis and Treatment in Pediatrics,* larger and richer than the second edition, with trusted distinguishing characteristics and associated findings as ever with each illustration and now the added ICD-10 codes and interactive e-book embellishment, leading the busy reader (without any sting at all) to a fast and accurate answer.

There was, in past times, description of pathologic or physical variation accomplished with extensive phrases and words defining as well as possible the size, color, comparative nature, and whatever else might be available in language to transmit to the reader what the writer felt and saw. Drawings and often detailed chromatic paintings were added to great advantage. In time, with the development of photography, and color photography in particular, the capacity to transfer this image was marvelously improved, gaining in detail much more than the old anatomist masters might have ever imagined might be possible to display.

Now with this third edition, which, like a third child, represents once more the attempt to create, as close to perfection as possible, an improvement on what had heretofore been considered a very fine work, there is the convenience of having, with the fingertip turning pages, thousands of messages that could never have been sent before. Here is help to identify, with a historical hint, distinguishing characteristics, associated findings, complications, predisposing factors, and treatment guidelines, the answer for which the clinician searches.

Gary G. Carpenter, MD
Associate Professor of Pediatrics
Sidney Kimmel Medical School
of Thomas Jefferson University
Nemours DuPont Pediatrics
Philadelphia, Pennsylvania

Preface

Pediatrics is an exciting field, full of the wonder of children and the joys that parents experience. Being a pediatrician has been a terrific honor and privilege. As I approach a quarter-century of being a doctor and a half-century of being a person, I look back in awe of the families that I have met. This book cannot capture all of the visual images that the contributors have seen or the essence of the children they have met. *Visual Diagnosis and Treatment in Pediatrics* is simply meant to capture important images in order to help today's busy clinician. Clinicians have little time to seek guidance from a book and are in need of quick, well-organized information. To address these needs, we developed a user-friendly format with differential diagnoses for a problem listed in a single table and photographs of these diagnoses placed side-by-side for comparison. We focused on providing pearls and approaches, rather than exhaustive descriptions or detailed lists. Available worldwide, the previous editions of this book have been translated into Chinese, Indonesian, and Portuguese.

The third edition of this book has improved readability with respect to format and layout, new photographic images, and many new contributors. As in the second edition, all chapters pertaining to the newborn are now organized into a single section, "Visual Diagnoses in the Newborn." A new addition is a chapter on Child Physical Abuse that includes photographs and pearls to help clinicians identify and address child abuse.

A major goal for this edition, and the first two, was to include photographs demonstrating the breadth of pediatrics and the ethnic diversity of patients living in the United States and abroad. We have photographs demonstrating marks found after "coining," a practice performed by some East Asian cultures, and we show classic "Mongolian" spots that are found in many people with pigmented skin. Bear in mind that these photographs are of people—someone's child, grandchild, nephew, or niece—to whom we are indebted. This book would not have been possible without them and the generosity of their families, who allowed us to care for and take photographs of them.

I am grateful for the opportunity to work with such a talented group of dedicated and experienced clinicians. Their willingness to gather photographs and to write chapters stems from their commitments to education and to improving the clinical care of patients. Our contributors, from academic medicine and private practice, have spent hours that extended well into the night.

I am grateful that a talented and committed associate editor, Dr. Lee R. Atkinson-McEvoy, returned to make our third edition better than the first two. Dr. Naline Lai and Dr. Michelle Terry, our newest associate editors, have recruited new authors and have worked tirelessly. Special thanks are due to Dr. Steven Handler, who provided many of the otolaryngology photographs in all editions of this book, and Dr. George A. Datto, who helped conceptualize the first edition of this book and whose photographs are found throughout all editions.

Wolters Kluwer—Lippincott Williams & Wilkins, our publisher, continues to produce books of the highest quality, thanks to their well-trained and professional staff, particularly Ashley Fischer and Alicia Jackson. Anitha Murugaiyan at S4Carlisle Publishing Services was extremely responsive and professional. Medical books continue to be an important source of information even during a time when many medical facts can be found by simply entering a few words into a computer search engine. We hope that you find this visual diagnosis book to be a valuable addition to the resources used in your clinical practice.

Esther K. Chung, MD, MPH,
Editor-in-Chief

Table of Contents

Section 7 MOUInt MOUTH

Section 8 NECK

Section 9 CHEST

Section **13** GENITAL AND PERINEAL REGION

Section **14** PERIANAL AREA AND BUTTOCKS

Section 15 SKIN

Section 1

VISUAL DIAGNOSES IN THE NEWBORN

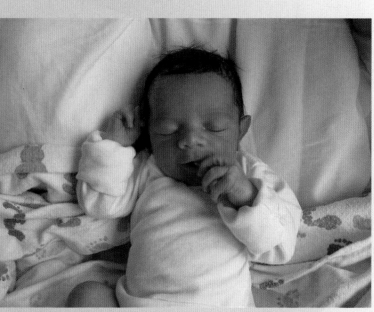

(Courtesy of Lee R. Atkinson-McEvoy, MD.)

Breastfeeding

Lourdes Forster and Lee M. Sanders

Approach to the Problem

Assessing a nursing infant requires careful attention to the mother and the child during each clinical encounter. Effective diagnosis and treatment of breastfeeding problems cannot be accomplished without the clinician's observation of the infant at the mother's breast.

Unlike most other pediatric encounters, the mother becomes an important subject of a focused history and physical examination. In the mother's medical and social history, critical findings can help the clinician easily identify treatable conditions or more difficult challenges to successful breastfeeding. Similarly, examination of the mother's breast can reveal tell-tale signs of underlying problems. First-time mothers will usually feel their milk "come in" by 72 hours after delivery. Infrequent or inadequate drainage of the breasts in the first days of life can result in greater pain from engorgement and ultimately affect the volume of milk produced.

While the infant is breastfeeding or attempting to breastfeed, the clinician can observe critical features—including infant feeding cues, position, and latch—that can help diagnose common problems or determine the need for further assistance from a lactation consultant.

The clinician's goals should be three-fold: (1) to encourage breastfeeding for all mothers and infants; (2) to assess and treat breastfeeding-related problems early; and (3) to provide a positive, nonjudgmental environment for promoting infant nutrition and growth.

Key Points in the History

Mother

- **Delivery Complications.** C-section incisions are often associated with increased pain during breastfeeding.

- **Medications.** Sedatives, antihistamines, diuretics, or exogenous estrogen (oral contraceptives) contribute to low milk synthesis. Even a single dose of barbiturates during labor (often given for a C-section delivery for failure to progress) has been shown to impede the milk intake of infants in the first days of life.

- *Medical History.* Hypothyroidism, peripartum infection, or retained placenta may impair breastfeeding success. Mothers who were overweight or obese (Body Mass Index >24) prior to pregnancy are less likely to initiate breastfeeding or to continue breastfeeding through 6 months. Preexisting or pregnancy-related back pain or hemorrhoids may also complicate the pain associated with certain breastfeeding positions.

- *Surgical History.* Breast reduction surgery may lead to a significant reduction in milk production. By contrast, most mothers who have breast implants can successfully nurse.

- *Tobacco Use.* Smoking has been shown to interfere with the milk let-down reflex. There is a direct relationship between the amount a woman smokes and decreased milk production.

- *Maternal Support.* Traditionally, women have relied on their spouses, mothers, and grandmothers for support and instruction. If these support figures are not available, mothers are more likely to benefit from thorough lactation instruction and support.

- *Depressive Symptoms.* Peripartum depression is common, often undiagnosed, and a significant contributor to other common maternal stressors in the first months of an infant's life. Depression and anxiety may impede milk production and successful infant latch.

Infant

- *Gestational Age.* Preterm and near-term (<37 weeks' gestation) infants are at higher risk for breastfeeding difficulty because of problems with latch and coordinated suckling.

- *Apgar Scores.* A 5-minute Apgar score less than 6 has been associated with decreased rates of successful breastfeeding initiation.

- *Medical History.* Significant metabolic, renal, or cardiac disorders may increase infant losses or metabolic demand. In addition to impairing adequate weight gain, these conditions may make breastfeeding more difficult for the infant or require supplementation with high-calorie formulas. Infants with Trisomy 21 syndrome often exhibit impaired oromotor skills that may make breastfeeding more challenging.

- *Feeding Pattern.* Infrequent feedings because of mother–infant separation, pacifier use, or supplementation with water, teas, or juices will interfere with milk production. Diaphoresis or tiring with feedings may be a sign of an undiagnosed cardiac or metabolic disease.

- *Use of Infant Formula.* Use of infant formula in the newborn nursery is a predictor of early discontinuation of breastfeeding and considered a red flag for insufficient milk production.

Key Points in the Physical Examination

Mother

- *Nipple.* Cracks or fissures of the nipple may indicate problems (see below). Nipple inversion is a common problem that may be corrected with the use of a nipple shield.

- *Maternal Mood.* Fatigue and stress are the most common causes of inadequate milk supply. Maternal–infant emotional attachment is crucial for the breastfeeding dyad to succeed. The mother's ability to identify and respond to her infant's feeding cues will ensure frequent and timely feeds. This, in turn, promotes continued milk production.

Nursing Process

- *Infant Feeding Cues.* Common infant feeding cues include wriggling with eyes wide open, hands to mouth or face, rooting with an open mouth, and smacking lips. Assess the mother's facility in identifying and acting on these cues.

- *Infant Feeding Position.* Four common positions (cradle hold, football hold, cross-cradle hold, and lying) are illustrated in Figures 1-1 to 1-4. Assess the mother's comfort and confidence in trying at least two different positions to accommodate her and her infant.

- *Infant Latch.* Nipple cracks, fissures, and pain may be caused by superficial latches that do not reach the infant's soft palate, where the infant's lower lip is curled inward, where mother is taking the infant off the breast without breaking suction or leading with the baby's nose instead of the chin. Appropriate infant latch should include the following:

  - Wide-open mouth immediately prior to bringing the baby to breast

  - The baby's lips should be flanged, "fish-like"

  - The mother holds her breast with her thumb on top and four fingers beneath ("C" hold)

  - Audible or visible swallowing, with about two to three sucks per swallow

- *Maternal Comfort.* During effective breastfeeding, the mother may experience tingling within the breast, but she should not experience sharp pains. After nursing, her breasts should feel softer without any soreness. Pain during breastfeeding is one of the most common causes of poor milk production and discontinuation of breastfeeding.

Infant

- Normal weight gain is a good sign of successful breastfeeding. Weight loss of greater than 10% from birth weight or other signs of failure to thrive merit further investigation, including increased attention to the breastfeeding history and examination of the nursing process.

- Moist mucous membranes, flat anterior fontanelle, and adequate peripheral perfusion are good signs of adequate oral hydration.

- Cleft lip or palate, high-arched palate, tight lingual frenulum, or micrognathia may impair a successful latch. Absence of a strong suck reflex may indicate poor oromotor development or an underlying neurologic abnormality that would impair breastfeeding.

- Abnormal motor tone or reflexes may indicate an underlying neurologic abnormality that may also impair oromotor development and, therefore, breastfeeding.

PHOTOGRAPHS OF SELECTED DIAGNOSES

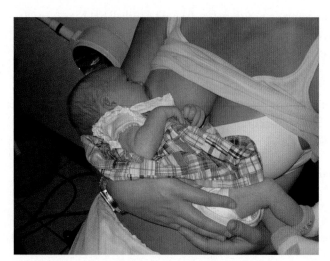

Figure 1-1 Cradle hold. (Courtesy of Lourdes Forster, MD, FAAP.)

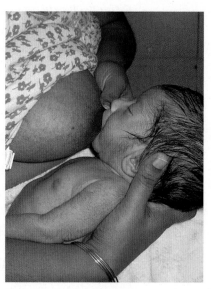

Figure 1-2 Football hold. (Courtesy of Lourdes Forster, MD, FAAP.)

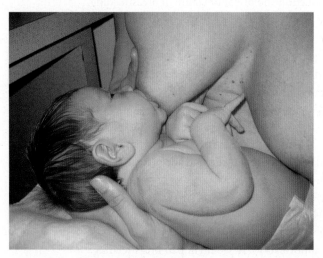

Figure 1-3 Cross-cradle hold. (Courtesy of Lourdes Forster, MD, FAAP.)

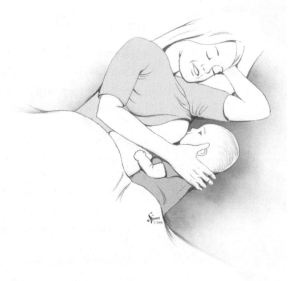

Figure 1-4 Lying position. (Drawing by Satyen Tripathi, MA.)

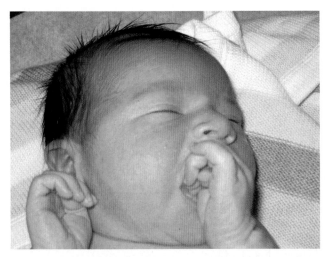

Figure 1-5 **Feeding cue (hand in mouth).** (Courtesy of Lourdes Forster, MD, FAAP.)

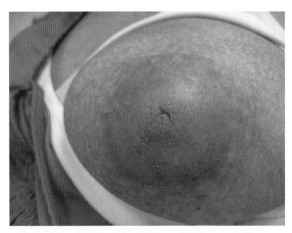

Figure 1-6 **Nipple fissure.** Note fissure from the 2 o'clock to 8 o'clock position. Such a fissure indicates an improper latch (i.e., "nipple latch"). (Courtesy of Lourdes Forster, MD, FAAP.)

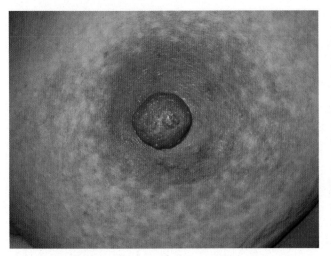

Figure 1-7 **Nipple fissure.** Note fissure from the 11 o'clock to 5 o'clock position. Such a fissure indicates an improper latch (i.e., "nipple latch"). (Courtesy of Lourdes Forster, MD, FAAP.)

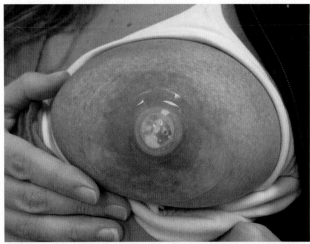

Figure 1-8 **Infant nursing on a retracted nipple covered with a nursing shield.** (Courtesy of Lourdes Forster, MD, FAAP.)

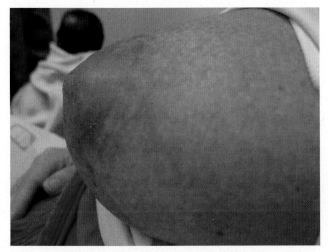

Figure 1-9 **Breast engorgement.** Signs of breast engorgement include a flat nipple. (Courtesy of Lourdes Forster, MD, FAAP.)

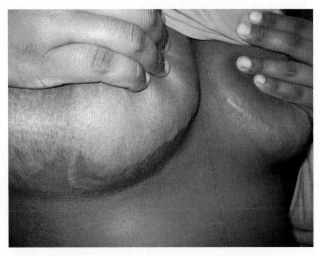

Figure 1-10 **Breast reduction.** Note scars from breast reduction surgery. (Courtesy of Lourdes Forster, MD, FAAP.)

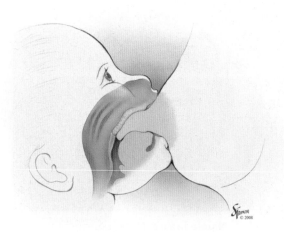

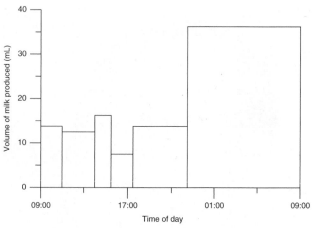

Figure 1-11 Cross section of infant latch. Note two critical features of a successful latch: the nipple protrudes to make contact with the infant's soft palate, and the infant's lower lip is folded outward. (Drawing by Satyen Tripathi, MA.)

Figure 1-12 Milk supply, over time. (Drawing by Satyen Tripathi, MA.)

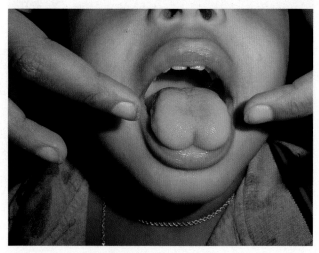

Figure 1-13 Ankyloglossia. Note the notched or heart-shaped tongue visible on protrusion. (Courtesy of Michael Lemper, DDS.)

DIFFERENTIAL DIAGNOSIS

DIAGNOSIS	ICD-10	CHARACTERISTICS	DURATION	ASSOCIATED FINDINGS	COMPLICATIONS	PRECIPITATING FACTORS	TREATMENT GUIDELINES
Breast Pain	N64.4	Nipple fissure, cracking	Variable	Pain	Infection	Fissures or cracks	Pain management Evaluate latch
Cracked Nipple Fissured	N64.0	Usually in first week, often worsening	Variable	Pain, bleeding	Mastitis Abscess	Poor latch, position	Counseling, repositioning
Nipple, Sore	O92.2	First indication of poor latch Up to 96% of mothers	Variable	Scabbing of the nipple	Infrequent feeds	Poor latch, position	Counseling, repositioning
Neonatal Difficulty in Feeding at Breast	P92.5	Poor weight gain, fussy Decreased stool and urine output	Variable	Apparently normal latch without rhythmic suck/ swallow	Poor weight gain Failure to thrive	Near-term infant Oral–motor dysfunction	Lactation consultant referral Supplement with expressed breast milk
Breast Engorgement	O92.29	Congestion or distension of the breast tissue Up to 85% of mothers	Peaks at 3–4 days after birth but can last up to 14 days	Breast tissue is tight and shiny. Milk flow is difficult.	Mastitis Decreased milk production	Supplemental feeding Infrequent feedings Mother–infant separation	Frequent feedings Heat application Cold therapy
Ankyloglossia	Q38.1	Sore nipple Slow weight gain despite frequent feedings	Variable	Infant unable to extend tongue beyond lower lip	Poor weight gain		Frenulotomy

Other
Diagnoses
to Consider

Maternal Causes of Poor Milk Supply

- Peripartum depression

- Retained placenta

- Postpartum hemorrhage

- Eating disorder

- Primary mammary glandular insufficiency

- Polycystic ovary syndrome

- Systemic lupus erythematosus

- Autoimmune disease or connective tissue disorder

- Other chronic illness

Infant Diagnoses That May Impair Breastfeeding

- Viremia/Viral syndrome

- Serious bacterial illness, including urinary tract infection, pneumonia, enteritis, sepsis, and meningitis

- Gastroesophageal reflux

- Prematurity

- Cleft lip or palate

- Ankyloglossia

- Gastroesophageal malformations

- Metabolic disorder

- Renal disease

- Hypocalcemia

- Hypothyroidism

- Oral–motor dysfunction

- Central nervous system abnormality

When to Consider Further Evaluation or Treatment

Failure to thrive is the most important indication for further evaluation by the pediatrician in partnership with a lactation consultant. Concerns for failure to thrive would include the following:

- Weight loss of greater than 10% in the first week of life

- Failure to regain birth weight by day 14

- Average daily weight gain of less than 20 g/day

- Infrequent stools, less than four stools per day, by the end of the first week

- Concentrated urine, less than six wet diapers per day, by the end of the first week

SUGGESTED READINGS

Ahluwalia IB, Morrow B, Hsia J. Why do women stop breastfeeding? Findings from the Pregnancy Risk Assessment and Monitoring System. *Pediatrics*. 2005;116:1408–1412.

Ballard JL, Aver CE, Khoury JC. Ankyloglossia: Assessment, incidence, and effect of frenuloplasty on breastfeeding dyad. *Pediatrics*. 2002;110:e63.

Brent N, Rudy SJ, Redd B, et al. Sore nipples in breast-feeding women. *Arch Pediatric Adolesc Med*. 1998;152:1077–1082.

Centers for Disease Control and Prevention. *Strategies to Prevent Obesity and Other Chronic Diseases: The CDC Guide to Strategies to Support Breastfeeding Mothers and Babies*. Atlanta: U.S. Department of Health and Human Services; 2013. http://www.cdc.gov/breast-feeding/pdf/BF-Guide-508.PDF. Accessed December 15, 2013.

Ip S, Chung M, Raman G, et al. *Breastfeeding and Maternal and Infant Health Outcomes in Developed Countries*. Evidence Report/Technology Assessment No. 153 (Prepared by Tufts-New England Medical Center Evidence-based Practice Center, under Contract No. 290–02–0022). AHRQ Publication No. 07-E007. Rockville, MD: Agency for Healthcare Research and Quality; 2007.

Lawrence RA and Lawrence RL. *Breastfeeding—A Guide for the Medical Profession*. 7th ed. Philadelphia, PA: Elsevier Mosby; 2011.

Riordan J. *Breastfeeding and Human Lactation*. 4th ed. Sudbury: Jones and Bartlett; 2009.

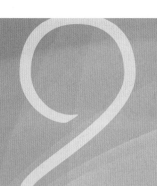

Scalp Swellings in Newborns

Kathryn T. Stroup and Hans B. Kersten

Most newborn scalp swellings are related to the forces exerted on the head by the birth canal or assistive equipment during delivery. These problems are usually self-limited, and they resolve within a couple of days to weeks, although some may require close monitoring. Swelling may occur despite skilled obstetric and neonatal care. Cesarean deliveries are associated less frequently with swelling. Fixed abnormalities in the skull shape and skin lesions of the head are described in chapters 3 and 4.

- Molding and caput succedaneum are usually evident right after birth, but a cephalohematoma or subgaleal hemorrhage may take hours to form or become evident.

- Obesity, diabetes, and short stature are maternal risk factors for molding, caput, cephalohematoma, or subgaleal hemorrhage.

- Macrosomia, cephalopelvic disproportion, and instrumented vaginal deliveries are newborn risk factors for molding, caput, cephalohematoma, or subgaleal hemorrhage.

- Caput succedaneum results from local subcutaneous edema and fluid collection, most commonly in the parieto-occipital region following a vaginal birth.

- Caput succedaneum and molding usually resolve in the first few days of life.

- Cephalohematoma, a hemorrhage that occurs between the periosteum and the skull bone, occurs in 1%–2% of all deliveries, and may take weeks to resolve.

- Five percent to twenty-five percent of patients with cephalohematomas may have an accompanying skull fracture.

- Subgaleal hemorrhage is a worrisome type of bleeding caused by trauma to the diploic veins under the galea aponeurotica that may occur with particularly traumatic deliveries. There is an increased incidence of subgaleal hemorrhage with vacuum extraction.

**Key Points
in the Physical
Examination**

- The swelling in caput succedaneum crosses suture lines because it is above the cranium in the subcutaneous tissue.

- The scalp with a caput succedaneum, unlike with a cephalohematoma, tends to have pitting edema.

- A caput succedaneum may be associated with a "halo scalp ring" of alopecia as a result of prolonged pressure of the scalp against the cervical os.

- Cephalohematomas are tense and do not extend across suture lines because they are limited by the boundaries of the periosteum.

- Skull fractures may underlie a cephalohematoma, but can be difficult to detect on physical examination.

- A cephalohematoma may leave a palpable calcification upon the skull as it resolves, which is typically small and nontender.

- There is no discoloration of the scalp with a cephalohematoma unless there is an overlying caput or bruising in the subcutaneous tissue.

- Subgaleal hematomas are fluctuant masses that cross suture lines, may be associated with a fluid wave or ecchymoses behind the ear, and may extend to other areas of the scalp.

- The ecchymoses associated with caput succedaneum and the bleeding seen with cephalohematomas and subgaleal hematomas can contribute to neonatal jaundice.

- Cranial meningoceles and encephaloceles are pulsatile midline masses that may present as cyst-like structures or a small sac with a pedunculated stalk. They will both transilluminate with a light, and neural tissue may be seen with an encephalocele.

PHOTOGRAPHS OF SELECTED DIAGNOSES

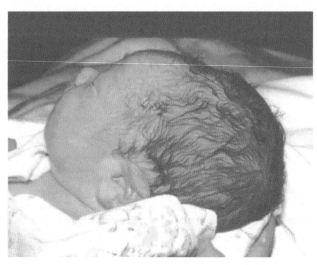

Figure 2-1 Molding. Note the superior and posterior displacement of the skull bones. (Courtesy of Joseph Piatt, MD.)

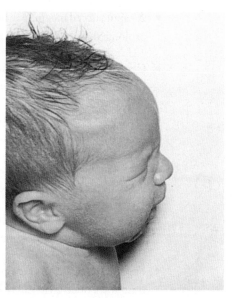

Figure 2-2 Caput succedaneum. Caput succedaneum shows pitting on pressure. (Used with permission from O'Doherty N. *Atlas of the Newborn*. Philadelphia, PA: JB Lippincott Co.; 1979:136.)

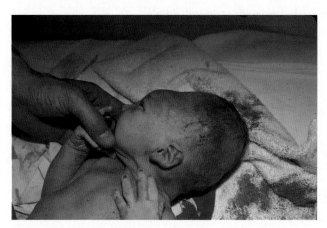

Figure 2-3 Caput succedaneum. Large soft swelling over the vertex, not confined to suture lines. (Courtesy of the late Peter Sol, MD.)

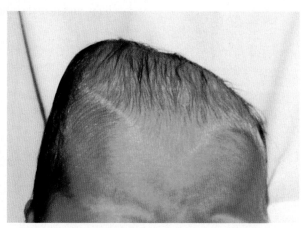

Figure 2-4 Cephalohematoma. Note the swelling over the right parietal area. (Used with permission from Fletcher MA. *Physical Diagnosis in Neonatology*. Philadelphia, PA: Lippincott–Raven Publishers; 1998:185.)

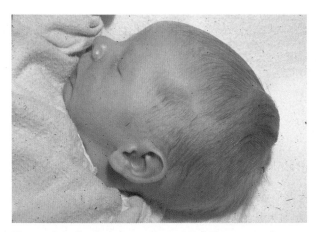

Figure 2-5 **Cephalohematoma.** Well-demarcated swelling over the left parietal bone. (Courtesy of the late Peter Sol, MD.)

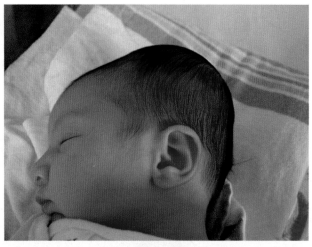

Figure 2-6 **Cephalohematoma.** Note the prominence of the left parieto-occipital area in this newborn with a cephalohematoma. (Courtesy of Esther K. Chung, MD, MPH.)

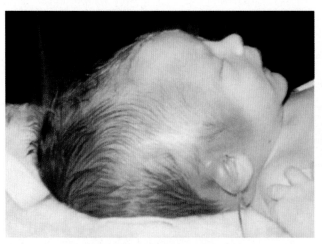

Figure 2-7 **Subgaleal hematoma.** Discoloration and swelling extends across suture lines onto the neck, even onto the ear, causing protuberance of the pinna. (Used with permission from Fletcher MA. *Physical Diagnosis in Neonatology.* Philadelphia, PA: Lippincott–Raven Publishers; 1998:185.)

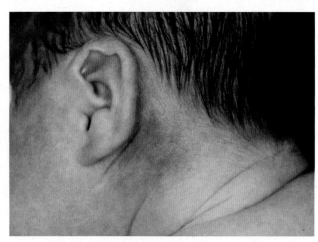

Figure 2-8 **Ecchymosis after subgaleal hemorrhage.** The bilateral location of this blood collection away from the site of forceps application suggests a wide area of involvement typical of a moderately large subgaleal hematoma. (Used with permission from Fletcher MA. *Physical Diagnosis in Neonatology.* Philadelphia, PA: Lippincott–Raven Publishers; 1998:128.)

DIFFERENTIAL DIAGNOSIS

DIAGNOSIS		ICD-10	DISTINGUISHING CHARACTERISTICS	DISTRIBUTION	DURATION/ CHRONICITY
Molding		P13.1	Overlapping bones along suture lines	Along suture lines	Present at birth Resolves in first few weeks of life
Caput Succedaneum		P12.81	Soft-tissue swelling that crosses suture lines; irregular borders	Parieto-occipital or diffuse swelling May see dependent edema on one side	Present at birth Resolves in the first few days of life
Cephalohematoma		P12.0	Subperiosteal hemorrhage Swelling that does not cross suture lines Tense swelling	Focal swelling Usually the parietal area May be bilateral	Develops incrementally during first 24 hours of life May take 2–3 months to resolve
Subgaleal Hematoma		P12.2	Fluctuant to tense scalp swelling that crosses suture lines	Focal or diffuse swelling Fluid wave	Develops shortly after birth May last weeks, could progress
Cranial Meningocele		Q01.9	CSF-filled meningeal sac Pulsatile Increased pressure when crying	Midline cranium	Present at birth
Cranial Encephalocele		Q01.9	CSF-filled meningeal sac plus cerebral cortex, cerebellum, and/or portions of the brain stem	Midline cranium, most commonly at the occiput	Present at birth Resolution after surgical correction

ASSOCIATED FINDINGS	COMPLICATIONS	PREDISPOSING FACTORS	TREATMENT GUIDELINES
Caput succedaneum	Hemorrhage Fracture	Vaginal birth	Observation Rare cause of shock requiring blood transfusion
Swelling develops during birth process Scalp ecchymoses Discoloration and distortion of the face with face presentations	Hemorrhage Fracture Jaundice	Vaginal delivery Vertex delivery Vacuum suctioning	Observation
Palpable rim Calcifications may develop Rare association with skull fracture, coagulopathy, and intracranial hemorrhage	Hemorrhage Skull fracture Jaundice Calcification Superinfection	Vaginal delivery Vacuum suctioning	Observation Monitor for neonatal jaundice. Consider evaluation for fracture if significant involvement.
Swelling Ecchymosis develops shortly after birth Ecchymoses behind ear	Hemorrhage Shock Severe anemia Death	Caused by bleeding from the diploic veins under the galea aponeurotica during traumatic delivery Vacuum suctioning	Observation Requires observation in an NICU for progressive enlargement and associated anemia, hypovolemia, shock, or jaundice
Fluctuant midline mass Transilluminates Occasional tethering, syringomyelia, and diastematomyelia	Good prognosis	Embryologic defect causing herniation of meninges through defect in the skull/cranial sutures	X-ray of the skull and cervical spine to define anatomy
Elevated α-fetoprotein levels in utero Midline mass, hydrocephalus due to aqueductal stenosis Chiari malformation or Dandy–Walker syndrome	Visual problems, mental retardation, craniofacial anomalies, and epilepsy	Embryologic defect causing herniation of meninges and other neural tissues through defect in the skull/cranial sutures	X-ray of the skull and cervical spine to define anatomy Ultrasound or neuroimaging to determine the contents and extent of the sac Neurosurgery consultation to assess need for removal or decompression

SECTION 1 • VISUAL DIAGNOSES IN THE NEWBORN

Other Diagnoses to Consider

- Plagiocephaly

- Craniosynostosis

- Skull fractures

- Porencephalic or leptomeningeal cyst

When to Consider Further Evaluation or Treatment

- A cephalohematoma with an accompanying skull fracture should be referred to neurosurgery, and neuroimaging should be considered, particularly if the fracture is depressed.

- Cephalohematomas, subgaleal hematomas, and caput succedanea may be complicated by anemia or jaundice severe enough to require phototherapy or blood transfusions.

- Subgaleal hematomas require observation in a neonatal ICU for progressive enlargement and associated anemia, hypovolemia, shock, or jaundice.

- If a cranial meningocele is a consideration, an x-ray must be done to confirm if there is a skull defect, and additional neuroimaging should be pursued to evaluate for associated complications.

- If a cranial encephalocele is a consideration, prompt neurosurgical consultation should be arranged for possible decompression.

SUGGESTED READINGS

Bickley L and Szilagi P, eds. *Bates' Guide to Physical Exam and History Taking*. 11th ed. Philadelphia, PA: JB Lippincott Co.; 2013:775–812.
Kliegman RM, Stanton B, Schor N, St Geme J, Behrman R, eds. *Nelson Textbook of Pediatrics*. 19th ed. Philadelphia, PA: WB Saunders; 2011:565–573.
Moczygemba C, Paramsothy P, Meikle S, et al. Route of delivery and neonatal birth trauma. *Am J Obstet Gynecol*. 2010;202:361.e1–6.
Nicholson L. Caput succedaneum and cephalohematoma: The Cs that leave bumps on the head. *Neonat Network*. 2010;26(5):277–281.
Parker L. Part 1: Early recognition and treatment of birth trauma: Injuries to the head and face. *Adv Neonat Care*. 2005;5(6):288–297.

Newborn Facial Lesions

Roy Benaroch

Approach to the Problem

Facial lesions on newborns are often the result of transient, self-limited conditions. However, some may have a lasting cosmetic impact or may herald serious underlying disease. Serious lesions need to be identified for appropriate and timely referral. Benign lesions can be safely watched, and healthcare providers can offer reassurance and instructions for when to seek further care.

Key Points in the History

- Determine when the lesion was first noticed. Nevus simplex (often called a salmon patch, stork bite, or angel's kiss), nevus flammeus (port-wine stain), and nevus sebaceous are present at birth. Neonatal acne, erythema toxicum, pustular melanosis, eczema, and seborrhea develop in the days or weeks after birth, and often spread after they first appear. Most hemangiomata also become noticeable after birth, continuing to enlarge after they first appear.

- Ask about the delivery. Incidental trauma from a difficult delivery can lead to bruising or subcutaneous fat necrosis. Forceps marks or a small laceration from the placement of a scalp electrode will heal over time.

- Though most newborn facial lesions cause no symptoms, eczema or rarely seborrhea can be pruritic. Newborns may "scratch" themselves by rubbing their cheeks against their bedding.

- Any lesion that obscures vision needs to be evaluated by an ophthalmologist urgently.

Key Points in the Physical Examination

- Blanching, flat, pale pink lesions on the forehead, eyelids, or nape of the neck are likely nevus simplex.

- Nevus flammeus, also known as a port-wine stain, appears deeply red or red-purple. About 8% of newborns with facial port-wine stains have Sturge–Weber syndrome, a neurocutaneous disorder that can involve the eyes or brain, causing complications, including glaucoma and seizures.

- Erythema toxicum includes poorly demarcated, splotchy red areas often with a white or yellow pustule in the center. Pustular melanosis appears as scattered pustules that fade into small brown freckles.

- Erythema toxicum appears one to several days after birth, and pustular melanosis may be present at birth.

- "Milia" are scattered white papules, present at birth. They are often confused with sebaceous hyperplasia, which appears as yellow-to-white raised lesions typically on the nose. "Miliaria" may be red (miliaria rubra or "prickly heat") or have clear superficial vesicles (miliaria crystallina).

- Red papules and pustules on the cheeks appearing at 2–4 weeks are commonly called "neonatal acne," also known as neonatal cephalic pustulosis.

- Eczema in newborns is worse on the cheeks and spares the nasolabial folds. Seborrhea is usually worse in the nasolabial folds, behind the ears, and in the eyebrows and scalp.

- Herpes simplex lesions appear as vesicles or papulovesicles on a red base.

- A yellowish, warty appearing lesion on the face or scalp may be a nevus sebaceous.

- Annular, round lesions on the scalp and face may be neonatal lupus, even if the mother has no history of systemic lupus erythematosus.

PHOTOGRAPHS OF SELECTED DIAGNOSES

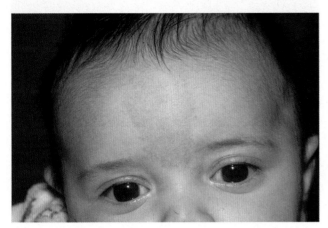

Figure 3-1 Nevus simplex. A pale pink, blanching macule on the face of an infant. These are also called "salmon patch," "angel's kiss," or "stork bite." (Used with permission from Goodheart HP. *Goodheart's Photoguide of Common Skin Disorders.* 2nd ed. Philadelphia, PA: Lippincott Williams & Wilkins; 2003:1.)

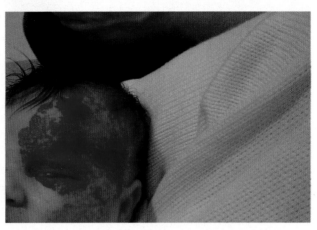

Figure 3-2 Nevus flammeus (port-wine stain). The involvement of the ophthalmic division of the trigeminal nerve necessitates neurological evaluation and an ophthalmic exam in this neonate. (Courtesy of Brian Forbes, MD.)

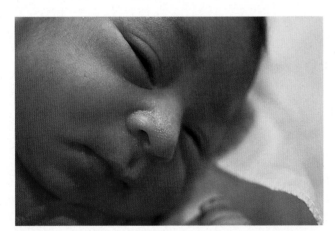

Figure 3-3 Sebaceous hyperplasia. Numerous tiny yellow-white papules on this infant's nose will gradually fade without treatment. (Courtesy of George A. Datto, III, MD.)

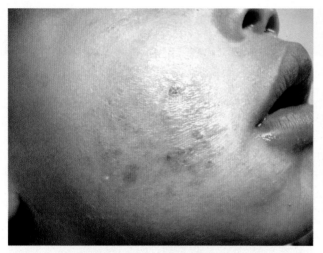

Figure 3-4 Infantile eczema. Dry excoriated skin progressing to weeping lesions is common in neonatal acne. (Courtesy of Paul S. Matz, MD.)

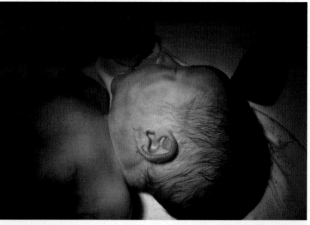

Figure 3-5 Forceps marks. Forceps marks are generally seen on the head and face and may mimic the shape of the forceps themselves. (Courtesy of the late Peter Sol, MD.)

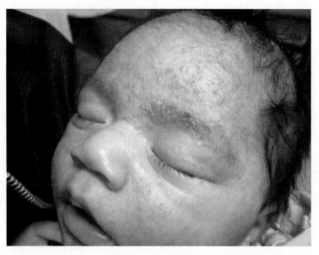

Figure 3-6 Seborrhea. The yellow crusting and scale overlying salmon-colored lesions are especially prominent on the eyebrows of this African American infant. (Courtesy of Paul S. Matz, MD.)

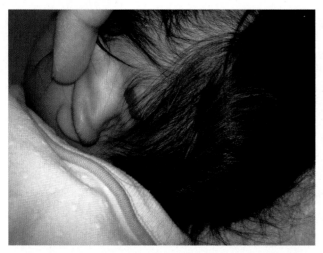

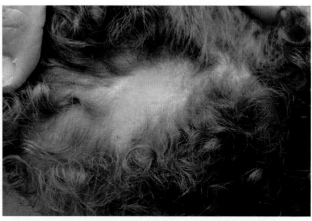

Figure 3-7 Hemangioma. These bright red lesions, here shown behind the ear of a 2-week-old newborn, appear shortly after birth anywhere on the body. They are sometimes referred to as "strawberry" or "cherry" hemangiomata. (Courtesy of Roy Benaroch, MD.)

Figure 3-8 Nevus sebaceous (also called nevus sebaceous of Jadassohn). Usually occurring on the face or scalp, these warty-appearing lesions are present at birth. (Courtesy of Roy Benaroch, MD.)

DIFFERENTIAL DIAGNOSIS

DIAGNOSIS		ICD-10	DISTINGUISHING CHARACTERISTICS	DISTRIBUTION	DURATION/CHRONICITY
Nevus Simplex		Q82.5	Flat pink macules or patch that darken with crying	Lids, forehead, nape of neck	Present at birth; slowly fades over months
Nevus Flammeus		Q82.5	Deep red or purplish	Typically unilateral, most often on face or neck	May deepen in color. Will not disappear
Erythema Toxicum Neonatorum		P83.1	Yellowish papulovesicular lesions with irregular surrounding erythema	Face, trunk, proximal extremities; spares palms and soles	Begins 1–14 days after birth and generally fades by 2–3 weeks
Sebaceous Hyperplasia		L73.9	Yellow to white papules	Typically on the nose and cheeks	Resolves in 1–2 weeks
Seborrhea		L21.1	Waxy red or yellow scale	Scalp, near nose, eyebrows	Usually resolves in infancy
Hemangioma		D18.0	Raised, bright red	Anywhere	Not present at birth; peaks in size at 6–9 months, many involute after this
Neonatal Acne (Neonatal Cephalic Pustulosis)		L70.4	Comedones, papules, pustules	Face (especially cheeks)	Resolves by 3–4 months of life
Infantile Eczema		L20.8	Scaly, red, often pruritic	Cheeks	May resolve quickly or remain present for years
Pustular Melanosis		P83.8	Initially pustules, becoming hyperpigmented macule after rupture	Anywhere, but especially chin, neck, trunk, buttocks	May be seen at birth, resolves within 3 months
Nevus Sebaceous (a.k.a. Nevus Sebaceous of Jadassohn)		I78.1	Warty, yellow	Face or scalp	May become thicker and/or more prominent in time

ASSOCIATED FINDINGS	COMPLICATIONS	PREDISPOSING FACTORS	TREATMENT GUIDELINES
None	None	None	No therapy needed
May be associated with genetic syndromes, including Sturge–Weber or Klippel-Trenaunay-Weber	May occur if underlying syndrome	None	Depends on underlying condition and cosmetic impact of the lesion
None	None	None	No therapy needed
None	None	None	Self-resolving
None	None	None	Medicated shampoos, topical antifungals, topical steroids
None	Cosmetic impact may be considerable, may interfere with vision	None	If treatment necessary, propranolol is rapidly becoming treatment of choice.
None	None; very rarely nodular/scarring	Typically none; if very severe consider hyperandrogenism.	If treatment necessary, benzoyl peroxide Some evidence for use of topical antifungals
May later be associated with atopic disease	Pruritus Secondary infection	Family history of atopy	Emollients; topical steroids
None	More common in families with darker skin	None	No therapy needed
None	Later in life, possible carcinoma	None	Removal at puberty

Other Diagnoses to Consider

- Neonatal lupus

- Herpes simplex virus infection

- Miliaria rubra or miliaria crystallina

- Subcutaneous fat necrosis

When to Consider Further Evaluation or Treatment

- Nevus flammeus (port-wine stain) lesions in the ophthalmic distribution of the trigeminal nerve require evaluation for Sturge–Weber syndrome, including referrals to neurology and ophthalmology. If necessary, an MRI of the brain can identify possible underlying vascular malformations; an ophthalmologic exam should be performed to measure intraocular pressure. Sturge–Weber syndrome should be especially suspected when there is port-wine staining of the lower or both the upper and the lower eyelids. It can be bilateral or unilateral.

- Suspected neonatal lupus should prompt evaluation with an electrocardiogram and tests for anti-Ro and anti-La antibodies.

- Any suspicion of neonatal herpes simplex infection should lead to immediate evaluation and appropriate infection control measures.

- A nevus sebaceous may develop areas of carcinoma after puberty. Nonurgent referral is indicated.

SUGGESTED READINGS

Conlon JD and Drolet BA. Skin lesions in the neonate. *Pediatr Clin North Am.* 2004;51:863–888.
O'Connor NR, McLaughing MR, Ham P. Newborn Skin: Part I. Common Rashes. *Am Fam Physician.* 2008;77(1):47–52.
Paller A and Mancini A. *Hurwitz Pediatric Dermatology: A Textbook of Skin Disorders of Childhood and Adolescence.* 4th ed. Philadelphia, PA: Saunders; 2011:10–36.
Zitelli BJ, McIntire SC, Nowalk AJ. *Zitelli and Davis' Atlas of Pediatric Physical Diagnosis.* 6th ed. Philadelphia, PA: Saunders; 2012:45–78.

Abnormal Head Shape

Laura E. Smals-Murphy

Approach to the Problem

Atypical skull shapes can occur in as many as 20% of infants. Abnormal head shape may be the result of genetic disorders, metabolic abnormalities, or improper positioning of the head. The infant skull is a moldable structure composed of seven unfused cranial plates that are separated by suture lines. Shaping of the skull can be disrupted by internal, external, or intrinsic forces. Internal forces include abnormalities of the brain and surrounding tissues such as abnormally poor brain growth and hydrocephalus. External forces include intrauterine compression and prolonged positioning of the head against a firm surface. Intrinsic forces include craniosynostosis (premature closure of one or more cranial sutures).

Key Points in the History

- Positional plagiocephaly, often a "flattened head," is the most common cause of abnormal head shape and is frequently due to having the head in the same position with supine sleep positioning. Obtaining a history of time spent in the supine position, frequency of "tummy time," and gross motor skill developmental history, is helpful in determining those at risk for positional plagiocephaly.

- History of head tilt with flattening of one side of the head may be a sign of congenital torticollis.

- Prematurity may lead to dolichocephaly because of positional molding of the scalp while in the neonatal intensive care unit.

- Perinatal injury or trauma may cause intracranial bleeding, which can lead to hydrocephalus and subsequent macrocephaly.

- Prolonged labor can result in severe, although transient, molding of the skull.

- Intrauterine fibroids or oligohydramnios can lead to cranial compression and abnormal head shape at birth.

- Developmental delays may indicate abnormal brain development as a cause of abnormal head shape or may be the result of craniosynostosis.

- Signs of increased intracranial pressure include vomiting, lethargy, and poor head control.

- Craniosynostosis can occur in isolation or in association with genetic syndromes. A family history of a syndrome or craniosynostosis may help to identify the etiology of an abnormal head shape.

Key Points in the Physical Examination

- When assessing the head shape, look at the skull from multiple angles: the top of the head from above, upward from below the chin, from the side to view the profile, and from the front and back.

- Evaluate symmetry of the forehead, eyes, nose, cheeks, mouth, and ears. Facial asymmetry may be noted at birth from in utero positioning, and later from positional plagiocephaly or craniosynostosis.

- Measure head circumference to see whether macrocephaly or microcephaly is present in addition to the abnormal head shape. Assess the anterior fontanelle for evidence of increased intracranial pressure or premature closure.

- Positional plagiocephaly may be accompanied by alopecia along the affected area of scalp.

- Suspect congenital torticollis when the child has a palpable nodule within the sternocleidomastoid muscle, a preference to look in one direction, and decreased range of neck rotation.

- In craniosynostosis, the smaller or flattened side of the skull is where the suture has prematurely fused. A palpable ridge may be appreciated over the fused suture line.

- Cloverleaf skull (Kleeblattschädel) occurs as the result of multiple suture synostosis and is rare.

- Dysmorphic facial features, such as a small midface and hypertelorism, may indicate a genetic syndrome as the cause of craniosynostosis.

- Craniosynostosis with associated cleft palate, hearing loss, and limb abnormalities such as syndactyly and cervical spine fusion may also be indicative of a genetic syndrome.

- Unilateral lambdoid craniosynostosis and positional plagiocephaly may be difficult to distinguish clinically. Positional plagiocephaly is common and associated with anterior positioning of the ipsilateral forehead and ear. Lambdoid craniosynostosis is rare and associated with posterior positioning of the ipsilateral ear and prominence of the contralateral forehead and parieto-occipital region.

PHOTOGRAPHS OF SELECTED DIAGNOSES

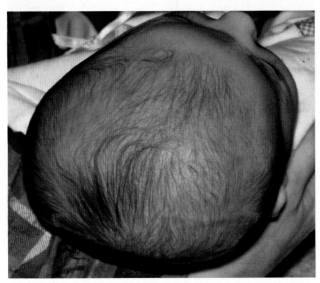

Figure 4-1 Positional plagiocephaly. Flattening of the right posterior skull and anterior positioning of the ipsilateral forehead and ear. (Courtesy of Joseph Piatt, MD.)

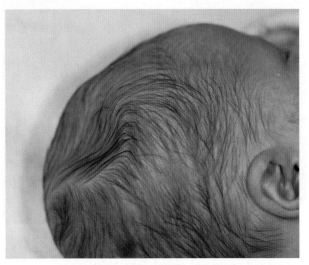

Figure 4-2 Neonatal ping-pong fracture. Note the cup-shaped depression in the head contour of this newborn. This skull defect is thought to be due to in utero positioning. (Courtesy of Esther K. Chung, MD, MPH.)

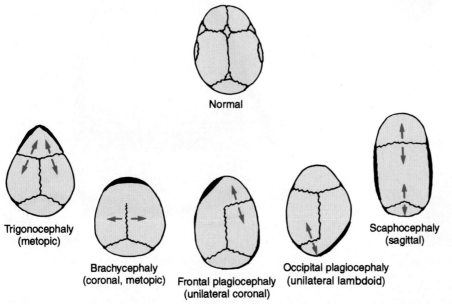

Normal

Trigonocephaly (metopic)

Brachycephaly (coronal, metopic)

Frontal plagiocephaly (unilateral coronal)

Occipital plagiocephaly (unilateral lambdoid)

Scaphocephaly (sagittal)

Figure 4-3 Skull shapes associated with craniosynostosis. The heavy line denotes the area of maximal flattening. The arrows indicate the direction of continued growth across the sutures that remain open. Growth perpendicular to the fused suture line is halted. (Used with permission from Fletcher MA. Physical diagnosis in neonatology. Philadelphia, PA: Lippincott–Raven; 1998:186.)

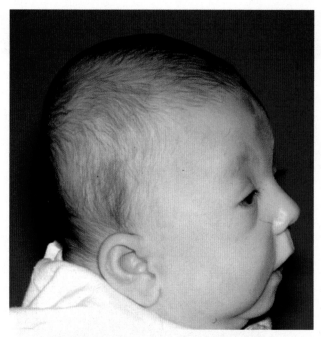

Figure 4-4 Brachycephaly. The short anteroposterior skull diameter results in shallow orbits and subsequent proptosis. (Courtesy of Joseph Piatt, MD.)

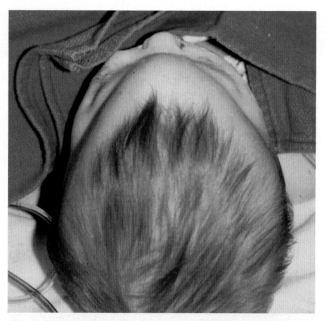

Figure 4-5 Trigonocephaly. Prominent ridge at the metopic suture line. (Courtesy of Scott VanDuzer, MD.)

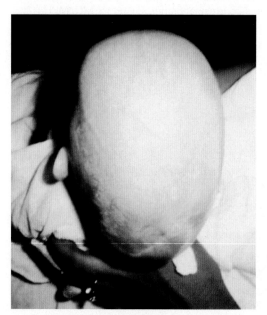

Figure 4-6 Scaphocephaly (Dolichocephaly), top view. Marked increase in head length with narrowed width resulting from premature fusion of the sagittal suture. Premature infants allowed to remain with the head in a side-lying position develop scaphocephalic changes but with more flattening of the sides of the skull. (Used with permission from Fletcher MA. Physical diagnosis in neonatology. Philadelphia, PA: Lippincott–Raven; 1998:186.)

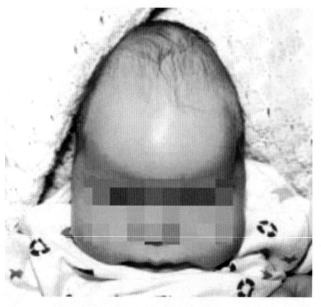

Figure 4-7 Sagittal synostosis. Narrow biparietal diameter. (Courtesy of Joseph Piatt, MD.)

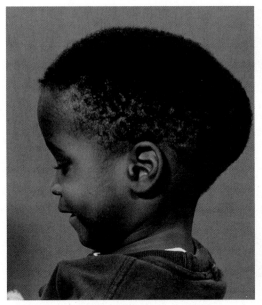

Figure 4-8 Sagittal synostosis. Severe, untreated presentation at 29 months. (Used with permission from Sabry MZ, Wornom IL, Ward JD. Results of cranial vault reshaping. Ann Plast Surg. 2001;47(2):123.)

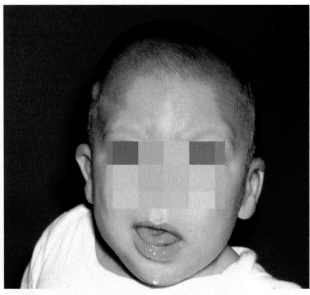

Figure 4-9 Metopic synostosis. Vertical ridge along the fused metopic suture line. (Courtesy of Joseph Piatt, MD.)

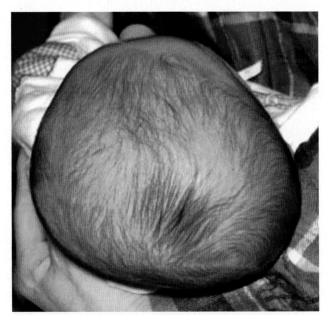

Figure 4-10 Unilateral lambdoid craniosynostosis, left sided. Prominence of the contralateral forehead and parieto-occipital region. (Courtesy of Joseph Piatt, MD.)

SECTION 1 • VISUAL DIAGNOSES IN THE NEWBORN

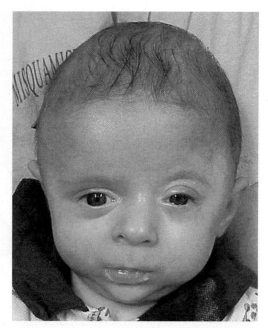

Figure 4-11 Left coronal synostosis. Compensatory growth of the right forehead with marked facial asymmetry. (Used with permission from Lui Y, Kadlub N, da Silva Freitas R, et al. The misdiagnosis of craniosynostosis as deformational plagiocephaly. *J Craniofac Surg.* 2008;19(1):133.)

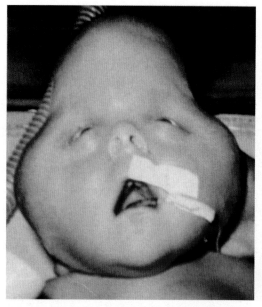

Figure 4-12 Cloverleaf skull (kleeblatt-schädel). Caused by craniosynostosis of all sutures, forcing brain growth through the anterior and temporal fontanels. This most severe form of restricted skull growth has the poorest prognosis because of a combination of craniostenosis and hydrocephalus. (Used with permission from Fletcher MA. Physical diagnosis in neonatology, Philadelphia: Lippincott—Raven; 1998:186.)

DIFFERENTIAL DIAGNOSIS

DIAGNOSIS	ICD-10	DISTINGUISHING CHARACTERISTICS	DISTRIBUTION	ASSOCIATED FINDINGS	PREDISPOSING FACTORS	TREATMENT GUIDELINES
Positional Plagiocephaly	Q 67.3	Flattened area of the skull with history of lying with the head in one position routinely	Usually posterior occiput Can be unilateral, especially when associated with torticollis Bilateral elongation of skull can be seen in premature infants with prolonged side positioning	Alopecia in area of flattening Congenital torticollis	Prolonged supine position, slow achievement of motor milestones, less than three times per day of "tummy time" and more common in first-born or male infants	"Tummy time," prone positioning in the infant when awake only several times per day Repositioning of the head Physical therapy Molding helmets only in severe cases
Congenital Deformity of the Skull	Q75.8	Abnormal head shape seen in a newborn in the absence of trauma May range from a mildly misshapen head to a cup-shaped depression, as with neonatal ping-pong fracture	Variable	May be isolated finding or associated with other abnormalities	Multigestation Aberrant fetal positioning Oligohydramnios	For major deformities, evaluation by pediatric neurosurgery as surgery may be necessary.
Craniosynostosis	Q75.0	Abnormal head shape secondary to premature closure of one or more cranial sutures	Varies with type (see subtypes below)	May have papilledema, increased intracranial pressure, vision and hearing problems, and/or developmental delay, if detected late Look for limb abnormalities, cleft palate, dysmorphic features to suggest an associated genetic syndrome	Genetic syndrome, defects in the fibroblast growth factor receptor (FGFR) gene	Treatment is surgical, including laparoscopic surgery, ideally within the first year of life Refer to a pediatric neurosurgeon. Early referral is optimal for best outcome.
Brachycephaly	Q75.0	Broad head with recessed forehead secondary to premature closure of the coronal suture	Shortened AP diameter	More common in girls Associated with syndromes, especially if bilateral	Genetic syndromes: Apert, Crouzon, Muenke, Jackson–Weiss	Same as other forms of craniosynostosis
Trigonocephaly	Q75.0	Triangular shaped forehead due to the premature closure of the metopic suture	Forehead	The second most common form of craniosynostosis May have papilledema, developmental delay	Genetic syndromes, defects in FGFR genes	Same as other forms of craniosynostosis
Scaphocephaly	Q75.0	Anteroposterior elongation with bitemporal narrowing due to premature closure of the sagittal suture. Must be distinguished from positional elongation that can be seen in premature infants	Long narrow skull	Risk of developmental delay	Genetic syndromes, defects in FGFR genes	Same as other forms of craniosynostosis

- Dandy–Walker malformation

- Cerebral agenesis

- Hydrocephalus

Syndromes associated with craniosynostosis:

- Antley Bixler

- Apert

- Jackson–Weiss

- Baller Gerold

- Carpenter

- Crouzon

- Pfeiffer

- Muenke

- Saethre–Chotzen

Diseases associated with secondary craniosynostosis:

- Ataxia–telangiectasia

- Hyperthyroidism

- Mucopolysaccharidoses

- Rickets

- Sickle cell disease

- Thalassemia major

When to Consider Further Evaluation or Treatment

- Positional plagiocephaly does not require imaging. Repositioning of the head away from the flattened side and "tummy time," prone positioning of the infant when awake only, should resolve the deformity over several weeks to months. Refractory cases may respond to molding helmets.

- In congenital torticollis, physical therapy consultation and range of motion exercises for the neck are helpful.

- When craniosynostosis is suspected, imaging with a skull x-ray or CT scan is indicated.

- Neurosurgical evaluation for craniosynostosis should take place promptly, within the first few months of life. A delay in intervention results in complications such as increased intracranial pressure, impaired brain development, severe cosmetic deformity, vision loss, and hearing loss.

- Severe cases of craniosynostosis, especially when syndromic in etiology, require a multidisciplinary approach, which may include consultation with neurosurgery, otolaryngology, maxillofacial surgery, plastic surgery, ophthalmology, genetics, orthopedics, social work, developmental pediatrics, and psychiatry.

SUGGESTED READINGS

Cunningham ML and Heike CL. Evaluation of the infant with an abnormal skull shape. *Curr Opin Pediatr*. 2007:645–651.

Fletcher MA. *Physical Diagnosis in Neonatology*. Philadelphia, PA: Lippincott–Raven; 1998:186.

Gartner JC and Zitelli BJ. *Common and Chronic Symptoms in Pediatrics*. St. Louis, MO: C.V. Mosby; 1997:102–109.

Laughlin J, Luerssen TG, Dias MS. Prevention and management of positional skull deformities in infants. *Pediatrics*. 2011:1236–1241.

Peitsch WK, Keefer CH, LaBrie RA, Mulliken JB. Incidence of cranial asymmetry in healthy newborns. *Pediatrics*. 2002;110(6):e72.

Ridgway EB and Weiner HL. Skull deformities. *Pediatr Clin North Am*. 2004;51(2):359–387.

Swiss Society of Neonatology. *Neonatal ping-pong fracture*. 2006;1–12. http://www.neonet.ch/assets/cotm/2006-11/COTM-2006-11.pdf. Accessed February 8, 2014.

Van der Meulen. Metopic synostosis. *Childs Nerv. Syst.* 2012;28:1359–1367.

Zitelli BJ and Davis HW. *Atlas of Pediatric Physical Diagnosis*. Philadelphia, PA: Mosby; 2012:892–900.

Newborn Lower Extremity Abnormalities

Holly M. Romero

Holly M. Romero

Approach to the Problem

Appreciation of the differences between the lower extremities of the normal newborn as compared with those of the older child is important in the detection of abnormalities. When compared with older children, normal newborns have greater mobility of the hip, varus alignment of the knee, flatter feet, greater ankle range of motion, and less defined bony prominences.

Lower extremity abnormalities can involve the hip, leg, foot and/or toes and can be positional or structural. While many abnormalities are isolated, some occur with other lower extremity abnormalities or in association with congenital disorders such as myelomeningocele or a congenital myopathy.

It is helpful to think about lower extremity abnormalities as intrinsic or extrinsic. Intrinsic abnormalities are due to characteristics of the infant such as genetic conditions like achondroplasia or osteogenesis imperfecta. Conversely, extrinsic abnormalities are due to in utero conditions such as breech positioning that limit fetal movement, a critical contributor to proper musculoskeletal development. Intrinsic abnormalities are more likely to be due to underlying pathology, whereas most extrinsic abnormalities are positional and resolve spontaneously or respond to surgical correction.

Key Points in the History

- Female gender, breech positioning, and family history of developmental dysplasia of the hip (DDH) are significant risk factors for DDH.

- 80% of cases of DDH occur in females.

- DDH is more common in first-born infants owing to the relative inelasticity of the primigravid uterus and abdominal wall.

- Native Americans and Laplanders are the ethnic groups at highest risk for DDH, with an incidence of up to 50 in 1,000 live births.

36

- History of diminished fetal movement for significant periods of time as reported by the mother may be associated with lower extremity abnormalities caused by intrauterine mechanical factors or intrinsic disease of the fetus such as a myopathy, chromosomal abnormality, or myelomeningocele.

- Congenital talipes equinovarus (clubfoot) occurs two to four times more often in males than in females.

- Maternal smoking during pregnancy is a significant risk factor for clubfoot.

- Though polydactyly is most likely to be an isolated trait, it can be inherited in an autosomal dominant manner with variable penetrance.

- Some teratogenic medications taken during pregnancy such as warfarin, methotrexate, and thalidomide are associated with limb anomalies.

Key Points in the Physical Examination

- A positive exam for DDH is the palpable "clunk" elicited by the Barlow maneuver (detects the hip subluxing or dislocating from the acetabulum) or Ortolani maneuver (detects reduction of the subluxed or dislocated hip).

- Benign, high-pitched soft tissue hip "clicks" are common and should not be confused with true clunks.

- Asymmetry of the inguinal, gluteal, and posterior thigh creases, although nonspecific, is common in DDH. Up to 20% to 30% of normal newborns may have thigh crease asymmetry.

- The malposition seen with metatarsus varus (metatarsus adductus) and positional calcaneovalgus foot are most often correctable with passive motion.

- Metatarsus adductus is distinguished from skewfoot (angled flat foot) by the ability to palpate the head of the talus in the arch of the skewfoot.

- The malposition in talipes equinovarus (clubfoot) is fixed and cannot be passively corrected.

PHOTOGRAPHS OF SELECTED DIAGNOSES

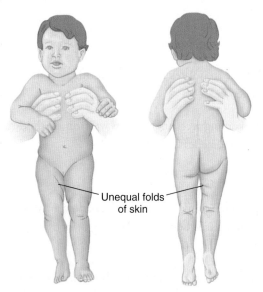

Unequal folds
of skin

Figure 5-1 Developmental dysplasia of the hip. Asymmetry of skin folds are common findings in DDH. (Used with permission from Anatomical Chart Co.)

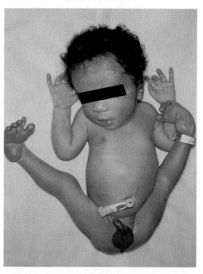

Figure 5-2 Hip flexion contracture. A newborn presents with bilateral hip flexion contracture after breech presentation. (Courtesy of Gerardo Cabrera-Meza, MD.)

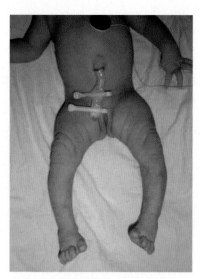

Figure 5-3 Physiologic bowing of the legs. Normal newborn knee alignment is 10–15 degrees varus, creating the bowlegged appearance. (Courtesy of Gerardo Cabrera-Meza, MD.)

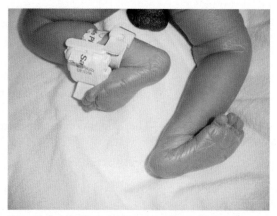

Figure 5-4 Talipes calcaneovalgus. The right foot is hyperdorsiflexed with the dorsal surface contacting the anterior tibial surface. (Courtesy of Gerardo Cabrera-Meza, MD.)

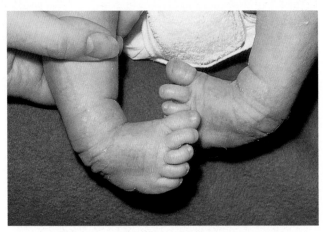

Figure 5-5 Talipes equinovarus (clubfoot). The heel is varus, and the forefoot is adducted and inverted. (Used with permission from Jim Stevenson/SPL/Science Source/Photo Researchers.)

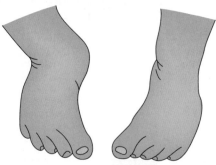

Figure 5-6 Metatarsus adductus. (Used with permission from Frank J Frassica, Paul D Sponseller, John H Wilckens. 5-Minute Orthopaedic Consult. 2nd edition. Philadelphia, PA: Lippincott Williams & Wilkins; 2006.)

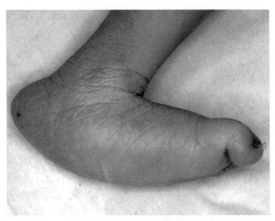

Figure 5-7 Congenital vertical talus (rocker bottom foot). The forefoot is dorsiflexed and abducted with a convex plantar surface. (Courtesy of Gerardo Cabrera-Meza, MD.)

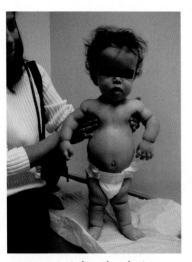

Figure 5-8 Achondroplasia. This infant with achondroplasia has tibial bowing, frontal bossing, rhizomelia (the proximal limb segment is shorter than the distal segment), and brachydactyly (short fingers). (Courtesy of Paul S. Matz, MD.)

SECTION 1 • VISUAL DIAGNOSES IN THE NEWBORN

DIAGNOSIS	ICD-10	DISTINGUISHING CHARACTERISTICS	DISTRIBUTION	DURATION/ CHRONICITY
Developmental Dysplasia of the Hip (DDH)	Q65.0 (unilateral dislocation) Q65.1 (bilateral dislocation) Q65.3 (unilateral subluxation) Q65.4 (bilateral subluxation)	Hip clunk on Barlow or Ortolani maneuver (indicates true subluxation or dislocation)	• Unilateral or bilateral • Left hip most commonly affected when unilateral	Most cases detected at birth and correctable by 2 months of age
Genu Varum (Physiologic Bowing of the Legs)	Q74.1	• Greater than 10 degrees of varus femoral–tibial alignment bilaterally • Bowing throughout the femur, proximal tibia and distal tibia	Bilateral	Remodels to neutral alignment by 14 months of age
Talipes Calcaneovalgus	Q66.4	• Hyperdorsiflexion contracture • Dorsal foot surface often lies against the anterior lower leg	Unilateral or bilateral	Spontaneous resolution over time
Congenital Talipes Equinovarus (Clubfoot)	Q66.0	• Equinus of hindfoot • Adduction of mid- and forefoot • Varus through subtalar joint • Cavus deformity of midfoot • Deep posterior and medial creases • Thick ligaments • Most cases are isolated • Males up to 4 times more affected	Unilateral or bilateral (evenly divided)	Persistent without correction
Metatarsus Varus (Metatarsus Adductus)	Q66.2	• Most common foot deformity in newborns • C-shaped foot due to medial forefoot deviation • Deep medial crease • Most are flexible • Can be inflexible or rigid	• Often bilateral • Left foot most commonly affected when unilateral	>90% of cases spontaneously resolve over time
Toes—Polydactyly	Q69.2	• Extra digit(s) ± duplication of the corresponding metatarsal • Preaxial: medial duplication (15%) • Postaxial: lateral duplication (79%) • Central (6%)	• Bilateral in 50% of cases • When bilateral, more than 60% are symmetric	Persistent without correction
Toes—Syndactyly	Q70.3 (without fusion of bone) Q70.2 (with fusion of bone)	• Fusion ("webbing") of adjacent digits • Simple: fused by skin only • Complex: fused by bone and skin	• Often bilateral • Most common fusion is between second and third toes	Persistent without correction
Achondroplasia (Heterozygous)	Q77.4	Tibial bowing Rhizomelia (the proximal limb segment is shorter than the distal segment). Brachydactyly (short fingers)		Increased mortality in first 5 years of life (particularly in first year) because of sudden death due to cervicomedullary compression

ASSOCIATED FINDINGS	COMPLICATIONS	PREDISPOSING FACTORS	TREATMENT GUIDELINES
• Leg-length discrepancy • Asymmetric inguinal, gluteal or posterior thigh folds Associated disorders: • Myelomeningocele • Arthrogryposis	If untreated: • Limited hip abduction • Femoral shortening • Abnormal gait • Lumbar hyperlordosis • Joint degeneration	• Female gender • Breech position • First-born • Family history • Ethnicity (Native American, Laplander)	• Consult pediatric orthopedics if hip clunk present • Pavlik harness before 6 months of age
In-toeing gait when ambulatory	• None, if truly physiologic • If persistent, unilateral and/or >16 degrees of varus, should rule out Blount disease	None: normal newborn knee alignment is 10–15 degrees varus	No treatment required
Flexible flatfoot (benign)	Only if not distinguished from more serious conditions: • Paralytic calcaneous foot deformity • Associated posteromedial tibial bowing • Congenital vertical talus	• Female gender • First-born • Any condition causing intrauterine crowding	Casting only if the foot cannot be passively flexed to neutral
• Deviant or absent dorsalis pedis artery Associated disorders: • Arthrogryposis • Prune Belly syndrome • Opitz syndrome • Möbius syndrome • Pierre Robin sequence • Larsen syndrome	Impaired mobility	• Maternal smoking • Family history • Combined effect of the above is more than additive	• Consult pediatric orthopedics • Ponseti method: serial manipulation and casting • French method: exercise, taping and continuous passive motion
In-toeing gait when ambulatory	Pain with shoe-wearing	• Family history • Twin gestation	• Flexible: None • Inflexible: Serial manipulation and casting before 1 year of age for best result
• About one-third of cases have polydactyly of the fingers as well • May be accompanied by syndactyly • Preaxial polydactyly can be associated with congenital hallux varus or short fifth metatarsal	• Pain with shoe-wearing • Progressive angular deformity of the toe	• Usually an isolated trait • Can be genetic by autosomal dominant transmission with variable penetrance	• Surgical treatment for any malaligned digit, especially preaxial • Surgical treatment for any duplication causing significant foot widening
Rarely associated with angular deformities unless associated with polydactyly	None, unless associated with polydactyly	Family history	None, unless associated with polydactyly
Frontal bossing and head circumference greater than 97th percentile Hypotonia Normal intelligence Hydrocephalus Spinal cord compression Pulmonary hypertension Sleep-disordered breathing	See other columns	Autosomal dominant inheritance 90% of cases arise de novo, likely to be exclusively inherited from the father and associated with advanced paternal age	Management of associated findings

<table>
<tr><td>

Other Diagnoses to Consider

</td><td>

- Arthrogryposis multiplex l

- Congenital myopathies (most commonly nemaline myopathy)

- Fibular hemimelia

- Klippel–Trenaunay–Weber syndrome

- Skeletal dysplasias (most commonly osteogenesis imperfecta and achondroplasia)

</td></tr>
<tr><td>

When to Consider Further Evaluation or Treatment

</td><td>

- Any infant with a positive exam for DDH (i.e., clunk on Barlow or Ortolani maneuver) should be referred directly to a pediatric orthopedic surgeon.

- All breech-born females without a positive exam should be referred for hip ultrasonography at 6 weeks of age in view of the high incidence of DDH and variable physical exam sensitivity.

- Any leg-length discrepancy should be further evaluated with plain radiography (at or after 4 months of age) for underlying cause and qualitative bone abnormalities.

- Talipes calcaneovalgus that cannot be passively flexed to neutral should be imaged with plain radiography to exclude congenital vertical talus (rocker bottom foot) and then referred for casting.

- Metatarsus adductus that cannot be passively corrected to neutral (i.e., inflexible metatarsus adductus) should be referred to a pediatric orthopedic surgeon for serial casting.

- All patients with rocker bottom feet should undergo MRI of the brain and spine to evaluate for possible underlying neuromuscular disorder.

</td></tr>
</table>

SUGGESTED READINGS

American Academy of Pediatrics, Committee on Quality Improvement, Subcommittee on Developmental Dysplasia of the Hip. *Clinical practice guideline: Early detection of developmental dysplasia of the hip. Pediatrics.* 2000;105(4 Pt 1):896–905.

Furdon SA and Donlon CR. Examination of the newborn foot: Positional and structural abnormalities. *Adv Neonatal Care.* 2002;2(5):248–258.

Gore AI and Spencer JP. The newborn foot. *Am. Fam. Physician.* 2004;69(4):865–872.

Kasser JR. The foot. *Lovell & Winter's Pediatric Orthopaedics.* 6th ed. Vol 2. Philadelphia, PA: Lippincott Williams & Wilkins; 2006:1258–1328.

Schoenecker PL and Rich MM. The lower extremity. *Lovell & Winter's Pediatric Orthopaedics.* 6th ed. Vol 2. Philadelphia, PA: Lippincott Williams & Wilkins; 2006:1158–1211.

Weinstein SL. Developmental hip dysplasia and dislocation. *Lovell & Winter's Pediatric Orthopaedics.* 6th ed. Vol 2. Philadelphia, PA: Lippincott Williams & Wilkins; 2006:988–1037.

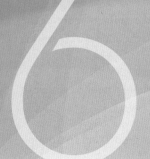

Imperforate Anus

Rebecca G. Taxier and Lauren Wilson

Approach to the Problem

Imperforate anus falls within a spectrum of congenital anomalies of the anus and rectum that are termed anorectal malformations (ARMs). These abnormalities occur with an incidence of 1 in 4,000 to 5,000 live births. Though the exact genetic and embryologic factors contributing to the development of imperforate anus are not completely understood, it is believed that there is a disturbance between the third and eighth gestational week during the development of the hindgut. The variations of ARM may be related to the timing at which the abnormality occurred.

Key Points in the History

- A prenatal diagnosis of imperforate anus is uncommon unless associated anomalies are detected on ultrasound.

- Delayed passage of meconium is often the initial presentation.

- When assessing for delayed passage of meconium, check the delivery room record for the presence of meconium in the amniotic fluid. This may be the only evidence of stooling in the first 24 hours of life.

- Parents or newborn nursing staff may report passage of meconium through another opening, such as the urethra or vagina.

- Assess for symptoms of bowel obstruction, including distended abdomen, emesis, and feeding intolerance.

- If a fistula from the rectum to the urethra or bladder is present, a urinary tract infection may be the initial presentation of an anorectal malformation.

- Hirschprung disease (congenital aganglionic megacolon) may present as a failure to pass meconium in the first days after birth, but this diagnosis does not present as an anatomic malformation of the anus or rectum.

Key Points in the Physical Examination

- Most anorectal malformations are detectable on routine physical examination during the neonatal period; however, it is important to check for patency of the anus as a depression or dimpling in the anal area does not imply a patent anus.

- High-level anomalies have the appearance of a flat perineum without a midline groove or anal dimple.

- Low-level anomalies have the appearance of a prominent midline groove and anal dimple.

- The bowel is not distended at birth; therefore, signs of obstruction may not be detectable in the first 24 hours after birth, but should be present by 72 hours of life.

- Assess for signs of fistula, including meconium staining on the urethral meatus.

- Assess for other congenital anomalies or dysmorphic features.

PHOTOGRAPHS OF SELECTED DIAGNOSES

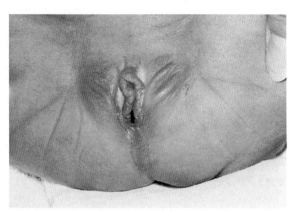

Figure 6-1 **Cloaca.** Cloaca is a high-level anomaly with the vagina, urethra, and rectum sharing a single perineal opening. (Courtesy of Kevin P. Lally, MD.)

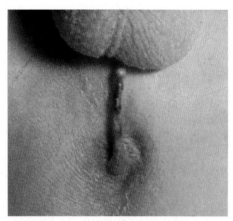

Figure 6-2 **Imperforate anus without fistula.** The visible meconium streak along the raphe is consistent with a low imperforate anus. (Courtesy of Kevin P. Lally, MD.)

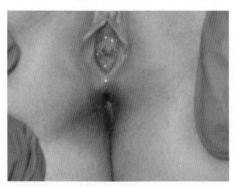

Figure 6-3 **Perineal fistula.** Opening into the perineum just posterior to the fourchette. (Courtesy of Christine Finck, MD.)

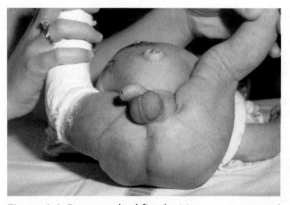

Figure 6-4 **Rectourethral fistula.** Meconium is passed through a fistula opening into the urethra, and there is no visible anal orifice. (Courtesy of Kevin P. Lally, MD.)

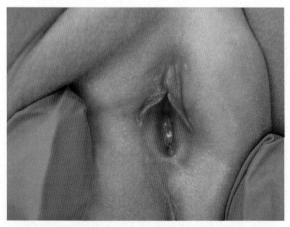

Figure 6-5 **Rectovestibular fistula.** Although there may be a normal appearing vagina and urethra, the rectum opens through the vestibule and causes meconium to pass through the vagina. There is no visible anal orifice. (Courtesy of Mary L. Brandt, MD.)

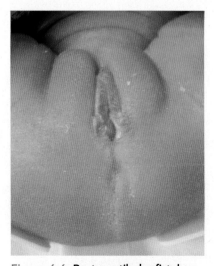

Figure 6-6 **Rectovestibular fistula.** The rectum opens through the posterior fourchette, and there is no visual anal orifice. (Courtesy of Mary L. Brandt, MD.)

DIFFERENTIAL DIAGNOSIS

DIAGNOSIS	ICD-10	DISTINGUISHING CHARACTERISTICS	ASSOCIATED FINDINGS	COMPLICATIONS	TREATMENT GUIDELINES
Cloaca	Q43.7	Single opening for urethra, vagina, and rectal fistula. Abnormally large vagina filled with mucous secretions	Bifid uterus	Pre-repair: hydrocolpos, hydronephrosis, cystitis Post-repair: urethrovaginal fistula, vaginal stricture, fibrosis	Referral to a pediatric surgeon. Length of common channel of structures dictates type of surgery and prognosis (shorter channel = better)
Imperforate Anus Without Fistula	Q42.3	Perineum covered without any identifiable anal opening	Around 50% of these patients have Trisomy 21	Long-standing issues with constipation even post repair	Referral to a pediatric surgeon for colostomy vs primary repair
Rectal Atresia	Q42.1	Externally normal in appearance	Failure to pass meconium	Associated defects rare	Referral to a pediatric surgeon
Rectoperineal Fistula	Q42.2	Majority of rectum in normal position with most distal portion located anteriorly to site of expected anal opening	"Bucket-handle" or "black ribbon" anomaly, which is a subepithelial fistula filled with meconium	Associated defects rare	Referral to a pediatric surgeon for primary repair in newborn period
Rectourethral Fistula	Q64.73	Rectum opens through the lower (bulbar) urethra or upper (prostatic) urethra	Meconium is passed through the urethra.	Low serum bicarbonate secondary to urine back-flowing to rectum	Referral to a pediatric surgeon and/or urologist Typically multistage surgery with initial diverting colostomy
Rectovesical Fistula	Q64.79	Rectum opens through the bladder neck	Meconium is passed through the urethra.	Incontinence	Referral to a pediatric surgeon and/or urologist
Rectovestibular Fistula (Female)	N82.4	Rectum opens through the vestibule, outside the hymenal orifice. Three distinct openings: urethra, vagina, and rectal fistula	Meconium is passed through the vagina.	Most with good functional outcome	Referral to a pediatric surgeon Typically caregivers can do dilations at home with definitive repair when the infant is >3 months old.

<table>
<tr><td>

Other Diagnoses to Consider

</td><td>

- Kidney and urinary tract anomalies plus sacral abnormalities such as caudal regression syndrome, which is seen in association with Trisomy 21.

- Cardiac anomalies

- Limb defects

- Tracheal and esophageal defects

- Urinary tract abnormalities

- VATER (vertebral, anal, trachea-esophageal fistula, rectal anomalies) or VACTERL (vertebral, anal, cardiac, trachea-esophageal fistula, rectal, limb anomalies) association

</td></tr>
<tr><td>

When to Consider Further Evaluation or Treatment

</td><td>

- Imperforate anus and most anorectal malformations require immediate referral to a pediatric surgeon for correction.

- Delay in treatment could result in intestinal perforation.

</td></tr>
</table>

SUGGESTED READINGS

Cho S, Moore SP, Fangman T. One hundred three consecutive patients with anorectal malformations and their associated anomalies. *Arch Pediatr Adolesc Med.* 2001;155:587–591.

Gourlay DM. Colorectal considerations in pediatric patients. *Surg Clin North Am.* 2013;93(1):251–272.

Herman RS and Teirelbaum DH. Anorectal malformations. *Clin. Perinatol.* 2012;39(2):403–422.

Kim HL, Gow KW, Penner JG, et al. Presentation of low anorectal malformations beyond the neonatal period. *Pediatrics.* 2000;105:E68.

Seattle Children's Hospital. Imperforate Anus. http://www.seattlechildrens.org/medical-conditions/digestive-gastrointestinal-conditions/imperforate-anus/. Accessed June 2013.

SECTION 1 • VISUAL DIAGNOSES IN THE NEWBORN

Newborn Skin Abnormalities

Denise A. Salerno

Denise A. Salerno

Approach to the Problem

Concerns about the skin are a common chief complaint during the initial newborn visit in the hospital and the outpatient setting. A recent study of hospitalized neonates found that only 4.3% of the newborns had no dermatological findings. Most newborn skin findings are transient and very rarely require treatment, but it is important to distinguish benign skin lesions from cutaneous manifestations of more serious disorders, such as infections. Therefore, a thorough inspection of the skin for rashes and skin abnormalities is an essential part of the newborn examination.

New parents are often concerned about their baby's skin. Knowledge and recognition of common, benign lesions of the newborn are important for counseling parents about the natural course of these dermatological lesions.

Key Points in the History

- A maternal history of primary active genital herpes simplex virus infection perinatally puts the infant at the highest risk of developing herpes neonatorum. A negative maternal history does not exclude the possibility of this diagnosis.

- A history of cyanosis of the hands and feet is often benign, while cyanosis of the lips and mouth is a sign of hypoxia.

- A rare condition involving transient erythema on one half of the body with a sharp demarcation down the midline is called harlequin color change. It is thought to be benign and subsides after the third week of life.

- Physiologic cutis marmorata, a transient rash brought on by exposure to cold or distress, resolves once the baby is warmed.

- Cutis marmorata telangiectatica is always visible.

- Dermal melanocytosis (a.k.a Mongolian spot) is present at birth in more than 90% of African Americans, 80% of Asians, and rarely in Caucasians.

- Pigmentation is first noted in the periungual and genital areas, which will often appear hyperpigmented at birth in dark-skinned newborns.

- The lesions of epidermolysis bullosa heal slowly, whereas sucking blisters often heal within 48 hours.

Key Points in the Physical Examination

- Infants who appear ill should have skin lesions cultured to rule out viral, bacterial, or yeast infections.

- Dermal melanocytosis consists of nontender, gray-blue macular lesions primarily located on the lumbosacral area, but may be seen over the entire back and on the shoulders and extremities. Familiarity with these lesions will enable a clinician to distinguish these from ecchymoses.

- Miliaria crystallina are pinpoint vesicles containing clear fluid. The lesions are easily denuded with pressure.

- The lesions of erythema toxicum, the most common transient rash in healthy term newborns, are often absent at birth and will often appear during the first few days of life.

- Erythema toxicum spares the palms and soles, while clusters of pustular melanosis may appear on pressure areas.

- Pustular melanosis may present at birth with small hyperpigmented macular lesions if the pustular phase occurred in utero.

- Neonatal pustulosis of transient myeloproliferative disorder has been reported in neonates with Trisomy 21. It presents with pustules and vesicles on a red base predominantly on the face, as part of congenital leukemia or transient myeloproliferative disorder. The lesions also occur at sites of trauma or adhesive usage. There is an associated leukocytosis. Pustules resolve over a few weeks as the leukocytosis resolves.

- Milia are isolated or scattered white pinhead-sized papules that usually occur on the face.

- Sebaceous hyperplasia is often found on the tip of the nose and is often mistaken as milia.

- Initially, neonatal acne may resemble milia, but the lesions become larger and more pustular in the first month of life.

- Acropustulosis of infancy consists of extremely pruritic lesions concentrated on the palms and soles.

- Neonatal seborrhea usually involves the ears, back of the neck, and shoulders. Neonatal eczema spares these areas.

- The vesicles of herpes simplex virus infection often occur on the presenting body part of the infant during birth.

- Cultures of pustular or vesicular lesions can help distinguish benign cutaneous lesions from those of infectious etiology.

PHOTOGRAPHS OF SELECTED DIAGNOSES

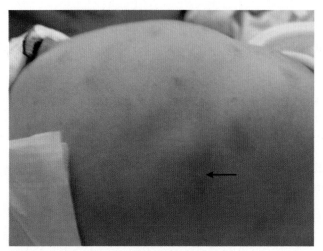

Figure 7-1 **Erythema toxicum.** Note the central papule with surrounding erythema. (Courtesy of Esther K. Chung, MD, MPH.)

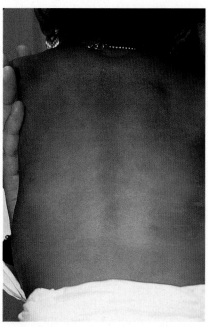

Figure 7-2 **Dermal melanocytosis.** Bluish-gray macular pigmentation on the back of a neonate. (Courtesy of George A. Datto, III, MD.)

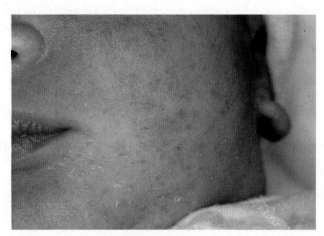

Figure 7-3 **Pustular melanosis.** Hyperpigmented macules with adherent white scale seen after the pustular lesions have ruptured. (Courtesy of Paul S. Matz, MD.)

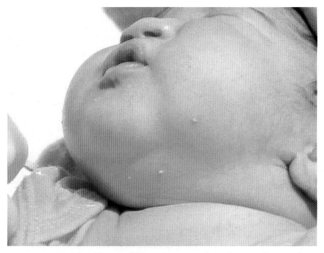

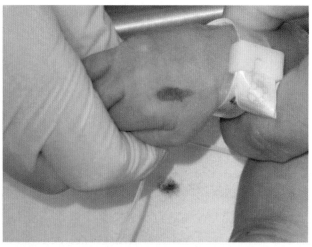

Figure 7-4 Pustular melanosis. Pustular phase of pustular melanosis located on the chin of a newborn. (Courtesy of Denise A. Salerno, MD, FAAP and Hanah Raverby, MD, BS.)

Figure 7-5 Sucking blister. The lesion on the left hand of this newborn is the result of sucking that occurred in utero. (Courtesy of Denise A. Salerno, MD, FAAP.)

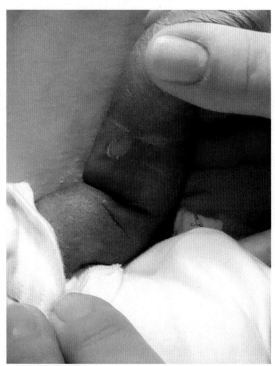

Figure 7-6 Sucking blister. The lesion on the right arm of this newborn resulted from sucking in utero. (Courtesy of Denise A. Salerno, MD, FAAP and Hanah Raverby, MD, BS.)

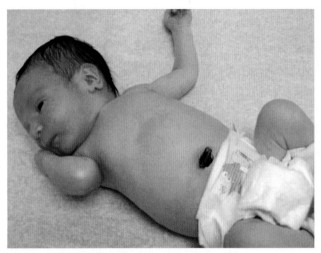

Figure 7-7 Jaundice. Physiologic jaundice. (Courtesy of Denise A. Salerno, MD, FAAP.)

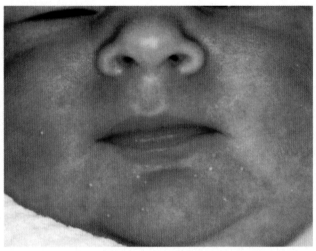

Figure 7-8 Milia. Milia on the cheek and chin of a newborn. (Courtesy of Denise A. Salerno, MD, FAAP.)

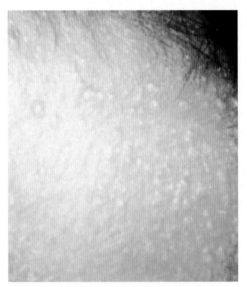

Figure 7-9 Miliaria crystallina alba. (Used with permission from Fletcher MA. *Physical diagnosis in neonatology*. Philadelphia, PA: Lippincott Williams & Wilkins; 1998:124.)

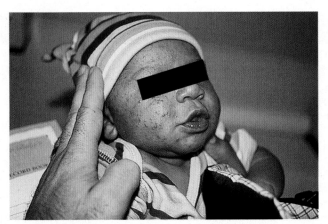

Figure 7-10 Neonatal acne. Erythematous pustular rash on cheeks of a 3-week-old neonate. (Courtesy of George A. Datto, III, MD.)

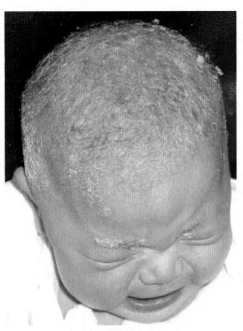

Figure 7-11 Seborrhea. Greasy, scaly lesions of scalp and eyebrows. (Courtesy of the Benjamin Barankin Dermatology Collection.)

DIFFERENTIAL DIAGNOSIS

DIAGNOSIS		ICD-10	DISTINGUISHING CHARACTERISTICS	DISTRIBUTION
Erythema Toxicum		P83.1	Small white-yellow papules with surrounding flare of erythema Onset first 48 hours of life	Trunk Arms Legs Face Palms and soles spared Few to several hundred
Dermal Melanocytosis		D22.5	Bluish-gray macular lesions Varying sizes Resulting from accumulation of melanocytes Incidence varies with ethnicity No risk of malignancy	Lumbosacral area Extensor surfaces Spares face, palms, and soles Single or multiple
Pustular Melanosis		R21	Pustules present in utero or at birth Fragile pustules unroof leaving brown macules surrounded by scale (a "collarette" of peeling skin)	Chin Face Lower back Nape of neck
Sucking Blister		T14.0	Bullous lesion or erosion	Finger Hand Wrist Lip
Neonatal Jaundice (Physiologic)		P59.9	Usually noted at 48–72 hours Yellow discoloration of skin Spreads cephalo-caudally as the bilirubin level increases	Skin Mucous membranes Sclera
Cutis Marmorata (Physiologic)		R23.8	Reticulated mottling of skin Disappears with re-warming	Arms Legs Torso
Milia (Epidermal Inclusion Cyst)		L72.3	Results from retention of keratin and sebaceous material within sebaceous glands Grouped whitish pinhead-sized papules Not denuded by pressure	Forehead Chin Cheeks Nose
Miliaria		Rubra L74.0 Crystillina L74.1	Crystallina • Clear thin-walled pinpoint vesicles • Appear as early as first day of life Rubra • Erythematous papules or vesicles • Appear after first week	Around hairline Face Nape of neck Upper trunk Intertriginous areas Occluded areas
Acne, Neonatal		L70.8	Comedones	Cheeks Forehead
Seborrhea "Cradle Cap"		L21.9 Infantile L20.83 Dermatitis L21.1	Greasy Red scaling Yellow crusting Nonpruritic	Scalp Diaper area Face Postauricular area Shoulder
Acropustulosis of Infancy		L40.3	Pruritic papulopustules or vesiculopustules Appear in crops Recur every few weeks	Hands Feet Wrists Ankles

DURATION/ CHRONICITY	ASSOCIATED FINDINGS	COMPLICATIONS	PREDISPOSING FACTORS	TREATMENT GUIDELINES
Self-limited Few days to few weeks	None	None	More common in full-term infants	Gram stain from fluid in lesions shows eosinophils. No treatment necessary
Fade during childhood Seldom last into adulthood	None	None	N/A	No treatment necessary
Pustular phase—24–48 hours Melanosis stage—few weeks to few months	None	None	N/A	Gram stain from fluid in pustules shows neutrophils. No treatment necessary
Resolves in 24–48 hours	None	None	Results from vigorous sucking on affected body part in utero	No treatment necessary
Depends on severity	May be associated with polycythemia, ABO incompatibility, Rh incompatibility, infection, or liver disease	Kernicterus—if level of bilirubin gets too high	ABO or Rh incompatibility Excessive bruising Breastfeeding	Depends on level of bilirubin and age of infant Resolution can be accelerated by phototherapy
Lasts until 6 months of life	None	None	Physiologic response to cold environment	No treatment necessary
Few weeks to few months	None	None	N/A	No treatment necessary
Resolves with elimination of excessive heat	None	None	Hot, humid weather Over-bundled infants	No treatment necessary
Resolves spontaneously over a few months	None	None	Placental transfer of maternal androgens	No treatment necessary
Seborrhea may be seen in newborns and young children up to age 3 years	None	Scales can become quite thickened and are cosmetically undesirable at times. Associated erythematous papular rash can be noted	N/A	Baby oil-rub on affected area, let sit for 10 min, comb out with fine-toothed baby comb Antiseborrheic shampoos Ketoconazole shampoo Topical steroids
Crops last 2–3 weeks Disorder resolves by 2 years of age	Intense pruritus interferes with sleep	Erosions Crusting Postinflammatory hyperpigmentation	N/A	Topical steroids and antihistamines relieve itch.

Other Diagnoses to Consider

- Herpes simplex neonatorum

- Ecchymoses

- Blue nevus

- Bug bites

- Staphylococcal skin infection

- Bullous impetigo

- Candidal skin infection

- Infantile atopic dermatitis

- Scabies

When to Consider Further Evaluation or Treatment

- Elevated bilirubin levels in the first 24 hours of life, or above the recommended American Academy of Pediatrics algorithm, should promptly be identified and when indicated treated with phototherapy and/or exchange transfusion.

- When neonatal herpes infection is suspected, cultures from multiple sites should be obtained, including any blisters, mucosal surfaces, serum, and cerebrospinal fluid (if indicated). Liver function tests should be obtained as well.

- Infants with bullous impetigo or suspected staphylococcal infections should be promptly treated with antibiotics. Strong consideration should be given to obtaining blood cultures and giving parenteral antibiotics pending culture results.

SUGGESTED READINGS

American Academy of Pediatrics, Committee on Fetus and Newborn. Technical report: phototherapy to prevent severe neonatal hyperbilirubinemia in the newborn infant 35 or more weeks of gestation. *Pediatrics.* 2011;128(4):e1046–e1052.

American Academy of Pediatrics, Committee on Infectious Disease, Committee of Fetus and Newborn. Clinical report: Guidance on management of asymptomatic neonates born to women with active genital herpes lesions. *Pediatics.* 2013;131(2):e635–e646.

Boralevi F and Taïeb A. Common transient neonatal dermatoses. In *Harper's Textbook of Pediatric Dermatology.* Vol 1, 2, 3rd ed. (eds Irvine, AD, Hoeger PH, Yan AC). Oxford, England: Wiley-Blackwell; 2011:6.1–6.12.

Burns T, Breathnach S, Neil C, et al. *Rook's Textbook of Dermatology.* 8th ed. Chichester, West Sussex, England: Wiley-Blackwell, 2010:17.1–17.48.

Ferahbas A, Utas S, Akcakus M, et al. Prevalence of cutaneous findings in hospitalized neonates: a prospective observational study. *Pediatr Dermatol.* 2009;26(2):139–142.

Fletcher MA. *Physical Diagnosis in Neonatology.* Philadelphia, PA: Lippincott Williams & Wilkins; 1998:124.

O'Connor N, McLaughlin M, Ham P. Newborn skin: Part I common rashes. *Am Fam Physician.* 2008;77(1):47–52.

GENERAL
APPEARANCE

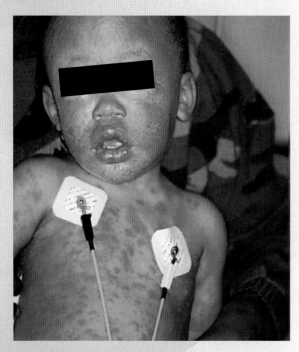

(Courtesy of Joseph Lopreiato, MD.)

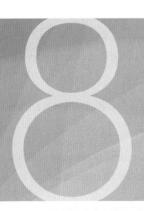

General Appearance

Evan J. Weiner

Approach to the Problem

A patient's general appearance is considered one of the most important elements of the physical examination. It represents a subjective impression of the patient's state of being. First and foremost, this impression informs about the patient's overall degree of wellness, distinguishing whether or not the patient is ill-appearing. In addition, one can assess specific aspects of the patient's presentation ranging from the obvious to the more subtle. Specifically, one can examine such patient characteristics as alertness level, nutritional status, facial expression, consolability, developmental ability, respiratory effort, personal interaction, behavior, hygiene, coloring, movement, and gait.

Key Points in the History

- It is essential to ascertain whether the observed general appearance is consistent with that noted by the caregivers.

- Obtaining a patient's baseline status is crucial.

- A changing story, or one inconsistent with physical findings or developmental ability, raises the suspicion of child abuse.

- In the case of a critically ill or injured patient, elicit a SAMPLE history—as described by Pediatric Advanced Life Support—**S**igns and symptoms, **A**llergies, **M**edications, **P**ast medical history, **L**ast meal, and **E**vents leading to presentation.

- When pain is present, assess the patient's subjective degree of pain, or preferably utilize a facial or numerical pain scale.

- When evaluating a febrile child, response to and timing of antipyretics, consolability, and willingness to feed help to determine the severity of illness. Reevaluation following defervescence is also helpful.

- When evaluating children of non-English-speaking families, all efforts should be made to communicate in their preferred language to avoid missing crucial elements in the history and physical examination.

- A social smile is rarely present in a child with meningitis or other invasive serious bacterial infections. However, it may be present in occult bacteremia.

- Absent tears, dry mucous membranes, ill general appearance, and delayed capillary refill are reliable external clues of dehydration.

- Tachypnea, nasal flaring, grunting, and accessory muscle use are signs of *respiratory distress*. Depressed sensorium, apnea, bradycardia, and cyanosis are signs of *respiratory failure*.

- Shock can be clinically diagnosed with evidence of poor organ perfusion, for example, altered sensorium, mottled skin, peripheral cyanosis, tachypnea, and decreased peripheral pulses. Septic or "warm" shock may lead to flushing and bounding pulses.

- Elements of a toxic general appearance include grunting, weak or persistent cry, sunken eyes, grey or mottled skin, depressed sensorium, and altered social response.

- Seizure activity may be evidenced by abnormal movements, posturing, extremity jerking, lip smacking, altered mental status, and staring eyes. Seizure activity in neonates may manifest as bicycling movements, chewing, blinking, and/or rigidity.

- A patient with peritoneal irritation lies flat and still. Patients with colicky abdominal conditions appear restless and uncomfortable. Paroxysms of irritability and drawing up of legs may indicate conditions such as intussusception.

- Children with epiglottitis appear toxic and may sit in a "tripod" position. Muffled voice, drooling, and stridor also indicate upper airway obstruction.

- Visual assessment of pain can be done via scales looking at a patient's cry, facial expression, torso position, and extremity movements.

PHOTOGRAPHS OF SELECTED DIAGNOSES

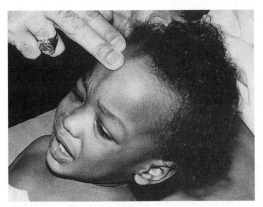

Figure 8-1 Meningitis. (Used with permission from Fleisher GR, Ludwig S, Baskin MN. *Atlas of Pediatric Emergency Medicine*. Philadelphia, PA: Lippincott Williams & Wilkins; 2004:183.)

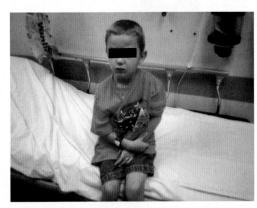

Figure 8-2 Well-appearing child with left supracondylar fracture. This well-appearing, but apprehensive, child's positioning informs of his supracondylar fracture of the left humerus. (Courtesy of Evan J. Weiner, MD, FAAP.)

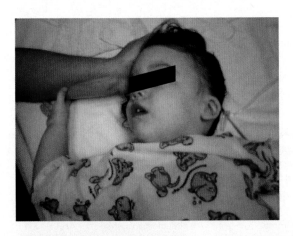

Figure 8-3 Ill-appearing child. This child appears weak and clingy but alert and active. Her ill appearance is the result of a mucocutaneous form of mycoplasma infection. (Courtesy of Evan J. Weiner, MD, FAAP.)

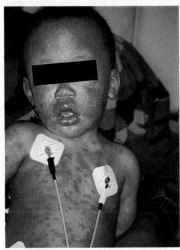

Figure 8-4 Ill-appearing child with Stevens–Johnson syndrome. (Courtesy of Joseph Lopreiato, MD.)

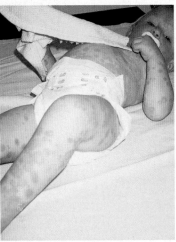

Figure 8-5 Ill-appearing child with urticaria. (Used with permission from Fleisher GR, Ludwig S, Baskin MN. *Atlas of Pediatric Emergency Medicine*. Philadelphia, PA: Lippincott Williams & Wilkins; 2004:88.)

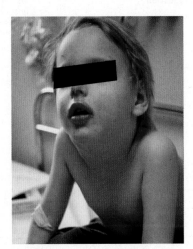

Figure 8-6 Epiglottitis and tripod positioning. This child's "tripod" positioning is indicative of epiglottitis. Note the child's toxic appearance. (Courtesy of M. Douglas Baker, MD.)

DIFFERENTIAL DIAGNOSIS

DIAGNOSIS	ICD-10	DISTINGUISHING CHARACTERISTICS	DISTRIBUTION	DURATION/ CHRONICITY
Bacterial Meningoencephalitis	G00.9 Bacterial meningitis, unspecified	Altered mental status Toxic appearance	Neurologic system	Acute to subacute
Hypovolemia	E86.1	Dry mucous membranes Absent tears Sunken eyes Lethargy	Mucosa Skin Eyes Vasculature	Acute to subacute
Congestive Heart Failure	I50.9 Heart failure, unspecified	Orthopnea Jugular venous distension Hepatomegaly Central cyanosis	Cardiac system Lungs Liver Extremities	Subacute
Increased Intracranial Pressure	G91 Hydrocephalus S09.90 Unspecified injury of head	Depressed sensorium Bulging fontanelle Cushing triad	Neurologic system	Acute to subacute
Acute Abdomen	R10.0 K56.1 (Intussusception)	Abdominal tenderness Irritability	Abdomen	Acute
Respiratory Distress	J80 Respiratory distress in child	Wheezing Stridor Retractions Nasal flaring Tachypnea	Pulmonary system	Acute to subacute
Toxic Ingestion	T65.94X Toxic effect of unspecified substance, undetermined, initial encounter	Toxidrome Evidence of substance ingested	Multiorgan system	Acute

ASSOCIATED FINDINGS	COMPLICATIONS	PREDISPOSING FACTORS	TREATMENT GUIDELINES
Fever Nuchal rigidity Kernig/Brudzinski signs Seizures Emesis Headache	Sepsis Hearing loss Encephalopathy	Immunocompromise Immunization delay	Broad-spectrum IV antibiotics Steroids prior to the first antibiotic dose
Poor perfusion Decreased urine output Decreased peripheral pulses Cool extremities	Electrolyte derangement Acidosis Renal failure Shock	Vomiting Diarrhea Hemorrhage Anorexia Polyuria	Oral rehydration therapy IV hydration
Respiratory distress Edema Growth failure Other malformations	Cardiac arrest Renal failure Hypoxia Shock	Congenital heart disease Cardiomyopathy Myocarditis Hypertension	Diuretics Inotropes Afterload reduction Surgery
Emesis Seizures Focal neurologic signs Apnea Sundowning	Cardiopulmonary arrest Traumatic brain injury	Trauma Hydrocephalus Tumor	Hyperventilation Mannitol Surgery Hypertonic saline
Fever Anorexia Vomiting Diarrhea Dehydration Tachypnea Peritoneal signs	Sepsis Bowel perforation	Appendicolith Intestinal obstruction For intussusception: • Meckel diverticulum • Viral illness	Broad-spectrum IV antibiotics Surgery Bowel rest Nasogastric tube For intussusception: • Air contrast enema • Surgery
Apnea Depressed sensorium Grunting Cyanosis	Cardiopulmonary arrest	Infection Bronchospasm Upper airway obstruction Foreign body aspiration	Oxygen IV access Bronchodilators Steroids Airway management Chest radiography
Vomiting Altered sensorium Respiratory distress Apnea Seizures	Arrhythmias Aspiration Brain injury	Lack of childproofing Suicidality Intentional poisoning	Naloxone Activated charcoal Specific antidotes Cardiac monitoring

Other Diagnoses to Consider

- Inborn error of metabolism

- Electrolyte derangement

- Hypoglycemia

- Adrenal crisis

- Hepatic encephalopathy

- Uremia

- Autoimmune disease

- Human immunodeficiency virus infection

- Supraventricular tachycardia

- Failure to thrive

- Child abuse and neglect

When to Consider Further Evaluation or Treatment

- Tachypnea and tachycardia may be subtle clues of a more serious underlying condition and future deterioration. They should prompt urgent evaluation.

- In patients with altered mental status, in addition to pursuing the etiology, one must ensure stability of the airway, even though a primary respiratory process may not be present.

- A shock state may be present, even when a normal blood pressure is maintained due to compensatory mechanisms. Ill general appearance should lead one to consider and treat shock.

SUGGESTED READINGS

Athreya B, Silverman B. Subjective observations. In: *Pediatric physical diagnosis.* Norwalk, CT: Appleton-Century Crofts; 1985:58–70.

Bang A, Chaturvedi P. Yale Observation Scale for prediction of bacteremia in febrile children. *Indian J Pediatr.* 2009;76:599–604.

Bass JW, Wittler RR, Weisse ME. Social smile and occult bacteremia. *Pediatr Infect Dis J.* 1996;15(6):541.

Gorelick M, Shaw K, Murphy K. Validity and reliability of clinical signs in the diagnosis of dehydration in children. *Pediatrics.* 1997;99(5):E6.

Hsiao AL, Chen L, Baker MD. Incidence and predictors of serious bacterial infections among 57- to 180-day-old infants. *Pediatrics.* 2006;117(5):1695–1701.

Levine DA, Platt SL, Dayan PS, et al. Risk of serious bacterial infection in young febrile infants with respiratory syncytial virus infections. *Pediatrics.* 2004;113(6):1728–1734.

McCarthy P, Sharpe M, Spiesel S, et al. Observation scales to identify serious illness in febrile children. *Pediatrics.* 1982;70(5):802–809.

HEAD

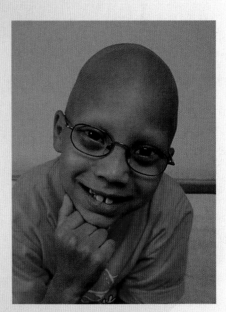

(Courtesy of Paul S. Matz, MD.)

THREE

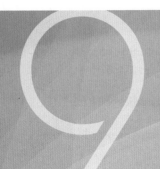

Hair Loss

Daniel R. Taylor

Approach to the Problem

Hair loss, or alopecia, may be congenital, hereditary, or acquired. The distribution of hair loss may be described as localized, as in alopecia areata, or more diffuse, as in telogen effluvium. Though hair loss often occurs in isolation, it may be a sign of systemic illness. Hair growth cycle disruption in the anagen (active), catagen (regressive), or telogen (resting) phases may cause hair loss. Also, any damage to the follicle or shaft may result in hair loss, as in trichotillomania. Some causes of hair loss, such as tinea capitis, may lead to scalp scarring and permanent hair loss if left untreated, which can be psychologically damaging to the parents and the child.

Key Points in the History

- Tinea capitis is the primary cause of alopecia in African American children.

- Home remedies for a child's scaling scalp, such as hair grease and oils, may mask the underlying scale of tinea capitis.

- Recent illness may cause the hair to enter the resting (telogen) phase and manifest as diffuse hair loss (telogen effluvium).

- Traction alopecia, from tight braiding, is a common cause of hair loss.

- Cutis aplasia and sebaceous nevus of Jadassohn may present at birth as well-circumscribed areas of the scalp devoid of hair.

- Hair loss in younger teens necessitates a search for autoimmune disorders, such as thyroid disorders or psychiatric problems.

- There may be a family history of hair loss or autoimmune disease, such as in systemic lupus erythematosus (SLE).

- Children with systemic symptoms, diffuse rash, and nail or teeth abnormalities may have hair loss as a manifestation of a more widespread disease, such as in acrodermatitis enteropathica.

- A prepubescent child with a scaly scalp should warrant a scalp culture to check for tinea capitis.

- The breakage of hair shafts close to the scalp in tinea capitis causes the "black dot" sign.

- Kerions and pustules, host inflammatory responses to fungal infections, usually do not represent bacterial superinfection.

- Trichophyton species, accounting for more than 90% of tinea capitis in North America, do not fluoresce under a Wood lamp.

- Intrinsic hair shaft defects, hair pulling, or tight braiding may cause hair breakage further away from the scalp.

- Older children with hair loss need to be assessed for psychological stress, if hair pulling, or trichotillomania, is the cause of their alopecia.

- Hair pulling tends to be biased toward the side of a patient's handedness.

- Major hair loss is often related to systemic widespread disease.

- The combination of considerable scalp erythema and hair loss should prompt an investigation into evolving psoriasis or lupus.

PHOTOGRAPHS OF SELECTED DIAGNOSES

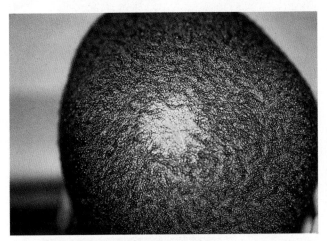

Figure 9-1 Tinea capitis. Circumscribed area of hair loss with scaliness of the scalp. (Courtesy of George A. Datto, III, MD.)

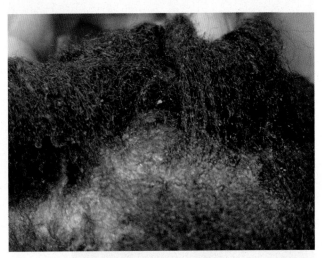

Figure 9-2 Tinea capitis. Diffuse scaling and pustules on the scalp. (Courtesy of Paul S. Matz, MD.)

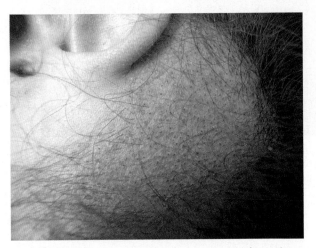

Figure 9-3 "Black dot" sign. Broken hair shafts at the scalp from tinea capitis. (Courtesy of Paul S. Matz, MD.)

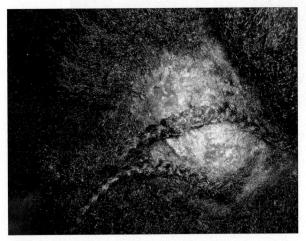

Figure 9-4 Kerion. Intense inflammatory response to tinea capitis. (Courtesy of Paul S. Matz, MD.)

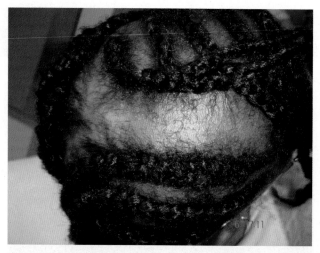

Figure 9-5 Traction alopecia. Alopecia where traction has been applied in association with hair braiding. (Courtesy of Carrie Ann Cusack, MD.)

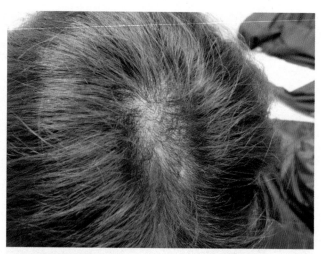

Figure 9-6 Trichotillomania. Broken hair shafts caused by pulling of one's hair. (Courtesy of George A. Datto, III, MD.)

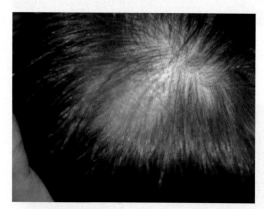

Figure 9-7 Sebaceous nevus of Jadassohn. Yellowish orange verrucous plaque on the scalp. (Courtesy of the Department of Dermatology, Drexel University College of Medicine.)

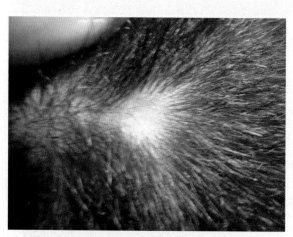

Figure 9-8 Cutis aplasia. Scar on the vertex of the scalp with complete hair loss secondary to cutis aplasia. (Courtesy of Paul S. Matz, MD.)

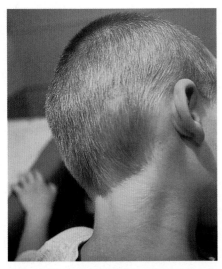

Figure 9-9 Discoid lupus. Oval area of hair loss associated with scalp erythema, scaling, and follicular plugging. (Courtesy of George A. Datto, III, MD.)

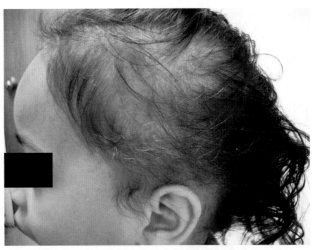

Figure 9-10 Telogen effluvium. Diffuse thinning of hair 3 months after febrile illness. (Courtesy of Paul S. Matz, MD.)

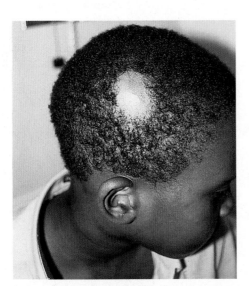

Figure 9-11 Alopecia areata. Localized circular patch of hair loss with normal scalp skin. (Courtesy of George A. Datto, III, MD.)

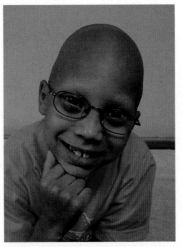

Figure 9-12 Alopecia universalis. Hair loss affecting the scalp, eyebrows, and eyelashes. (Courtesy of Paul S. Matz, MD.)

DIFFERENTIAL DIAGNOSIS

DIAGNOSIS		ICD-10	DISTINGUISHING CHARACTERISTICS	DISTRIBUTION
Tinea Capitis		B35.0	Alopecia, associated with scaling May present as diffuse dryness without alopecia "Black dot" sign	Focal or diffuse
Telogen Effluvium		L65.0	Abrupt hair loss with brushing or washing	Diffuse
Traction Alopecia		L66.8	Hair is thinned at edges of braids	Focal
Trichotillomania		F63.3	Broken hair shafts of varying lengths Irregular borders	Crown of head (Friar Tuck sign) Occipital Parietal
Sebaceous Nevus of Jadassohn		Q85.9	Orange Waxy Congenital	Focal
Cutis Aplasia		Q84.8	Congenital Oval-shaped alopecia	Midline
Alopecia Areata		L63.8	Absence of scaling or erythema in areas of hair loss "Exclamation mark" hairs (broken short hairs that taper proximally) Sharp borders	Parietal Occipital
Discoid Lupus		L93.0	Erythema Scaly	Focal
Syphilitic Alopecia		A51.32	Moth-eaten alopecia Generalized thinning	Focal or diffuse

ASSOCIATED FINDINGS	COMPLICATIONS	PREDISPOSING FACTORS	TREATMENT GUIDELINES
Occipital and posterior auricular lymphadenopathy Id reaction can occur and may worsen with treatment.	Kerion	*Trichophyton tonsurans* African American or Hispanic race/ethnicity	Scalp culture Oral antifungals—griseofulvin first line If resistant, consider terbinafine or fluconazole (need baseline liver function tests prior to and during treatment) Selenium sulfide shampoo to prevent spread Can return to school after initiation of treatment
N/A	Psychological	Acute illness in previous several months	Parental and patient reassurance
Small inflammatory papules Regional lymphadenopathy	Scarring of hair follicles	Tight braids or ponytails	Loosen hair braids and/or ponytails Topical antibiotics if infected
Anxious child Obsessive–compulsive disorder	Bezoars due to ingesting pulled hairs	Psychological stress	Cognitive behavioral therapy Selective serotonin reuptake inhibitors
N/A	Potential for basal cell carcinoma after puberty	N/A	Biopsy and removal usually recommended prior to puberty
Can be associated with congenital anomalies	Permanent hair loss, due to scarring	N/A	For large areas, plastic surgery revision may be needed
Eyebrow hair loss Nail changes Autoimmune diseases	Psychological	Autoimmune pathogenesis Atopy Genetic	Consider thyroid testing Watchful waiting Topical corticosteroids injectable corticosteroids Oral immunosuppressants
Similar lesions on sun-exposed skin	Permanent hair loss due to scarring	Autoimmune pathogenesis	17% chance of progression to SLE within 3 years Topical immunosuppressants
Skin manifestations on hands and feet Positive rapid plasma reagin	Progression to tertiary syphilis	Sexual activity	Penicillin G

SECTION 3 • HEAD

Other Diagnoses to Consider

- Monilethrix

- Pili torti

- Menkes kinky hair syndrome

- Trichorrhexis nodosa

- Loose anagen syndrome

- Ectodermal dysplasia

When to Consider Further Evaluation or Treatment

- Further evaluation and treatment should be considered for areas of intense scalp inflammation.

- Several months of treatment failure for tinea capitis with griseofulvin as first-line therapy warrant consideration of reinfection, resistance, or an alternate diagnosis, such as psoriasis.

- Consider referral to a psychologist for children with trichotillomania.

- Diffuse hair loss warrants a search for a systemic disorder, such as SLE, syphilis, thyroid disorders, or vitamin D deficiency.

SUGGESTED READINGS

Jabeen M, Mendiratta V. Hair loss and its management in children. *Expert Rev Dermatol*. 2011;6(6):581–590.

Shy R. Tinea corporis and tinea capitis. *Pedaitr Rev*. 2007;20(5):164–174.

Tay Y, Levy M, Metry D. Trichotillomania in childhood: Case series and review. *Pediatrics*. 2004;113(5):e494–e498.

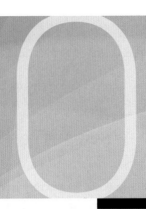

White Specks in the Hair

Benjamin W. Sanders and Hans B. Kersten

Approach to the Problem

White specks in the hair may be a manifestation of systemic disease or of localized scalp disease. It is important to check other parts of the body for signs of disease as white specks in the hair may not always be from disease limited to the scalp. Once properly identified, white specks in the hair can usually be treated effectively.

Key Points in the History

- Extensive application of hair products can present as white, nonpruritic flakes close to the scalp.

- Tinea capitis is a common cause of white specks in the hair and/or alopecia in children of African descent, but it is uncommon in children of other race/ethnicities.

- Tinea capitis is acquired through personal contact with spores from a lesion.

- Seborrheic dermatitis, also known as cradle cap in infants, may also occur in adolescents during puberty.

- Seborrheic dermatitis in infants usually involves the scalp but may extend to other areas of the body. It typically resolves by 7 to 8 months of age.

- Atopic dermatitis is common in infants and may involve the scalp. Patients often have a family history of asthma, allergies, or allergic rhinitis.

- Children with atopic dermatitis affecting the scalp often complain of itchiness or scratching.

- Head lice infestation, a relatively common cause of itchy scalp, is usually a disease of school-aged girls. It is uncommon in children of African descent, and occurs in all socioeconomic groups. Head lice are acquired through close contact with an infested person. Although less commonly than previously thought, acquisition may also occur through contact with infested items such as hats, headsets, combs, brushes, and bedsheets.

- Psoriatic lesions may occur over the entire body. Thirty to forty percent of affected patients have a family history of disease.

- Round patches of inflammation with flakiness and alopecia are typical with tinea capitis.

- Occipital lymphadenopathy is commonly seen with tinea capitis, which helps to distinguish it from other causes of white flakes.

- Diffuse tinea capitis may resemble seborrheic dermatitis and present as diffuse scalp dryness without alopecia or erythema.

- Wood lamp examination will produce a yellow-green fluorescence for microsporum dermatophyte species but not for trichophyton species, which account for 90% of tinea capitis cases.

- Scales on the scalp may not be seen on examination if family members are applying hair grease or other oily hair products to the scalp.

- Greasy, scaly, yellowish, or salmon-colored lesions on the scalp characterize seborrheic dermatitis. Lesions may also appear on the face, eyebrows, neck, shoulders, intertriginous areas, flexural areas of the extremities, or the diaper area.

- Atopic dermatitis, typically pruritic, may also involve the face and trunk. Popliteal and antecubital involvement distinguishes it from seborrheic dermatitis. Lesions are often accompanied by scabbing and excoriations.

- Lesions of seborrheic dermatitis usually are well circumscribed, while lesions of atopic dermatitis are more diffuse.

- The nits of head lice may be confused with dandruff. They can be distinguished from dandruff because nits are firmly attached to the hair shaft while dandruff is not.

- Nits more than 10 mm from the scalp are unlikely to be viable; their nymphs have hatched, leaving behind a casing. Using a nit comb to remove nits close to the scalp while the hair is wet may improve outcomes.

- The scalp is typically normal in appearance with head lice. With atopic dermatitis, seborrheic dermatitis, and tinea capitis, there is scaling of the scalp.

- Psoriasis may present with erythematous, thick, silver, scaly plaques.

PHOTOGRAPHS OF SELECTED DIAGNOSES

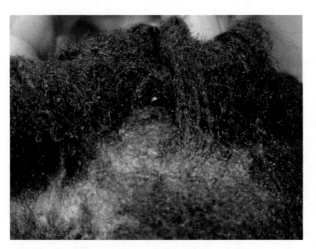

Figure 10-1 Tinea capitis. Note the dry, flaky appearance. (Courtesy of Paul S. Matz, MD.)

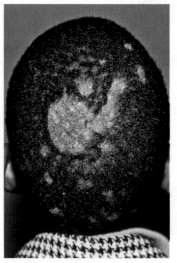

Figure 10-2 Tinea capitis. This photograph shows areas of black-dot alopecia. (Courtesy of Paul S. Matz, MD.)

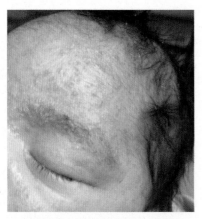

Figure 10-3 Seborrhea. Note the greasy appearance. (Courtesy of Paul S. Matz, MD.)

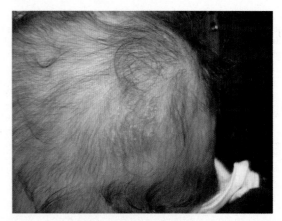

Figure 10-4 Scalp eczema. Note the area of erythema underlying the dry scale. (Courtesy of Paul S. Matz, MD.)

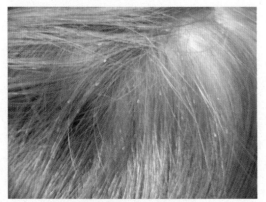

Figure 10-5 Pediculosis capitis. Note the whitish nits found along the hair shafts. (Courtesy of Hans B. Kersten, MD.)

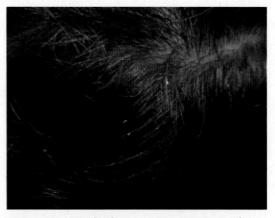

Figure 10-6 Pediculosis capitis. (Courtesy of Hans B. Kersten, MD.)

DIFFERENTIAL DIAGNOSIS

DIAGNOSIS		ICD-10	DISTINGUISHING CHARACTERISTICS	DISTRIBUTION	DURATION/CHRONICITY
Tinea Capitis		B35.0	Scaly scalp Black-dot sign Patches of alopecia with scales on scalp	Focal or diffuse	Resolves over weeks with systemic antifungal therapy Kerions may take weeks to improve even with proper treatment.
Seborrhea		L21.9	Salmon-colored macules with greasy, yellowish to brownish scale. Young infants and adolescents Rash on scalp, diaper, or intertriginous areas	Rash involves the face, eyebrows, neck, shoulders, flexural and intertriginous areas of the extremities, and/or diaper area	Usually resolves by 1 year of age Occurs also during puberty
Eczema		L30.9	Pruritus Fluctuating course Rash distribution changes with age Generally worse in the winter time Usually spares diaper area	Extensor surfaces and face in infancy; flexural surfaces in older children; may be diffuse	Symptoms wax and wane, but often persist throughout childhood
Head Lice (Pediculosis Capitis)		B85.0	Difficult to dislodge nits from the hair shaft Nits right next to the scalp Lice on the scalp Normal scalp	Diffuse nits in the hair near nape of the neck	Quickly eliminated with effective treatment Recurrence is common secondary to poor compliance and repeated exposures at school.
Psoriasis		L40.9	Overlying erythema, silvery thick scales with well-defined borders Commonly extends beyond hairline Auspitz's sign: punctate bleeding when scales are picked is a pathognomonic sign.	Scalp is initial site in 20%–40%	Chronic with recurrences

ASSOCIATED FINDINGS	COMPLICATIONS	PREDISPOSING FACTORS	TREATMENT GUIDELINES
Occipital or cervical adenopathy Id reaction—papulovesicular rash on trunk	Kerion—a boggy, edematous inflammatory reaction to tinea capitis Hair loss	Age—occurs almost exclusively in childhood Gender—boys affected five times more than girls	Systemic antifungal agents—may need to treat longer because of increased resistance Selenium sulfide shampoo two times per week to reduce spore transmission Oral corticosteroids—may hasten recovery with kerion, but not routinely recommended
None	Candidal infections in intertriginous areas Bacterial infections Intertrigo Blepharitis	Age—Infancy (birth—12 months) Adolescence—at onset of puberty	Scalp: • Attempt to clear scalp lesions. • Anti-seborrheic shampoo (containing sulfur or salicylic acid) • Topical mineral oil—loosens thick and adherent scales on the scalp • Topical corticosteroid lotion to scalp ONLY in difficult-to-treat cases Body: mild-potency corticosteroids
Diffusely dry skin (xerosis) Lichenification Dermatographism Atopic diseases Hyper-accentuated palmar creases Altered cell-mediated immunity Keratosis pilaris	Secondary infection Bleeding Lichenification Personality traits—active, restless, irritable, aggressive Kaposi varicelliform eruption with abrupt vesicular onset Cataracts—early onset in 4%–12% of affected individuals	Atopy—part of an allergic triad that also includes allergic rhinitis and asthma	Moisturizers/lubricants Mild soaps Antihistamines Soft, nonirritating clothing Topical corticosteroids—mainstay of treatment for flares Calcineurin inhibitors as second-line agents (note black box warning and potential risk of malignancies) Systemic corticosteroids—not routinely recommended unless cannot be controlled by other methods
Lice on the scalp or in the hair Normal scalp	None	Humans—exclusive reservoir for lice Close personal and crowded contact—schools, camps, institutions Rare in blacks; more common among whites	Permethrin 1%—nonprescription, repeated in 7–10 days (some evidence that most efficacious retreatment at 9 days) Examine and treat all household contacts with confirmed lice or sharing bed with an infested person. Permethrin cream 5%—prescription Spinosad Pyrethrins and piperonyl butoxide 4% Benzyl alcohol Malathion Lindane—no longer recommended Hot air treatment with an approved device may be an effective alternative. Other devices, commercial preparations, and home products such as olive oil, mayonnaise, or petroleum jelly have little data to support efficacy. Nit combing of wet hair after use of pediculocides may improve results.
Usually includes lesions beyond the scalp	May advance to other forms of psoriasis	Caucasian background Positive family history	Topical corticosteroids and scale removal using oil-based products Tar and keratolytics such as urea

SECTION 3 • HEAD

Other Diagnoses to Consider

- Acrodermatitis enteropathica

- Wiskott–Aldrich syndrome

- Langerhans cell histiocytosis

- Impetigo

When to Consider Further Evaluation or Treatment

- Further evaluation and treatment should be considered if scalp flaking fails to improve with standard treatment regimens above.

- Tinea capitis recalcitrant to first-line medical treatment requires a second treatment course or use of a different antifungal agent.

- Significant hair loss secondary to a kerion found in association with tinea capitis should prompt referral to a dermatologist.

- Severe atopic dermatitis unresponsive to frequent use of emollients and mid-potency topical steroids requires referral to a dermatologist.

- Severe atopic dermatitis accompanied by failure to thrive warrants further evaluation and possible referral to a dermatologist.

- Persistent weeping of lesions in seborrhea may signal a secondary candidal infection.

- Recurrent lice is common in school-aged children secondary to poor medication compliance and repeated exposures at school.

SUGGESTED READINGS

Ahuja A, Land K, Barnes CJ. Atopic dermatitis. *South Med J.* 2003;96:1068–1072.

Chen BK, Friedlander SF. Tinea capitis update: A continuing conflict with an old adversary. *Curr Opin Pediatr.* 2001;13:331–335.

Frankowski BL, Bocchini JA; Council on School Health and Committee on Infectious Diseases. Head lice. *Pediatrics.* 2010;126:392.

Gupta AK, Bluhm R. Seborrheic dermatitis. *J Eur Acad Dermatol Venereol.* 2004;18:13–26.

Paller AS, Mancini AJ. *Hurwitz Clinical Pediatric Dermatology: A Textbook of Skin Disorders of Childhood and Adolescence.* 4th ed. Philadelphia, PA: Elsevier Saunders; 2011:37–52, 56–57, 71–80, 391–395, 424–427.

Lumps on the Face

Kelly R. Leite

Approach to the Problem

Facial lumps cause concern for parents though many of these lesions are benign and self-limited. The more common pediatric facial lesions include dermoid cyst, epidermoid cyst, superficial and deep (subcutaneous) hemangioma, pilomatricoma, buccal cellulitis, pyogenic granuloma, Spitz nevus, and suppurative parotitis. Less common lesions include trichoepitheliomas, Pott puffy tumor, panniculitis, fat necrosis, juvenile xanthogranuloma, and mumps. Although many of these facial lumps do not require immediate therapy, it is important to correctly diagnose and identify those lesions requiring urgent medical attention.

Key Points in the History

- Trauma is usually associated with hematomas.

- Hemangiomas, juvenile xanthogranulomas, and dermoid cysts are present at birth or appear in early infancy.

- Epidermoid cysts can appear at any age but appear more commonly after puberty.

- Prolonged exposure to cold in the area of swelling suggests panniculitis. Fat necrosis often occurs secondary to cold trauma.

- Constitutional symptoms of fever and malaise may suggest mumps, suppurative parotitis, buccal cellulitis, or Pott puffy tumor.

- A history of recurrent parotid swelling or a family history of parotid swelling may indicate juvenile recurrent parotitis, a nonsuppurative parotid inflammation of unknown etiology.

- The history of an unimmunized child with parotid inflammation strongly suggests mumps.

- Chronic, nonpainful swelling of the parotid gland may be seen in patients with HIV infection.

- Swelling that obscures the angle of the jaw suggests parotid inflammation or parotitis.

- Children with mumps are rarely ill-appearing.

- Suppurative parotitis, most commonly caused by *Staphylococcus aureus,* is associated with an ill-appearing child with purulent discharge from Stensen duct.

- Buccal cellulitis, panniculitis, hematoma, parotitis, and Pott puffy tumor produce painful lumps.

- Swelling associated with erythema of the overlying skin suggests buccal cellulitis, panniculitis, fat necrosis, or suppurative parotitis.

- Friable lesions are characteristic of pyogenic granulomas.

- A Spitz nevus is a rapidly growing dome-shaped, erythematous papule commonly found on the face and extremities.

- Lumps with an associated bluish hue suggest a pilomatricoma or deep (subcutaneous) hemangioma.

- A pilomatricoma is typically a rock-hard papule due to its propensity to calcify.

- Fluctuant, tender, erythematous swelling over the frontal sinus suggests a frontal osteomyelitis with associated subperiosteal abscess, a condition known as Pott puffy tumor.

PHOTOGRAPHS OF SELECTED DIAGNOSES

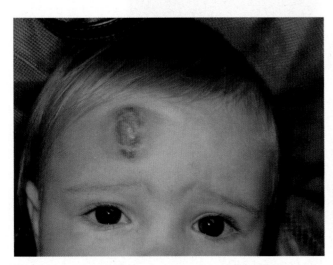

Figure 11-1 Mixed hemangioma. A rapidly growing mass with superficial and subcutaneous components. (Courtesy of Andrea L. Zaenglein, MD.)

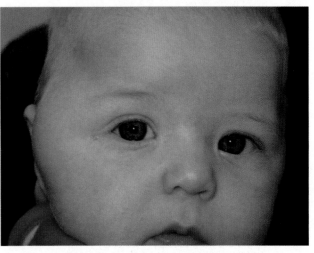

Figure 11-2 Deep or subcutaneous hemangioma. Note the normal overlying skin. (Courtesy of Andrea L. Zaenglein, MD.)

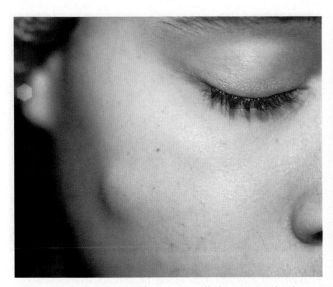

Figure 11-3 Epidermoid cyst. A well-demarcated solitary nodule on the face. (Used with permission from Goodheart HP. *Goodheart's Photoguide of Common Skin Disorders*. Philadelphia, PA: Lippincott Williams & Wilkins; 2003:4.)

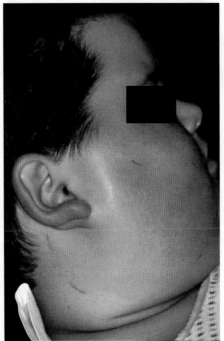

Figure 11-4 Parotitis. Dramatic edema, erythema, and induration of the face overlying the parotid gland. (Courtesy of Kathleen Cronan, MD.)

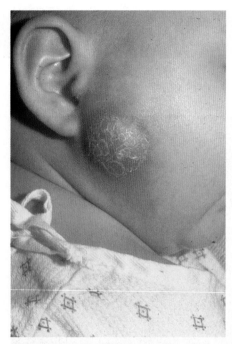

Figure 11-5 Parotid abscess. A well-demarcated fluctuant mass overlying the parotid gland. (Courtesy of the late Peter Sol, MD.)

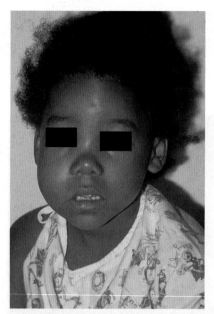

Figure 11-6 Buccal cellulitis. Diffuse unilateral facial swelling associated with dental caries. (Courtesy of the late Peter Sol, MD.)

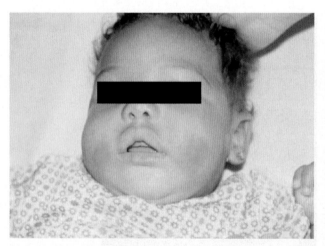

Figure 11-7 Panniculitis. Bilateral, erythematous firm subcutaneous nodules in the cheeks of this infant caused by cold trauma (popsicle). (Courtesy of Kathleen Cronan, MD.)

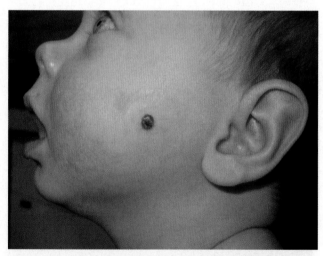

Figure 11-8 Pyogenic granuloma. Isolated erythematous nodule that easily bleeds. Note the annular "band-aid sign" around the lesion, showing evidence that a band-aid had been used for the bleeding. (Courtesy of Andrea L. Zaenglein, MD.)

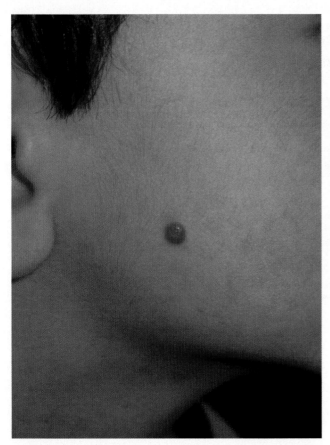

Figure 11-9 **Spitz nevus.** Erythematous, solitary, dome-shaped lesion on the cheek of this child. (Courtesy of Andrea L. Zaenglein, MD.)

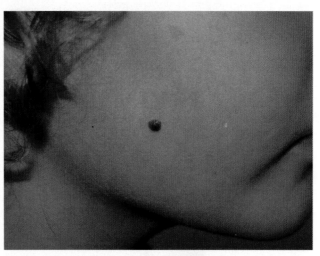

Figure 11-10 **Pigmented Spitz nevus.** Deeply pigmented, solitary, dome-shaped nodule. (Courtesy of Andrea L. Zaenglein, MD.)

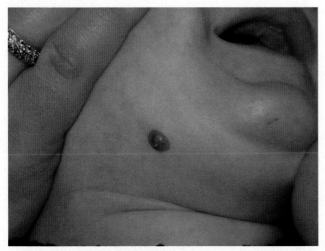

Figure 11-11 **Juvenile xanthogranuloma.** Isolated orange/brown firm papule on the chin of this child. (Courtesy of Andrea L. Zaenglein, MD.)

DIFFERENTIAL DIAGNOSIS

DIAGNOSIS	ICD-10	DISTINGUISHING CHARACTERISTICS	DISTRIBUTION
Hematoma	S00.93xa	Large, erythematous and/or bluish hue	Most commonly on forehead
Hemangioma	D18.01	Superficial or "strawberry" (pink/red) lesions Deep/subcutaneous (blue/skin-colored) lesions	Head and neck most common May occur on trunk, oral and genital mucosae
Fat Necrosis	P15.6	Multiple or single, erythematous, nontender nodules	Cheeks, buttocks, thigh Sites of trauma
Epidermoid Cyst	L72.0	Well-demarcated, solitary nodule or papule	Face, scalp, neck, trunk
Parotitis	B26.9 (mumps) K91.89 (suppurative)	Painful swelling of parotid that obscures angle of mandible	Parotid gland Mumps is usually bilateral. Suppurative type is unilateral.
Buccal Cellulitis	K12.2	Tender to palpation Salmon or violaceous color	Subcutaneous and dermal layers of cheek Unilateral
Popsicle Panniculitis	M79.3	Erythematous nodules Painful to palpation	Perioral subcutaneous fat Angle of mouth often bilateral
Pyogenic Granuloma	L98.0	Bright red, exophytic lesion Moist appearing	60% on head/neck Usually solitary
Spitz Nevus	I78.1	Red, dome-shaped papule Pigmentation may vary.	Face Extremities
Dermoid Cyst	D23.9	Firm, skin-colored nodules	Periorbital area lateral eyebrows, midline forehead
Pilomatricoma	D23.9	Bluish hue Hard nodule Nontender Female predominance	Face, head, and neck
Trichoepithelioma	D23.39	Smooth, flesh-colored papules Irregular borders	Nasolabial folds, upper lip, forehead
Juvenile Xanthogranuloma	D23.3 (Benign neoplasm of face)	Arise abruptly on head/neck Yellow/orange color Various size nodules	Head/neck
Pott Puffy Tumor	J32.1	Erythematous, painful fluctuant mass	Frontal scalp edema

DURATION/CHRONICITY	ASSOCIATED FINDINGS	COMPLICATIONS	TREATMENT
Rapid resolution of edema with remaining bruise	Associated trauma Pain to palpation	Subcutaneous nodule with slow resolution	Ice to lesion and pain control at time of initial trauma
Rapidly enlarge in first year of life Involution by 6 years of age	Rapidly enlarging lesions seen in Kasabach–Merritt or PHACE syndrome	Bleeding after trauma Obstruction of airway, vision, or genitourinary tract	Reassurance Oral propranolol or intralesional/oral steroids for obstructive lesion Pulse dye laser
Appears in first weeks of life Heals spontaneously	Associated trauma	Calcification Ulceration Infection	Self-limited Dermatology consult if calcification
Slow-growing Persists for life	Normal overlying skin Central dimple	Recurrent inflammation Lesions may rupture.	Surgical excision
Viral type in childhood Suppurative type in neonates/older children	Brief prodrome with mumps Increased amylase level in 70% cases	Rarely: orchitis, encephalitis, pancreatitis, deafness, nephritis, myocarditis	Supportive (mumps) Antistaphyloccocal antibiotics for suppurative cases
Acute onset Peak incidence at 9–12 months Resolves with treatment	Acute otitis media commonly seen Generally ill-appearing child	Bacteremia, meningitis intracranial extension, cavernous sinus thrombosis	Parenteral antibiotics
Lesions persist 2–3 weeks Lesions not immediately apparent	Well-appearing child Caused by cold trauma	N/A	No treatment required as this self-resolves
Most commonly in childhood Persists unless excised	Associated trauma	Profuse bleeding Infection Postexcision lesions	Curettage and cauterization
Rapidly growing	Increased melanin creates a brown or black lesion	N/A	Simple excision
Congenital	Intracranial extension in midline lesions	Risk of meningitis/infection, if communication with underlying structures	Surgical excision
Unlikely to regress	Multiple lesions less common	Calcification often occurs	Excision of lesion
Slow-growing	Multiple lesions suggest familial association	Disfigurement with presence of multiple lesions	Simple excision Dermabrasion, curettage for multiple lesions
Most present in first year Spontaneous regression by 6 years of age	Extracutaneous involvement—most commonly ocular	Hyphema, glaucoma—ocular involvement is most common Organ involvement is rare.	Corticosteroids, radiation, and surgical excision for systemic involvement or symptomatic lesions
Generally responds to treatment once properly identified	Headache, fever, frontal sinus pain	May progress to intracranial abscess formation	Surgical drainage Antibiotics

Other Diagnoses to Consider

- Metastasis of malignant tumor

- Idiopathic neuroma

- Multiple mucosal neuromas (multiple endocrine neoplasia type 2B)

- Lymphocytoma cutis

When to Consider Further Treatment

- Enlarging hemangiomas at risk for obstructing the nose or eye should be referred to a dermatologist.

- Hemangiomas in a "beard" distribution require evaluation by a dermatologist due to the risk of airway complications.

- Lesion consistent with fat necrosis may require dermatology referral if calcification or ulceration occurs.

- Epidermoid cysts with recurring inflammation may require surgical excision.

- Prompt medical attention is required if parotid or buccal mucosal swelling is accompanied by fever or an ill appearance.

- Pyogenic granulomas with frequent or profuse bleeding require urgent surgical excision.

- Dermoid cysts communicating with underlying structures may evolve into serious infections requiring antibiotics.

- A deeply pigmented Spitz nevus warrants a dermatology evaluation to rule out a more significant lesion such as malignant melanoma.

- Multiple xanthogranulomas on the face should prompt a referral to ophthalmology to assess for extracutaneous involvement.

- Pott puffy tumor can lead to significant morbidity if not diagnosed and treated promptly.

SUGGESTED READINGS

Haggstrom A, Drolet B, Baselga E. Prospective study of infantile hemangiomas: Clinical characteristics predicting complications and treatment. *Pediatrics*. 2006;118(3):882–887.
Kinsey EN, Wilson BB. Pyogenic granuloma. *Consultant*. 2012;52:82.
Krowchuk D, Mancini A. *Pediatric Dermatology*. 2nd ed. Elk Grove Village, IL: American Academy of Pediatrics; 2012:321–339, 417–419.
Miller T, Frieden IJ. Hemangiomas: New insights and classification. *Pediatr Ann*. 2005;34(3):179–190.
Nahlieli O, Shachem R, Shlesinger M, et al. Juvenile recurrent parotitis: A new method of diagnosis and treatment. *Pediatrics*. 2004;114(1):9–12.
Pickering LK, Baker CJ, Kimberlin DW, et al., eds. *Red Book: 2012 Report of the Committee on Infectious Diseases*. 29th ed. Elk Grove Village, IL: American Academy of Pediatrics; 2012:653–668.
Suwan PT, Mogal S, Chaudhary S. Pott's puffy tumor: An uncommon clinical entity. *Case Reports in Pediatrics*. 2012;2012, Article ID 386104, 4 pages.
Pride H, Yan A, Zaenglein A. *Requisites in Pediatric Dermatology*. London/GB: Elsevier; 2008:120–136.

EYES

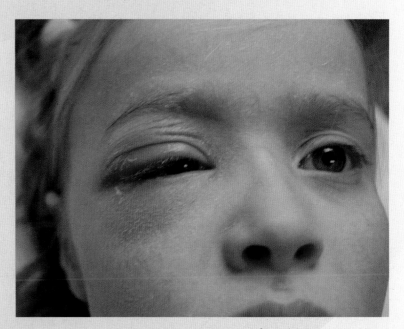

(Courtesy of Parul P. Soni, MD, MPH.)

FOUR

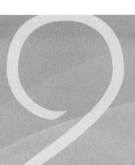

Red Eye

Parul P. Soni and Steven M. Selbst

Approach to the Problem

A red eye is an eye with vascular congestion of the conjunctiva resulting from inflammation, trauma, conjunctivitis, or glaucoma. Redness may also be secondary to eyelid pathology. Conjunctivitis is the most common cause of a red eye, whereas glaucoma is rare in pediatrics. Conjunctivitis is commonly referred to as "pink eye" when it is caused by a viral or bacterial infection. Conjunctivitis may also have an allergic etiology. Trauma to the eye can cause eye redness in association with corneal abrasions, iritis, and subconjunctival hemorrhage. Red eye may be related to eyelid pathology such as blepharitis and periorbital (preseptal) or orbital (postseptal) cellulitis (see Chapter 13). Red eyes may also be seen in some systemic diseases such as Kawasaki disease.

Key Points in the History

- A history of atopy, allergen exposure, or seasonality will often help distinguish viral from allergic conjunctivitis.

- Pruritus is a common complaint with allergic conjunctivitis.

- While viral and bacterial conjunctivitis may have purulent discharge, early morning lid crusting or gluey eyes usually points to a bacterial etiology.

- The time of presentation is very important in the neonate with conjunctivitis; chemical conjunctivitis usually occurs in the first 24 hours, conjunctivitis secondary to gonococcal infection usually appears within 1 week after birth, and conjunctivitis secondary to chlamydial infection usually appears 1 to 2 weeks after birth.

- Ocular pain with eye movement suggests orbital cellulitis rather than preseptal cellulitis.

- Pain after trauma suggests corneal abrasion or iritis, while subconjunctival hemorrhages are usually painless.

- Decreased vision and marked photophobia suggest a more serious diagnosis, such as glaucoma.

- Consider Kawasaki disease when an irritable child with fever has red eyes but no eye discharge.

- Chemosis is swelling of the conjunctiva due to allergy or irritation.

- Conjunctivitis associated with pharyngitis is often caused by adenovirus.

- A palpable, preauricular lymph node in association with conjunctivitis is suspicious for viral conjunctivitis.

- Unilateral conjunctivitis with surrounding vesicular lesions is highly suspicious for keratoconjunctivitis resulting from herpes simplex virus.

- A history of gluey or sticky eyelids and physical findings of mucoid or purulent discharge are highly predictive of bacterial infection.

- Forty percent to fifty percent of those who have conjunctivitis in association with acute otitis media (formerly described as the otitis media–conjunctivitis syndrome) may have infection due to nontypeable *Haemophilus influenzae*.

- Visual acuity, because it may be impaired, should be tested whenever orbital cellulitis is suspected.

- Signs of orbital cellulitis, such as limited eye movement and decreased vision, may mimic those of orbital pseudotumor and neoplasm.

- Fluorescein examination is extremely helpful in diagnosing a corneal abrasion. Holding the fluorescein strip near the outer canthus, while having the patient blink, allows the dye to taint the tears. To further limit discomfort, fluorescein dye may be applied to the conjunctiva following the application of an ocular anesthetic.

- Consider other diagnoses, such as keratitis, iritis, or uveitis, when the limbus (the sclerocorneal junction) is involved.

PHOTOGRAPHS OF SELECTED DIAGNOSES

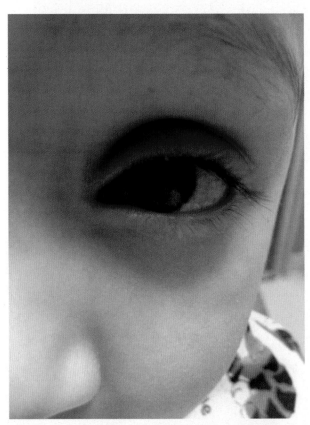

Figure 12-1 Allergic conjunctivitis with lid edema and conjunctival injection. (Courtesy of Parul P. Soni, MD, MPH.)

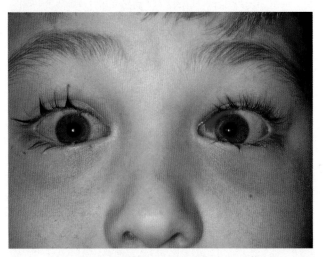

Figure 12-3 Conjunctivitis with a subconjunctival hemorrhage. Note the subconjunctival hemorrhage on the left. (Courtesy of Steven M. Selbst, MD, FAAP.)

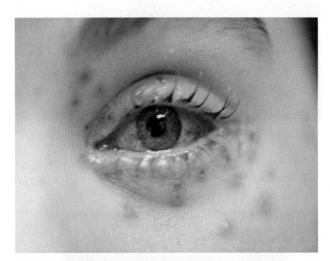

Figure 12-4 Herpes keratoconjunctivitis. Note the classic vesicular lesions around the eye. (Courtesy of Steven M. Selbst, MD, FAAP.)

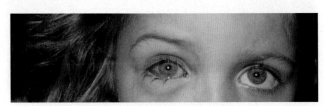

Figure 12-2 Viral conjunctivitis. Note the classic appearance of the red eye, absence of thick eye discharge. (Courtesy of Parul P. Soni, MD, MPH.)

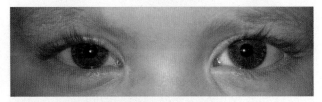

Figure 12-5 Bacterial conjunctivitis. The early-morning eyelid gluing and/or crusting may be absent on examination. (Courtesy of Steven M. Selbst, MD, FAAP.)

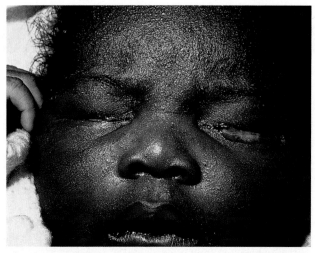

Figure 12-6 Gonococcal ophthalmia neonatorum. (Used with permission from Ostler HB, Maibach HI, Hoke AW, et al. *Diseases of the Eye and Skin: A Color Atlas.* Philadelphia, PA: Lippincott Williams & Wilkins; 2004:269.)

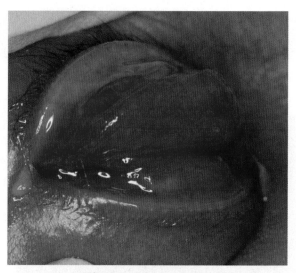

Figure 12-7 Chlamydia conjunctivitis. Note the severe chemosis and purulent discharge. (Courtesy of Parul P. Soni, MD, MPH.)

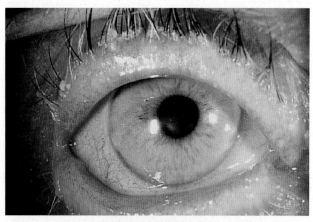

Figure 12-8 Blepharitis. Note the irritation of the eyelid margins. (Used with permission from Weber J, Kelley J. *Health Assessment in Nursing.* 2nd ed. Philadelphia, PA: Lippincott Williams & Wilkins; 2003:196.)

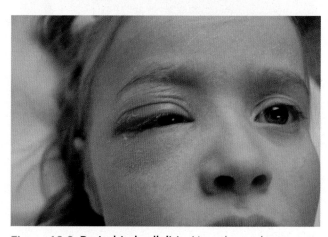

Figure 12-9 Periorbital cellulitis. Note the erythema and swelling of the eyelids. (Courtesy of Parul P. Soni, MD, MPH.)

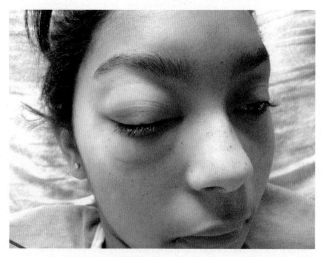

Figure 12-10 Orbital cellulitis. Note swelling and proptosis of the right. (Courtesy of Steven M. Selbst, MD, FAAP.)

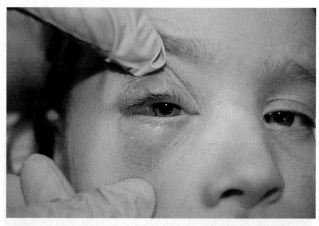

Figure 12-11 Chemosis. Note the impressive swelling of the conjunctiva. (Courtesy of Parul P. Soni, MD, MPH.)

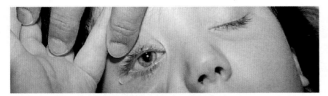

Figure 12-12 **Corneal abrasion.** Note the prominence of fluorescein medially. (Courtesy of Kathleen Cronan, MD.)

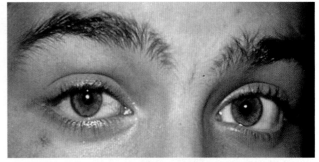

Figure 12-13 **Traumatic iritis.** Note the conjunctival injection that appeared the day after trauma. (Courtesy of Steven M. Selbst, MD, FAAP.)

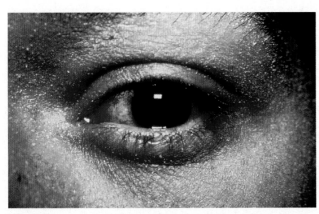

Figure 12-14 **Conjunctivitis seen with Kawasaki disease.** (Used with permission from Goodheart HP. *Goodheart's Photoguide to Common Skin Disorders.* 2nd ed. Philadelphia, PA: Lippincott Williams & Wilkins; 2003:198.)

DIFFERENTIAL DIAGNOSIS

DIAGNOSIS		ICD-10	DISTINGUISHING CHARACTERISTICS	DISTRIBUTION
Allergic Conjunctivitis		H10.10 Acute atopic conjunctivitis, unspecified eye H10.45 Other chronic allergic conjunctivitis	Seasonal or year-round Pruritic Conjunctival edema (chemosis) Usually watery discharge Bilateral	Diffuse (involves whole conjunctiva and sclera)
Viral Conjunctivitis		B30.9 Viral conjunctivitis, unspecified	History of exposure Ocular discomfort Watery discharge Tender preauricular lymph node Follicular aggregates	Diffuse (involves whole conjunctiva and sclera)
Herpes Keratoconjunctivitis		B00.52 Herpes simplex keratoconjunctivitis	Lid often swollen Watery discharge Painful Unilateral Photophobia Foreign body sensation Periorbital vesicles Dendritic (tree-like) pattern with fluorescent stain seen with slit lamp	Diffuse
Bacterial Conjunctivitis		H10.89 Other conjunctivitis	*Bacterial conjunctivitis* Usually mucopurulent discharge Early-morning crusty or "gluey" eye	Diffuse marked erythema
		A54.31 Gonococcal conjunctivitis	*Gonococcal conjunctivitis* Profuse purulent discharge Lids often swollen High risk in neonates usually less than 2 weeks old and sexually active adolescents	Diffuse hyperacute conjunctival injection
Blepharitis		H01.009 Unspecified blepharitis unspecified eye, unspecified eyelid	Redness and swelling of eyelid margins Scaly, flaky debris on lid margins Gritty, burning sensation Matting of eyelashes upon awakening	Eyelid margins
Periorbital (Preseptal) Cellulitis		H05.019 Cellulitis of unspecified orbit	Infection of the space anterior to the orbital septum Lid warmth, edema, erythema, and tenderness More common in children <5 years Usually unilateral	Eyelids, upper and lower
Orbital (Postseptal) Cellulitis		H05.01	Infection involving the orbital structures posterior to the orbital septum Lid warmth, edema, erythema, and tenderness Chemosis Proptosis Decreased extraocular movement Periocular pain Usually unilateral	Eyelids, upper and lower Mild, diffuse conjunctival injection

DURATION/ CHRONICITY	ASSOCIATED FINDINGS	COMPLICATIONS	PREDISPOSING FACTORS	TREATMENT GUIDELINES
Resolves with allergen removal and/or treatment	Atopy Teary eyes Photophobia	Usually none	Allergens including pollen, ragweed, dust, animal dander (usually airborne)	Oral or topical antihistamines
3–7 days Self-limited	Viral syndrome (fever, pharyngitis, adenopathy) Ocular discomfort Eyelid swelling	Infectious to others	Exposure from direct contact or from fomites	Self-resolving Emphasis on hand washing
Variable, depends on treatment May be recurrent	Mucocutaneous or predominantly periorbital vesicles Corneal ulceration Systemic involvement Sepsis-like picture or seizures in neonates	Systemic infection in neonates Infectious to others	Neonates of infected mothers are at risk Sexually active adolescents	Ocular antiviral in conjunction with oral acyclovir Consult ophthalmologist.
7–10 days Generally self-limited in infants and older children	Sometimes occurs with acute otitis media (usually due to nontypeable *H. influenzae*) Ocular discomfort	Infectious to others	Exposure from direct contact with other infected individuals	Ocular antibiotics Add oral antibiotics if suspecting *H. influenzae* Consult ophthalmologist if contact lens wearer
Variable, depends on treatment	Sepsis-like picture in neonates May be associated with disseminated gonococcal disease (arthritis, rash) or urethral discharge in adolescents	Loss of eye from abscess, corneal ulceration, and perforation when untreated Infectious to others	Vertical transmission (mother to baby) Sexually active adolescents Victims of sexual abuse Exposure to (direct contact) infected person	Consider full sepsis workup in neonates and admission for IV antibiotics Consult ophthalmologist.
Chronic/recurrent	Rosacea or seborrheic dermatitis	Hordeolum	Usually none	Keep eyelids clean. Warm compresses and light scrubbing with baby shampoo Consider ocular antibiotics.
Resolves after 7–10 days with oral antibiotic treatment	Fever and pain	Orbital cellulitis Bacteremia/sepsis Meningitis	Minor trauma or insect bite Localized lid infections Bacteremia because of *H. influenzae* type B	Oral antibiotics, IV antibiotics if ill appearing, not improving
Resolves after 10–14 days with IV and oral antibiotic treatment	Fever Associated URI (upper respiratory tract infection) symptoms Decreased visual acuity Malaise	Blindness Brain abscess Meningitis Cavernous sinus thrombosis	Sinusitis Minor trauma Dental abscess Periorbital (preseptal) cellulitis	CT scan of the orbits Ophthalmology consult Otolaryngology consult if sinus infection, abscess found IV antibiotics

SECTION 4 • EYES

(continued)

DIFFERENTIAL DIAGNOSIS *(continued)*

DIAGNOSIS		ICD-10	DISTINGUISHING CHARACTERISTICS	DISTRIBUTION
Subconjunctival Hemorrhage		H11.3	Painless Benign Spontaneous resolution	Localized rupture of small subconjunctival vessels
Corneal Abrasion		S05.00XA Injury of conjunctiva and corneal abrasion without foreign body, unspecified eye, initial encounter	Intense pain Tearing (+/−) photophobia	Localized
Glaucoma		H40	Cloudy or hazy cornea (because of corneal edema) Tearing but discharge is unusual Photophobia, blurred vision Irregular corneal reflex Rare in children except congenital variety The eye may appear large.	Circumcorneal injection (ciliary flush)
Conjunctivitis with Kawasaki disease		H10.89 Other conjunctivitis	Nonpurulent Nonulcerative Bilateral	Bulbar conjunctivitis (spares limbus)

DURATION/ CHRONICITY	ASSOCIATED FINDINGS	COMPLICATIONS	PREDISPOSING FACTORS	TREATMENT GUIDELINES
Resolves in 2–3 weeks	Periorbital trauma	None	Direct trauma Spontaneous Childbirth or birth trauma Increased intrathoracic pressure (as seen with coughing, vomiting)	Self-resolving
Improves within 24–48 hours	Facial trauma Other eye injury	Infection Ulceration (contact lens wearers)	Direct trauma Rubbing eyes Foreign body Insertion/removal of contact lenses	Ocular antibiotics Follow-up with ophthalmology if no improvement in 2 days or promptly if contact lens wearer Discontinue use of contact lenses
Variable	Increased intraocular pressure Acute periocular pain Nausea and vomiting with acute angle glaucoma	Blindness	Trauma Congenital Other ocular diseases	Consult ophthalmologist
1–2 weeks if untreated	Signs and symptoms of acute phase of Kawasaki disease (fever, irritability, rash, lymphadenopathy, mucous membrane and extremities changes) Acute iridocyclitis Punctate keratitis Subconjunctival hemorrhage	Coronary artery aneurysms, myocardial infarction, and/or death when Kawasaki disease is left untreated	Uncertain	Admission for IVIG, aspirin, echocardiogram, cardiology consultation

SECTION 4 • EYES

Other Diagnoses to Consider

- Dacryocystitis

- Keratitis

- Episcleritis/scleritis

- Chemical or toxin conjunctivitis

- Iritis (anterior uveitis or iridocyclitis)

When to Consider Further Evaluation or Treatment

- All patients suspected to have herpes simplex virus keratitis should follow up with an ophthalmologist.

- Neonates suspected of having gonococcal conjunctivitis should be hospitalized, and consideration should be given to conducting a full sepsis workup.

- Patients with orbital cellulitis should be admitted for intravenous antibiotics, an ophthalmology evaluation, and an orbital CT scan to rule out abscess formation.

- For patients with corneal abrasions, prescribe an ocular antibiotic such as erythromycin for prophylaxis against conjunctivitis.

- Corneal abrasions usually heal within 24 to 48 hours. Consultation with an ophthalmologist and a slit lamp examination may be necessary if symptoms persist. Prompt consultation is essential if the patient wears contact lenses.

- Avoid prescribing steroids to treat patients with red eye in the absence of an ophthalmology consultation.

SUGGESTED READINGS

Alessandrini EA. The case of the red eye. *Pediatr Ann.* 2000;29(2):112–116.
Coote MA. Sticky eye, tricky diagnosis. *Aust Fam Physician.* 2002;31(3):225–231.
Pasternak A, Irish B. Ophthalmologic infection in primary care. *Clin Fam Pract.* 2004;6(1):19–25.
Patel PB, Diaz MCG, Bennett JE, et al. Clinical features of bacterial conjunctivitis in children. *Acad EM.* 2007;14(1):1–5.
Rietveld RP, van Weert HCPM, ter Riet G, et al. Predicting bacterial cause in infectious conjunctivitis: Cohort study on informativeness of combinations of signs and symptoms *BMJ.* 2004;329:206–210.
Sethuraman U, Kamat D. The Red Eye: Evaluation and management. *Clin Pediatr.* 2009;48(6):588–600.
Teoh DL, Reynolds S. Diagnosis and management of pediatric conjunctivitis. *Pediatr Emerg Care.* 2003;19(1):48–55.

Swelling of/Around the Eye

Naline L. Lai

Approach to the Problem

The etiology of swelling of/around the eye ranges from benign, temporary irritation to more serious ophthalmological emergencies. Preseptal swelling can be broadly divided into two categories: conditions with diffuse swelling and those with discrete swelling. Diffuse swelling may be due to edema from localized extravasation of the capillary fluid as seen in allergies, or from hypoalbuminemia associated with nephrotic syndrome or reduced cardiac output. Discrete swelling results from growths such as hemangiomas, occlusion of the nasolacrimal duct system, or inflammation or infection of eyelid glands as seen with a hordeolum.

Key Points in the History

- Preseptal cellulitis often occurs after an insult to skin integrity as seen with an insect bite. Timing of the swelling in relation to timing of the bite helps distinguish between a superimposed infection and a simple bite. Generally, bacterial infections do not set in until 2 to 3 days after the initial bite.

- Preseptal cellulitis is often preceded by a history of a bacterial infection such as acute otitis media or sinusitis.

- In cases of IgE-mediated allergic reactions, consider not only airborne allergens but also contact irritants from substances rubbed into the eye. Sunscreen or lotion is a common irritant. Food allergies are unlikely to cause isolated, unilateral periorbital swelling.

- A history of pruritus suggests allergy; however, allergy-induced swelling can be deceivingly nonpruritic.

- Cardiac failure patients may report dyspnea or diaphoresis on exertion (e.g., infants during feeding, older children during exercise), orthopnea, nocturnal dyspnea, cyanosis, or respiratory distress. Look also for a history of failure to thrive.

- A history of abdominal pain may be associated with Henoch–Schönlein purpura (HSP) and hereditary angioedema.

- An intermittent history of swelling may be associated with hereditary angioedema (plasma protein C1 inhibitor deficiency). Tingling in the area may precede swelling.

- Sudden appearance of a tender eyelid mass suggests a hordeolum.

- Chalazia are generally painless and can be present for weeks prior to presentation.

- Hemangiomas and lymphangiomas often appear the same on physical examination. However, hemangiomas are not present at birth and tend to be more rapidly growing than lymphangiomas. Approximately half of all lymphangiomas are present at birth.

Key Points in the Physical Examination

- Unilateral diffuse swelling results from localized extravasation of the capillary fluid into the periorbital area in association with allergic, infectious, or traumatic causes.

- The presence of fever or tenderness on examination points toward infection. This is particularly important to note when differentiating between an insect bite and periorbital cellulitis. In periorbital cellulitis, look for the presence of other bacterial infections such as acute otitis media or sinusitis.

- Signs of orbital infection include proptosis, restriction of extraocular movements (usually inability to look up), visual changes, and pain with eye movement. Systemic symptoms such as fever, drowsiness, vomiting, or headache may be present and should raise the suspicion for bacteremia, meningitis, or brain abscess.

- In ocular trauma, look for decreased visual acuity, tearing, and pain. The presence of an orbital-rim step-off signals a fracture. Crepitus over the eyelids may be evident if there is a fracture in the paranasal sinuses. The presence of hyphema (blood in the anterior chamber) may result after blunt trauma. Photophobia can be a sign of traumatic iritis. Restricted eye movement and double vision are ominous signs for globe rupture, but may also be seen with a blow-out fracture.

- Bilateral diffuse swelling usually represents edema from hypoalbuminemia or low cardiac output states. Although less common, allergic reactions can sometimes present as bilateral diffuse swelling.

- In hypoalbuminemia and cardiac failure states, other areas of dependent edema should be present. In infants, look for sacral edema, and in children who can stand, look for ankle edema. In cardiac failure, hepatosplenomegaly or crackles on auscultation of the lung fields may be present. Tachycardia may be a sign of cardiomyopathy.

- A purpuric lower extremity rash raises suspicion for HSP.

- Most chalazia point toward the conjunctival surface, whereas hordeola may point toward or away from the conjunctival surface. When looking for hordeola or chalazia, palpate the eyelid for nodules and visualize beneath the eyelid.

- Deep hemangiomas often have a bluish hue. Superficial hemangiomas may be bluish but are more often "strawberry" red. Hemangiomas typically blanch with pressure.

- Congenital nasolacrimal duct obstruction (dacryostenosis) predisposes infants to dacryocystitis.

- Dermoids tend to be firm masses, whereas hemangiomas and lymphangiomas are soft.

PHOTOGRAPHS OF SELECTED DIAGNOSES

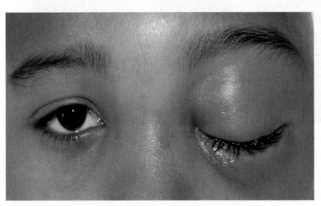

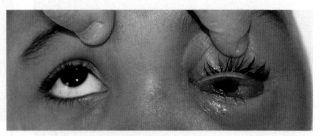

Figure 13-2 Orbital cellulitis. This is the same patient as in the previous photograph. Note the presence of ophthalmoplegia. (Courtesy of Scott Goldstein, MD.)

Figure 13-1 Orbital cellulitis. The swelling and erythema seen externally with orbital cellulitis may be similar to that seen with periorbital cellulitis. (Courtesy of Scott Goldstein, MD.)

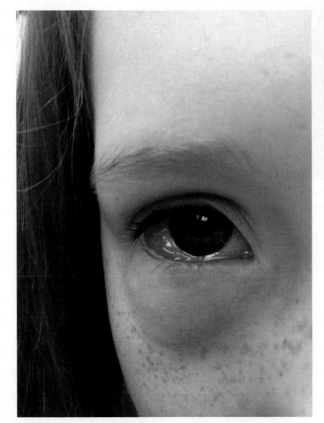

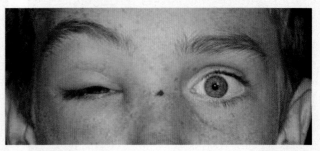

Figure 13-4 Insect bite. This patient was stung by an insect at dusk but did not notice any swelling until the next morning. (Courtesy of Naline L. Lai, MD.)

Figure 13-3 Allergic reaction. Springtime allergens caused swelling and subsequent chemosis in this school-age child. Note the gelatinous watery look of the exudate from chemosis. (Courtesy of Naline L. Lai, MD.)

SECTION 4 • EYES

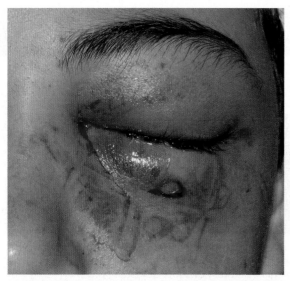

Figure 13-5 **Trauma.** This child was hit by a baseball. (Courtesy of Scott Goldstein, MD.)

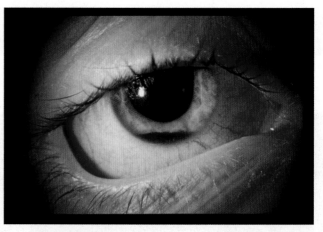

Figure 13-6 **Hyphema.** This photo illustrates the importance of ophthalmological consultation when an eye is too swollen to completely examine. This hyphema would have been missed if the lower half of the iris was obscured. (Courtesy of Monte Mills, MD, MS.)

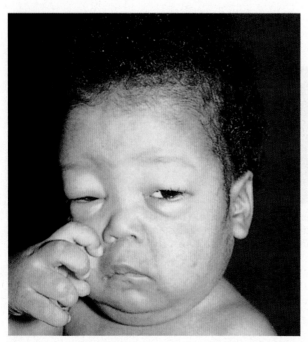

Figure 13-7 **Edema.** This child has nephrotic syndrome. For infants who do not stand, edema may be more prominent around the eyes rather than the feet. (Used with permission from Kyle T, Carman S. *Essentials of Pediatric Nursing.* 2nd ed. Philadelphia, PA: Lippincott, Williams & Wilkins; 2012.)

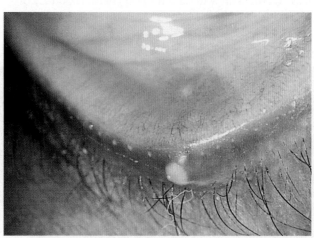

Figure 13-8 **Hordeolum.** This tender lesion points toward the conjunctival surface in this patient. A hordeolum may point either way, whereas a chalazion points inward. (Used with permission from Weber J, Kelley J. *Health Assessment in Nursing.* 2nd ed. Philadelphia, PA: Lippincott Williams & Wilkins; 2003:196.)

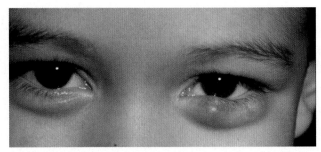

Figure 13-9 **Chalazion.** This is a relatively painless lesion. (Courtesy of Terri L. Young, MD.)

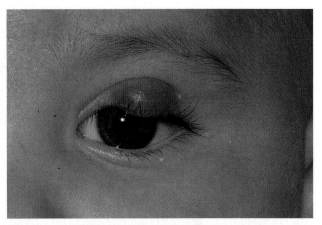

Figure 13-10 **Hemangioma.** This hemangioma is beginning to obscure this child's vision. (Courtesy of Scott Goldstein, MD.)

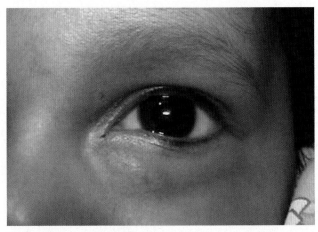

Figure 13-11 **Lymphangioma.** Note the bluish hue, which can also be seen in deep hemangiomas. (Courtesy of Barry Oppenheim, MD.)

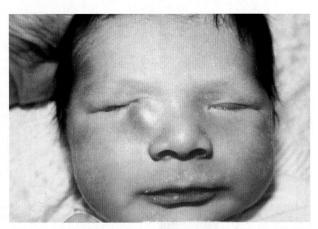

Figure 13-12 **Congenital dacryocystocele.** (Courtesy of Terri L. Young, MD.)

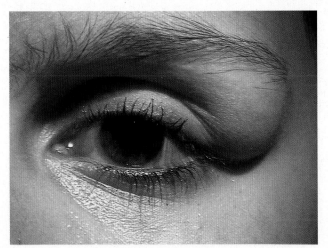

Figure 13-13 **Dermoid.** Note the swelling in the upper eyelid. (Courtesy of Barry Oppenheim, MD.)

DIFFERENTIAL DIAGNOSES

DIAGNOSIS	ICD-10	DISTINGUISHING CHARACTERISTICS	DISTRIBUTION	DURATION/ CHRONICITY
DIFFUSE SWELLING				
Periorbital (Preseptal) and Orbital Cellulitis	H00.0 (Abscess of eyelid) H05.0 (Cellulitis of orbit)	Both: warm, tender, erythematous, nonpruritic Orbital cellulitis: proptosis, ophthalmo-plegia, decreased visual acuity	Unilateral Upper and/or lower palpebrae	Acute onset
Allergic Reaction	H01.1 (dermatitis, allergic of eyelid)	Warm, nontender, ±erythematous, ±pruritic, diffuse swelling	Bilateral Periorbital	Acute onset Often appears on awakening after night time exposure
Insect Bite	T63.4	Warm, nontender, nondurated erythematous, pruritic, ±punctation, diffuse swelling	Unilateral	Acute onset Often appears on awakening after night time exposure
Trauma	S00.1 (other superficial injuries of eyelid and periocular area) S01.1 (open wound of eyelid and periocular area) S00.1 Black eye	Not warm, tender, ecchymosis/erythema, diffuse swelling	Unilateral	Acute onset
Edema from Hypoalbuminemia (Most Commonly Nephrotic Syndrome)	N04 (nephrotic syndrome)	Not warm, nontender, nonerythematous, nonpruritic, diffuse swelling	Bilateral	Acute or chronic onset
Edema from Cardiovascular Causes	I50.0 (congestive heart failure)	Not warm, nontender, nonerythematous, nonpruritic, diffuse swelling	Bilateral	Acute onset
Hereditary Angioedema	D84.1 (defects in the complement system)	Not warm, nontender, nonerythematous, nonpruritic, diffuse swelling	Unilateral or bilateral	Intermittent, usually presents in adolescence

ASSOCIATED FINDINGS	COMPLICATIONS	PREDISPOSING FACTORS	TREATMENT GUIDELINES
Prior insult to skin integrity Concomitant bacterial infection	Venous sinus thrombosis Meningitis	Bacterial infection, such as sinusitis, acute otitis media, or conjunctivitis Trauma	Oral antibiotics Include coverage for beta-lactamase-producing organisms in uncomplicated periorbital cellulitis. Consider coverage for methicillin-resistant *Staphylococcus aureus*. Admit if suspicion of orbital cellulitis, fever, not improving.
Chemosis (gelatinous-appearing reaction to allergen)	Bacterial superinfection	Exposure to environmental allergens Allergens often carried on hands and rubbed into eyes	Irrigate area well. Cool compresses Oral antihistamines Oral steroid Antihistamine and/or mast stabilizer ophthalmic drops
Other bites present on body	Bacterial superinfection	N/A	Oral antihistamines Cool compresses Over-the-counter pain medication Consider oral steroids.
N/A	Lens dislocation, retinal detachment, uveal hemorrhage, retinal artery occlusion with sudden increases in intraocular pressure, optic nerve compression, muscle entrapment	N/A	If suspicion of a ruptured globe, no further examination to be attempted except by ophthalmologist, protect the eye with a shield (paper or foam cup can be substituted). If there is visual impairment, an inability to fully examine an eye or any suspicion of anything beyond mild soft-tissue injury and corneal abrasion, an ophthalmologist should be consulted.
Edema over other dependent areas, bilateral ankles after standing or sacral edema after lying down In nephrotic syndrome urine with 3–4+ proteinuria	Renal failure if renal etiology	N/A	Manage underlying disease causing hypoalbuminemia.
Edema over other dependent areas, bilateral ankles after standing or sacral edema after lying down Signs of heart failure, including hepatosplenomegaly, dyspnea or diaphoresis on exertion, poor growth, orthopnea, nocturnal dyspnea, cyanosis, respiratory distress	Heart failure	N/A	Manage underlying cardiac disease.
May be associated with autonomic instability Usually one area involved but may involve several areas, including face, hands, arms, legs, genitalia, and buttocks Vomiting and/or abdominal pain may mimic a surgical emergency Upper airway obstruction may occur from laryngeal edema.	Airway obstruction, autonomic instability	N/A	Prophylaxis with androgens During attack may require respiratory support and intravenous fluids for maintenance of autonomic stability

(continued)

SECTION 4 • EYES

DIFFERENTIAL DIAGNOSIS *(continued)*

DIAGNOSIS		ICD-10	DISTINGUISHING CHARACTERISTICS	DISTRIBUTION	DURATION/ CHRONICITY
DISCRETE SWELLING					
Hordeolum (Common Name, Stye)		H00.0	Tender, discrete mass, firm May point toward or away from the conjunctival surface	Unilateral Infection of eyelid glands (meibomian gland in internal hordeolum or Zeis in external hordeolum)	Acute onset
Chalazion		H00.1	Nontender, discrete mass, firm Usually points toward the conjunctival surface	Unilateral meibomian gland dysfunction	Subacute or chronic onset
Hemangioma		D18.0	Nontender, discrete mass, soft or firm Bright red "strawberry" Deeper lesions have a bluish hue Blanches with pressure	Unilateral	Usually not present at birth, appears shortly thereafter Grows quickly in the first year of life, often involutes by age 6
Lymphangioma		D18.1	Nontender, smooth, discrete mass, soft	Unilateral	May be present at birth (~50%) Slow growth Often stabilizes in adulthood
Lacrimal Drainage System Infections (Dacryocystitis, Canaliculitis)		H04.3 (dacryocystitis, lacrimal canaliculitis) P39.1 (neonatal conjunctivitis and dacryocystitis)	Tender, discrete mass, soft or firm, erythematous	Unilateral, nasolacrimal area	Acute onset
Congenital Dacryocystocele (Mucocele)		H04.4 (lacrimal mucocele)	Bluish hue, discrete mass, firm	Unilateral, nasolacrimal area	At birth or shortly after
Dermoid		D23.1 (neoplasm benign, eyelid)	Nontender, smooth, discrete mass, firm, usually fixed	Unilateral Usually over the brow or upper eyelid	Congenital: may increase in size with age, usually recognized by age 16

ASSOCIATED FINDINGS	COMPLICATIONS	PREDISPOSING FACTORS	TREATMENT GUIDELINES
N/A	Periorbital cellulitis	Bacterial blepharitis	Usually caused by infection with *S. aureus* Warm compresses, gently wash with baby shampoo If inflamed beyond localized lesion, use topical antibiotic.
N/A	Corneal abrasions Astigmatism from mass effect causing pressure on the globe	N/A	Warm compresses Surgical intervention if present after 3–4 weeks or if mass effects present
N/A	Amblyopia if vision is occluded	N/A	Referral to ophthalmologist if occluding vision Topical beta-blockers, laser, surgical options
Other facial lymphangiomas may be present.	Occlusion of vision with resulting amblyopia, cosmetic issues	N/A	Surgical excision often must be repeated because lymphangiomas are difficult to remove in a single surgical procedure.
Congenital nasolacrimal duct obstruction (dacryostenosis) predisposes to dacryocystitis.	Periorbital cellulitis Orbital cellulitis	N/A	Oral antibiotics Massage nasolacrimal area, warm compresses
If bilateral, assess breathing for possibility of nasal obstruction.	Infection/abscess	Blocked nasolacrimal duct	Warm compresses, massage, antibiotic ointment, may need surgical intervention if recurring infection or abscess develops If bilateral, assess breathing for any associated nasal obstruction.
Eyelid, iris colobomas, microphthalmos, retinal and choroidal defects, first branchial arch defect Common in Goldenhar syndrome	Occlusion of vision with resulting amblyopia, cosmetic issues Risk of cyst rupture, which can produce secondary granulomatous inflammation	N/A	Complete surgical excision

SECTION 4 • EYES

Other Diagnoses to Consider

- Dermatomyositis

- Proptosis from Graves disease

- Infarction of orbital bones seen with sickle cell disease

- Ptosis

- Foreign body reaction from penetrating injury

When to Consider Further Evaluation or Treatment

- When there is minimal eyelid swelling with preseptal cellulitis in an afebrile, well-appearing, older child with reliable follow-up and no suspicion of orbital cellulitis, outpatient treatment with oral antibiotics is recommended. Although pneumococcus and hemophilus remain the most common causes of periorbital cellulitis, consideration must be given to the role of community-acquired methicillin-resistant *S. aureus*.

- In any case where there is visual impairment or an inability to fully examine the eye, consult an ophthalmologist. Even if benign, mass lesions large enough to obstruct vision may lead to amblyopia or induce astigmatism and should, therefore, be evaluated by a pediatric ophthalmologist. Dermoids are at high risk for rupture; therefore, the treatment is complete surgical excision.

- Chalazia may need surgical intervention if they persist beyond 3 to 4 weeks or if a mass effect is present.

- If dacryocystitis is recurrent, or if nasolacrimal duct obstruction continues beyond age 1 year, referral to a pediatric ophthalmologist is indicated.

SUGGESTED READINGS

Gerstenblith A, Rabinowitz M, eds. *The Wills Eye Manual. Office and Emergency Room Diagnosis and Treatment of Eye Disease.* 6th ed. Philadelphia, PA: Lippincott Williams & Wilkins; 2012:135–138, 144–149, 195.
Rafailidis PL, Falagas ME. Fever and periorbital edema: A review. *Surv Ophthalmol.* 2007;52(4):422–433.
Wald ER. Periorbital and orbital infections. *Infect Dis Clin North Am.* 2007;21:393–408.

14 Discoloration of/Around the Eye

Kimberly A. Neutze and Jonathan H. Salvin

Approach to the Problem

Discoloration around the eye, the periorbital skin and eyelids, and of the eye may result from multiple causes. Children and adults with darker skin pigmentation—those of African, Asian, or Hispanic descent—may also have increased pigmentation of the bulbar conjunctivae. This discoloration is often bilateral, but may be asymmetric and patchy and most noticeable in the interpalpebral area. Conjunctival hyperemia, injection, and inflammation, inclusively referred to as conjunctivitis, can occur from numerous causes, including infection, trauma, allergies, foreign bodies in the eye, reaction to drugs or other toxins, and mechanical irritation from eyelashes and eyelids. Discoloration below the eyes can be seen with "allergic shiners," which results from venous congestion due to sinus mucosal edema from systemic allergic inflammation. Chalazions are granulomas formed from blocked meibomian glands along the eyelash margin. They are not infectious and do not require antibiotic treatment. Cellulitis, orbital (postseptal) and periorbital (or preseptal), can cause discoloration and swelling of the periorbital skin as well as eyelids and can cause hyperemia of bulbar conjunctivae. In orbital cellulitis, the infection extends past the orbital septum, resulting in eye motility restriction, optic nerve compression and vision loss, and/or secondary extension into the central nervous system. Certain tumors can cause discoloration around and in the eyes. Neuroblastoma, a tumor of embryonic sympathetic neuroblasts typically originating in the abdomen, can cause unilateral or bilateral proptosis, periorbital swelling, and lid or infraorbital ecchymosis as part of the classic presentation for orbital metastasis. Rhabdomyosarcoma, the most common primary malignant orbital tumor in children, may present with rapidly progressive proptosis and eyelid redness not associated with localized warmth or fever, distinguishing it from cellulitis. Capillary hemangiomas are vascular orbital tumors of proliferating capillary endothelial cells. They can cause a bluish discoloration of the overlying skin or the classic strawberry mark. A nevus flammeus, or port-wine stain, which can be seen in Sturge–Weber syndrome, is a vascular malformation of dilated capillaries causing a reddish stain to the skin. Melanocytic lesions can affect conjunctiva as well as surrounding tissues of the eye and include

111

conjunctival nevus, congenital nevocellular nevus of skin, and oculodermal melanocytosis or nevus of Ota. Conjunctival nevi may be flat or elevated and are typically brown and commonly found at the temporal and nasal limbi. Congenital nevocelluar nevus of skin, which occurs on eyelids, has potential for malignant transformation. Ocular and oculodermal melanocytosis, or nevus of Ota, causes slate-gray or bluish discoloration to sclera, and can involve eyelid and adjacent skin producing a brown, bluish, or black discoloration. Icterus is a yellow discoloration of the sclera that occurs with jaundice and results from bilirubin binding to the bulbar conjunctiva. In some connective tissue disorders such as Ehler–Danlos syndrome, Marfan syndrome, and osteogenesis imperfecta, the sclera may appear blue because of the underlying blue-brown uveal tissue (retina and ciliary body) showing through the thinner and more transparent sclera. In blunt trauma to the eye, there can be significant swelling and bruising that affect surrounding tissues.

Key Points in the History

- Itching and tearing are the hallmark of allergic eye disease. Patients will often report other allergy symptoms of rhinorrhea and nasal congestion, and a history of other atopic diseases such as asthma and eczema. A family history of atopic disease may also be reported.

- Viral conjunctivitis usually occurs in epidemic outbreaks in schools and child care settings. It may also be associated with concurrent or recent viral upper respiratory tract infections.

- Periorbital cellulitis may follow superficial eyelid trauma, conjunctivitis, skin infection, or upper respiratory tract or sinus infection.

- Orbital cellulitis in children is most commonly associated with sinus disease. A history of rapid onset of swelling, blurred vision, and double vision is common.

- Capillary hemangiomas are typically not evident at birth, but exhibit rapid growth over the first several months to about 6 to 9 months of age. After the first year of life, they show signs of regression at a variable rate.

- Vision loss, eye pain, or double vision may be reported with trauma to the eye and its surrounding tissues.

- Poor and/or double vision may occur with infiltrative disease of the orbit and extraocular muscles.

Key Points in the Physical Exam

- Visual acuity should always be checked and documented with age appropriate tools when possible.

- Preauricular lymphadenopathy may be seen with viral conjunctivitis.

- If bullous mucosal lesions are seen with conjunctivitis, consider Stevens–Johnson syndrome in the differential diagnosis.

- Proptosis, decreased ocular movement, decreased vision, and/or abnormal pupillary response to light suggest orbital involvement and may help to distinguish orbital from periorbital cellulitis. In periorbital cellulitis, the periorbital skin becomes taut and inflamed, but there is no orbital involvement.

- The ecchymotic discoloration associated with metastatic neuroblastoma can precede diagnosis of the primary tumor, which is typically found in the thorax or abdomen.

- Computed tomography (CT) or magnetic resonance imaging (MRI) may be needed to distinguish hemangioma from plexiform neurofibroma, lymphatic malformation, and rhabdomyosarcoma, which all can exhibit rapid growth and proptosis.

- In evaluating traumatic injuries, it is important to rule out any intraocular injuries that may be present. Presence of subconjunctival hemorrhage along with hyphema raises concern for ruptured globe.

PHOTOGRAPHS OF SELECTED DIAGNOSES

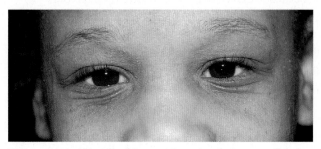

Figure 14-1 **Allergic shiners.** Note the darkening of the periorbital areas, the lichenification, and the characteristic double fold (Dennie–Morgan fold) that extends from the inner to the outer canthus of the lower eyelid. (Used with permission from Goodheart HP. *Goodheart's Photoguide of Common Skin Disorders.* 2nd ed. Philadelphia, PA: Lippincott Williams & Wilkins; 2003:48.)

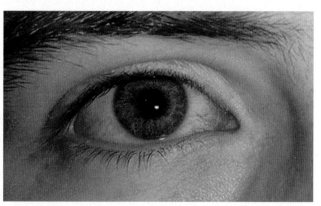

Figure 14-2 **Conjunctivitis, viral.** (Used with permission from McDonagh DO, Lereim I, Micheli LJ, et al. *FIMS Sports Medicine Manual.* Philadelphia, PA: Lippincott Williams & Wilkins; 2011.)

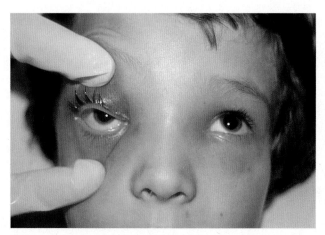

Figure 14-3 **Periorbital cellulitis.** Note the absence of proptosis and symmetric upward gaze. (Courtesy of James W. McManaway, III, MD, Hershey Pediatric Ophthalmology Associates.)

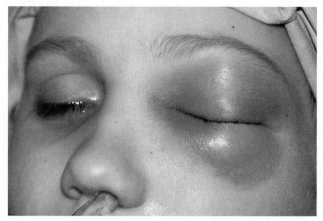

Figure 14-4 **Orbital cellulitis.** (Courtesy of the Penn State Hershey Eye Center.)

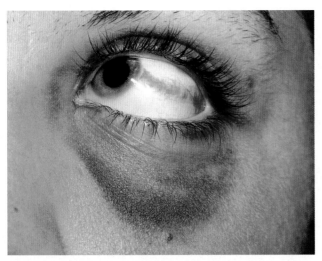

Figure 14-5 Subconjunctival hemorrhage and black eye from trauma. (Courtesy of Dean John Bonsall, MD, MS, FACS.)

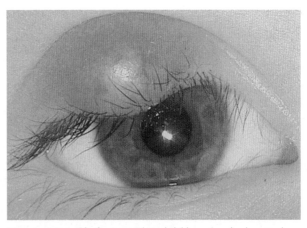

Figure 14-6 Chalazion. This child has a red, elevated, erythematous nodular mass located on lid margin. (Used with permission from Berg D, Worzala K. *Atlas of Adult Physical Diagnosis*. Philadelphia, PA: Lippincott Williams & Wilkins; 2006.)

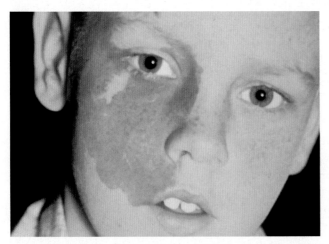

Figure 14-7 Nevus flammeus (port-wine stain). This child has a large, irregular, macular patch along the right side of his face that has the dark red appearance of port-wine stain. (Used with permission from Weber J, Kelley J. *Health Assessment in Nursing*. 2nd ed. Philadelphia, PA: Lippincott Williams & Wilkins; 2003.)

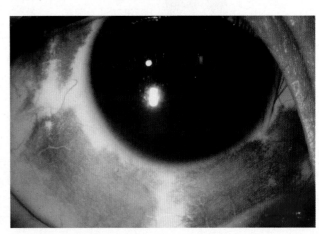

Figure 14-8 Nevus of Ota. This child has blue/gray macular patch involving most of their sclera and around the eyelid consistent with nevus of Ota. (Courtesy of Dean John Bonsall, MD, FACS.)

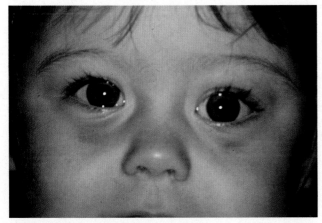

Figure 14-9 Metastatic neuroblastoma. (Courtesy of Julia L. Stevens, MD, University of Kentucky.)

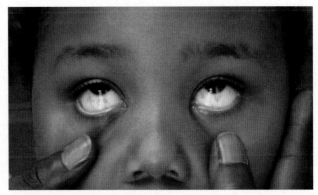

Figure 14-10 Scleral epithelial melanosis. (Courtesy of Julie A. Boom, MD.)

SECTION 4 • EYES

DIFFERENTIAL DIAGNOSIS

DIAGNOSIS	ICD-10	DISTINGUISHING CHARACTERISTICS	DISTRIBUTION	DURATION/ CHRONICITY
Allergic Eye Disease	H10.10 (Acute allergic conjunctivitis) H10.45 (Other chronic allergic conjunctivitis)	Bilateral darkening of the skin around the eyes; erythema and chemosis of conjunctiva, itching, and tearing	Periorbital skin, conjunctiva	May be concurrent with symptoms of rhinitis (not necessary) Seasonal (spring and fall)
Conjunctivitis	H10.9 (Unspecified conjunctivitis) B30.9 (Viral conjunctivitis, unspecified)	Conjunctival inflammation, burning, foreign-body sensation, matting of eyelids, discharge	Conjunctiva, unilateral or bilateral	Bacterial: Acute, rapid symptoms, 5–7 days Viral: Acute, may start unilaterally and spread bilaterally, 10–14 days
Periorbital Cellulitis	H05.019 (Cellulitis of unspecified orbit)	Erythema and edema of eyelids	Periorbital	Acute
Orbital Cellulitis	H05.011 (Right orbital cellulitis) H05.012 (Left orbital cellulitis)	Erythema and edema of eyelids; proptosis; irregular eye movements; diplopia	Periorbital, orbital	Acute
Capillary Hemangioma "Strawberry" Hemangioma	D18.00 (Hemangioma, unspecified site)	Can range from bright red appearance to more bluish hue	Any skin area, including eyelids Intraorbital	Rapid proliferation and growth during first year of life, then regression
Subconjunctival Hemorrhage	H11.30 (Conjunctival hemorrhage, unspecified eye)	Bright red patch on sclera due to broken subconjunctival blood vessel	Sclera	Acute; 7–10 days
Chalazion	H00.19 (Chalazion, unspecified eyelid)	Erythematous, firm nodular mass of the eyelid	Eyelid margin; can be external or internal	Can have rapid growth; many resolve with conservative treatment; can become chronic
Conjunctival Nevus	D31.00 (Benign neoplasm of the conjunctiva)	Flat or elevated; typically brown but can be amelanotic	Bulbar conjunctiva, most commonly	Can be present at birth; commonly develops during later childhood and adolescence
Nevus Flammeus (Port-wine Stain)	Q82.5	Flat red or pink skin lesion	Periorbital, often following trigeminal nerve distribution	Congenital Tend to get darker, thicker, and more nodular over time
Nevus of Ota	D22.30 (Melanocytic nevi of unspecified part of face)	Blue/gray skin discoloration on periorbital skin and sclera	Most are unilateral.	Congenital
Neuroblastoma (Metastatic)	C74.90 (Neuroblastoma, unspecified site)	Unilateral or bilateral ecchymosis Proptosis Periorbital swelling	Periorbital	Precedes, follows, or is concurrent with primary tumor

ASSOCIATED FINDINGS	COMPLICATIONS	PREDISPOSING FACTORS	TREATMENT GUIDELINES
Rhinitis, asthma, eczema	Of rhinitis: Epistaxis Infection Change in body structure of the face and palate	Exposure to allergens	Limit exposure Cool compresses and cool water flushes for comfort Topical antihistamine and mast cell inhibitors Systemic antihistamine and/or nasal corticosteroid if needed
URI Skin vesicles with herpes simplex virus (HSV)	Rarely corneal scarring with infiltrative etiologies (*Pseudomonas*, HSV)	Occurs in outbreaks; highly contagious (viral > bacterial)	Generally self-limited Topical antibiotics Supportive treatment with tears, cool compresses Hand washing and good hygiene to limit spread
Fever	Orbital extension (see above)	Eyelid trauma Skin and eye infections	Systemic antibiotics Close follow-up
Proptosis Decreased or painful extraocular movements Fever; Diplopia; Decreased vision	Orbital abscess Vision loss Cavernous sinus thrombosis Meningitis/Encephalitis	Sinus infection Retained foreign body Orbital trauma	Orbital CT Consult with ophthalmology and ENT Systemic antibiotics to cover *Staphylococcus aureus*, *Streptococcus pyogenes*, *Streptococcus pneumoniae*, and *Haemophilus influenzae* May require surgery
Ptosis Proptosis Irregular eye movements	Amblyopia Ptosis Orbital compression (rare)	Unknown	Observation Intralesional steroids Systemic steroids Propranolol Surgery
Look for concurrent eye injury if trauma suspected.	None	Eye infections Trauma Increased valsalva (coughing, vomiting) Diabetes/HTN Anticoagulation	Artificial tears for comfort Observe Self-limited
Blocked meibomian glands	Preseptal cellulitis	Blepharitis	Warm compresses Surgical drainage, if chronic
None	Rarely malignant change to melanoma	Unknown	Observation Surgical excision if large, unsightly or concern for irregularity
Sturge–Weber syndrome	Glaucoma Seizures	Unknown	Laser treatments can be done to reduce port-wine stain. Close observation by ophthalmologist to monitor for glaucoma
Pigmentation of oral mucosa	Increased risk of malignant choroidal melanoma Glaucoma	Unknown	Referral to ophthalmologist for observation, monitor for glaucoma
Opsoclonus myoclonus Ptosis Horner syndrome Palpated abdominal mass	Flushing Tachycardia Superior vena cava syndrome Airway and urinary obstruction	Unknown	Consultation with oncology and work-up including the following: Urinary catecholamines CT/MRI of chest and abdomen Bone marrow biopsy Bone scan Treatment based on tumor grade

Other Diagnoses to Consider

- Uveitis

- Episcleritis/scleritis

- Other orbital tumors, including metastatic disease or extraocular extension of intraocular tumors (retinoblastoma)

- Dacryocystitis

- Dacryoadenitis

- Mucocele

- Encephalocele

When to Consider Further Evaluation or Treatment

- Eye discoloration associated with decreased vision should be evaluated by an ophthalmologist promptly.

- Scleral icterus should be evaluated with serum total and direct bilirubin levels, and underlying causes of jaundice should be considered.

- Children with periorbital cellulitis may be treated with oral systemic antibiotics and closely monitored. If there are no signs of improvement within 48 to 72 hours, CT imaging and changing to IV antibiotics should be considered.

- Children with suspected orbital cellulitis should have an orbital CT and started on systemic antibiotics. Otolaryngology and/or ophthalmology should be consulted for evaluation of possible surgical drainage.

- Children with suspected orbital disease should be evaluated with CT and/or MRI.

- Suspected connective tissue diseases should be referred to genetics for further evaluation.

SUGGESTED READINGS

Helveston EM, Ellis FD. *Pediatric Ophthalmology Practice.* 2nd ed. St Louis, MO: Mosby; 1984.

Nelson LB, Olitsky SE, Harley RD, eds. *Harley's Pediatric Ophthalmology.* 5th ed. Philadelphia, PA: Lippincott Williams & Wilkins; 2005:201–216, 367–419.

Shields CL, Fasiudden A, Mashayekhi A, et al. Conjunctival nevi: Clinical features and natural course in 410 consecutive patients. *Arch Ophthalmol.* 2004;122:167–175.

Traboulsi E. Pediatric ophthalmology. In: McMillan JA, ed. *Oski's Pediatrics Principles and Practice.* 4th ed. Philadelphia, PA: Lippincott Williams & Wilkins; 2006:801–827.

Wright KW, Spiegel PH, eds. *Pediatric Ophthalmology and Strabismus.* 2nd ed. New York, NY: Springer; 2003.

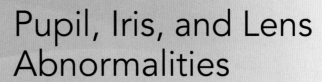

Pupil, Iris, and Lens Abnormalities

Renee M. Turchi and
Esther K. Chung

Approach to the Problem

There are various abnormalities of the pupils, iris, and lens in children. In most cases, timely diagnosis and management are critical. The assessment of visual acuity is the most integral facet of the ophthalmologic examination. More than half of the visual abnormalities in children are first discerned by their primary care physician. Many diagnoses, such as leukocoria, require prompt referral to an ophthalmologist. When in doubt, referral is a prudent approach in managing many of these diagnoses.

Key Points in the History

- Congenital cataracts are associated with intrauterine infections, such as congenital rubella and congenital varicella syndrome, and metabolic disorders. Congenital cataracts may be associated with Down, Edward, and Turner syndromes.

- One third of cataracts are hereditary, and nearly one third of cataracts in children have no identifiable etiology.

- Brushfield spots occur in up to 85% to 90% of children with Down syndrome, but they may be seen in normal children as well.

- Colobomas may occur in normal children or as part of genetic syndromes, such as CHARGE syndrome.

- Iritis and uveitis raise suspicion for conditions associated with systemic inflammation as in juvenile idiopathic arthritis (JIA).

- Hyphemas are often the result of blunt trauma to the globe.

Key Points in the Physical Examination

- Small, centrally located cataracts are often clinically stable without an impact on vision.

- Leukocoria, or a white pupillary reflex, is an important clinical sign of intraocular tumors, such as retinoblastoma. Retinoblastoma is the leading malignant ocular tumor in children.

- Leukocoria is bilateral in 30% to 40% of cases.

- It is important to rule out scleral rupture or the presence of a foreign body when chemosis is present.

- Kaiser–Fleischer rings are rims of brown-green pigment in the cornea. Although occasionally visible to the naked eye, slit lamp examination is sometimes necessary to visualize these rings.

- Iritis is characterized by pain, tearing, photophobia, and decreased visual acuity. Symptoms may be acute and develop rapidly over 1 to 2 days. Iritis may be asymptomatic in children with rheumatologic disease such as JIA.

- Blunt traumatic injuries to the eye warrant an inspection of the anterior chamber, the space between cornea and iris, for hyphemas.

- Small hyphemas require slit lamp examination, whereas larger ones may be visible to the naked eye.

- When blood pools in the inferior portion of the eye from a hyphema, it often causes elevated intraocular pressure and decreased visual acuity.

PHOTOGRAPHS OF SELECTED DIAGNOSES

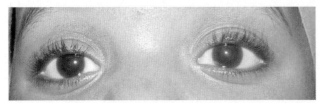

Figure 15-1 Aniridia. This photograph shows a child with bilateral aniridia. (Courtesy of Brian Forbes, MD.)

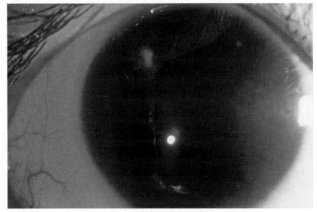

Figure 15-2 Aniridia. (Courtesy of Sophia M. Chung, MD.)

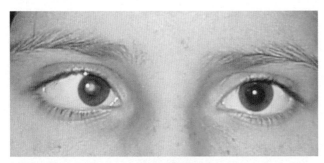

Figure 15-3 Cataract. Note the central haze in the right eye of this patient. (Courtesy of Brian Forbes, MD.)

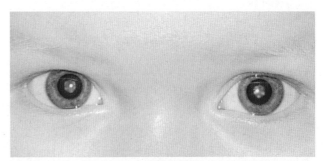

Figure 15-4 Bilateral central cataracts. (Courtesy of Brian Forbes, MD.)

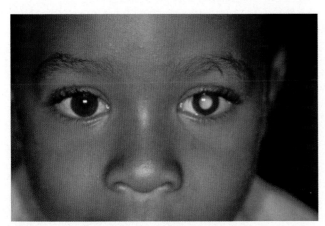

Figure 15-5 Leukocoria. (Used with permission from Rubin E, Farber JL. *Pathology.* 3rd ed. Philadelphia, PA: Lippincott Williams & Wilkins; 1999:765.)

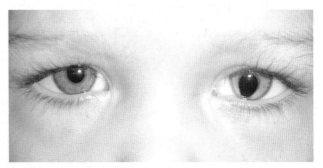

Figure 15-6 Coloboma in the left eye. (Courtesy of Brian Forbes, MD.)

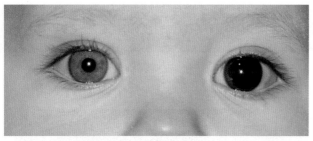

Figure 15-7 **Heterochromia iridium.** (Courtesy of Brian Forbes, MD.)

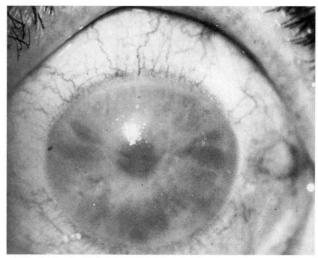

Figure 15-8 **Iritis.** (Used with permission from Harwood-Nuss AL, Wolfson AB, Linder CH, et al. *The Clinical Practice of Emergency Medicine.* 3rd ed. Philadelphia, PA: Lippincott Williams & Wilkins; 2001:66.)

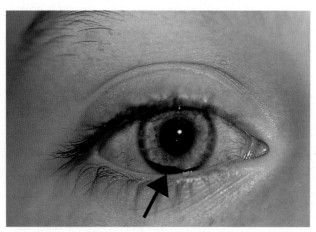

Figure 15-9 **Hyphema.** This 7-year-old girl was struck by a hard rubber ball and presented with blurred vision. The 1-mm hyphema was only visible when she was upright. (Used with permission from Fleisher GR, Ludwig S, Baskin MN. *Atlas of Pediatric Emergency Medicine.* Philadelphia, PA: Lippincott Williams & Wilkins; 2004:403.)

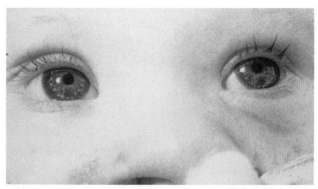

Figure 15-10 **Brushfield spots.** (Used with permission from Bickley LS, Szilagyi P. *Bates' Guide to Physical Examination and History Taking.* 8th ed. Philadelphia, PA: Lippincott Williams & Wilkins; 2003:771.)

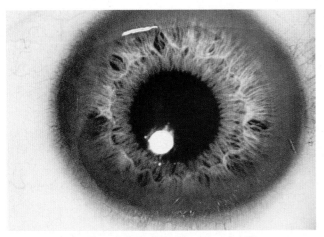

Figure 15-11 **Kaiser–Fleischer ring.** (Used with permission from Tasman W, Jaeger E. *The Wills Eye Hospital Atlas of Clinical Ophthalmology.* 2nd ed. Philadelphia, PA: Lippincott Williams & Wilkins; 2001:466.)

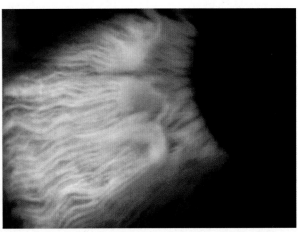

Figure 15-12 **Lisch Nodule.** Lisch nodule of iris characterized by its elevation, smooth contour, and soft translucency. (Used with permission from Gold DH, Weingeist TA. *Color Atlas of the Eye in Systemic Disease.* Baltimore, MD: Lippincott Williams & Wilkins; 2001).

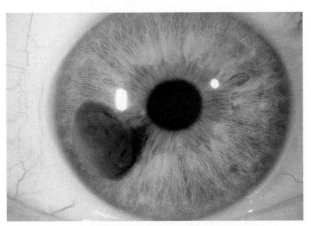

Figure 15-13 **Iris Melanoma.** (Used with permission from Tasman W, Jaeger E. *The Wills Eye Hospital Atlas of Clinical Ophthalmology.* 2nd ed. Philadelphia, PA: Lippincott Williams & Wilkins, 2001.)

DIFFERENTIAL DIAGNOSIS

DIAGNOSIS		ICD-10	DISTINGUISHING CHARACTERISTICS	DISTRIBUTION	DURATION/CHRONICITY
Aniridia		Q13.1 Absence of iris	Iris hypoplasia Pupil is same size as cornea Edge of lens visible Incidence 1:64,000 to 1:96,000	Usually bilateral Some cases asymmetrical	May employ pigmented contact lens to ameliorate symptoms
Anisocoria		H57.02	Unequal pupil size Change in light reactivity	N/A	Related to etiology
Cataract		Q12.0 Congenital cataract H26.0 Other cataract	Haze over eyes Apparent with red reflex testing	Location and density of cataract determine visual effects	Dense bilateral cataracts require urgent surgery. Partial cataracts removed after visual assessment
Leukocoria		H44.539	White pupillary reflex	May be unilateral or bilateral, depending on etiology (up to 40% of time bilateral in retinoblastoma)	Related to diagnosis and ability to treat
Coloboma		Q13.0 Coloboma of iris Q12.2 Coloboma of lens	Notch, hole, or defect in iris or choroid	Defect often located inferior and nasal May be unilateral or bilateral	Visual loss related to affected area
Heterochromia Iridium		Q13.2 Congenital heterochromia of the iris	Rare May be isolated finding	Iridium—different colors between irises Iridis—different colors within one iris	N/A
Iritis		H20.9 Iridocyclitis (inflammation of the iris and ciliary body)	Pain, redness, and photophobia In severe cases, may have vision disturbances and hypotonia of the eye	Inflammation of the iris	Pain, redness, and photophobia may last weeks in acute cases Chronic cases may have milder symptoms for months to years Blurred vision Poor pupillary light response
Hyphema		H21.0 Hyphema S05.1 Hyphema, traumatic	Collection of blood in anterior chamber of the eye	Superior located meniscus in anterior chamber	Clot often gone in 3–5 days Re-bleeding can occur if there is inadequate rest, unstable intraocular pressure; and is more prevalent in sickle cell disease

ASSOCIATED FINDINGS	COMPLICATIONS	PREDISPOSING FACTORS	TREATMENT GUIDELINES
Photophobia Nystagmus Cataracts Glaucoma Part of WAGR and Gillespie syndromes	Poor vision	May be genetically inherited (usually autosomal dominant—sporadic in one third)	• Depends on features present • Correct vision with glasses • Surgery, rarely • Regular follow-up
Horner syndrome Drugs Lesion of parasympathetic system, including CN III	Changes in vision with severe cases	Physiological, 20% Horner syndrome Drugs Tonic pupil Lesion of parasympathetic system, including CN III Trauma to pupil	• Treatment related to etiology • Nerve palsy, trauma, or mydriasis may require surgical intervention.
Decrease in visual acuity	Blindness Amblyopia Glaucoma Strabismus	Intrauterine infections Metabolic disorders, such as hypoglycemia, hypocalcemia Genetic disorders, such as Trisomy 21	• Medical management if no visual impairment • Surgery, often when >3 mm in diameter, or if associated with nystagmus, strabismus, or any visual impairment
Orbital tumors Proptosis, pain, diplopia, conjunctival edema	Blindness Myopia Cataracts	Retinoblastoma is most serious etiology. Other etiologies: • Congenital cataracts (most common) • Retinopathy of prematurity (ROP) • Retinal detachment • Persistent hyperplastic primary vitreous • Coat disease • Toxocariasis	• Dilating drops for better examination may require imaging if suspect retinoblastoma • Treatment of underlying condition—intraocular tumor, cataract, ROP, retinal detachment, infection
Small eye Glaucoma Retinal detachment Disc degeneration Cataracts	Poor vision	Dominant inheritance when present without systemic manifestations Associated syndromes: • Trisomy 13 and 18 • Cat eye syndrome • Wolf–Hirschhorn syndrome • Rieger syndrome • CHARGE association	• Usually no treatment • Cosmetic contact lenses and sunglasses may be used. • Vision correction, if vision impaired
Irises two different colors	Glaucoma (rare)	Trauma Congenital pigmented nevi Waardenburg syndrome Piebald trait Horner syndrome	• Treat underlying cause/disease, if applicable. • Cosmetic contact lenses, if desired
Cataract Glaucoma	Amblyopia Corneal changes and blurry vision Band keratopathy Macular edema Red eye Light sensitivity	JIA (most common) Trauma Kawasaki disease Infections (measles, mumps, varicella, Epstein–Barr virus, leprosy, Lyme) Spondyloarthropathies Sarcoidosis	• Mitigate cause of inflammation, if known • Topical steroid drops
Occasional blood staining of the cornea	Glaucoma (10%) Increased intraocular pressure Re-bleeding	Trauma (most common) Herpes zoster Iritis Orbital tumors Juvenile xanthogranulomatosis	• Topical corticosteroids • Antifibrinolytic agents • Usually outpatient management • Risk for re-bleeding and increased intraocular pressure

(continued)

DIFFERENTIAL DIAGNOSIS *(continued)*

DIAGNOSIS		ICD-10	DISTINGUISHING CHARACTERISTICS	DISTRIBUTION	DURATION/CHRONICITY
Brushfield Spots		Q13.2 Other congenital malformations of the iris	White and yellow spots evenly arranged around pupil in iris Iris looks speckled	Often bilateral	N/A
Kaiser–Fleischer Rings		H18.049	Corneal staining from copper that is brown to orange-green in color	Staining more common at upper pole or cornea	Often present after systemic disease treated
Lisch Nodules		H21.9 Unspecified disorder of iris and ciliary body Q85.01 Neurofibromatosis, type I	Well-defined melanocytic hamartomas, yellow to brown in color Dome-shaped elevations on surface of the iris Blurred margins	Usually bilateral Benign hamartomas, histologically identical to iris nevi	Usually arrive by age 10 By age 20, present in all patients with NF type 1
Iris Nevi/ Melanomas		H21.9 Unspecified disorder of iris and ciliary body	Brown or dark nodule in iris	Can be circumscribed or diffuse	Nevus often present in early childhood followed by rapid growth

ASSOCIATED FINDINGS	COMPLICATIONS	PREDISPOSING FACTORS	TREATMENT GUIDELINES
Most often seen in children with Trisomy 21 (90%)	N/A	Trisomy 21 (most often)	• Typically no intervention necessary
Liver disease, neurological impairment, and cognitive deficits in Wilson disease	No visual impairment Often fade with treatment	Wilson disease (defect in copper metabolism) Liver failure Carotenemia Multiple myeloma	• Treatment aims to manage copper metabolism as part of treatment for Wilson disease • Correct visual impairment.
Most common ocular involvement in neurofibromatosis type 1	Do not usually cause any ophthalmologic complications	Neurofibromatosis type 1	Usually do not require treatment
Criteria for the clinical diagnosis for melanoma: • The size is greater than 3 mm in diameter and 1 mm in thickness. • It replaces the stroma of the iris. • Three of the following five features are present: photographic documentation of growth, secondary glaucoma, secondary cataract, prominent vascularity, or ectropion irides	Pain with large lesions Diffuse lesions can cause heterochromia and glaucoma	Iris nevi may grow and evolve into iris melanoma More common in Caucasians and patients with light-colored irises	Patients need periodic examinations with photographs. Surgical excision may be needed for growing lesions.

SECTION 4 • EYES

Other Diagnoses to Consider

- Pupil abnormalities:
  - Horner syndrome
  - Adie syndrome
  - Third cranial nerve palsy
  - Persistent pupillary membrane
- Lens abnormalities:
  - Lens subluxation
  - Dystrophy
  - Cystinosis
  - Lenticular myopia
- Iris abnormalities:
  - Ocular albinism
  - Iridodialysis
  - Cyclodialysis

When to Consider Further Evaluation or Treatment

- Leukocoria is a diagnosis warranting immediate attention and referral as it may result in visual impairment and may be life threatening.

- Retinoblastoma, the most common intraocular tumor in childhood, typically presents with leukocoria. Mean age at diagnosis is 12 months for bilateral and 24 months for unilateral tumors.

- Iritis and uveitis require prompt attention and a slit lamp examination. In addition, patients should be evaluated for other systemic diseases to determine the cause of inflammation.

- An iris nevus that changes shape, size, or thickness requires prompt attention as iris nevi and melanomas are the most common primary tumors of the iris.

SUGGESTED READINGS

Halder S, Oureshia W, Ali A. Leukocoria in children. *J Pediatr Ophthalmol Strabismus.* 2008;45(3):179–180.

Krishnamurthy R, VanderVeen DK. Infantile cataracts. *Inter Ophthalmol Clin.* 2008;48(2):175–192.

Lai JC, Ferkat S, Barron Y, et al. Traumatic hyphema in children: Risk factors for complications. *Arch Ophthalmol.* 2001;119(1):64–70.

McLaughlin JP, Fung AT, Shields JA, Shields CL. Iris melanoma in children: Current approach to management. *Oman J Ophthalmol.* 2013;6:53–55.

Melamud A, Palekar R, Singh A. Retinoblastoma. *Am Fam Physician.* 2006;73(6):1039–1044.

Patel H. Pediatric uveitis. *Pediatr Clin North Am.* 2003;50:125–136.

Savar A, Cestari DM. Neurofibromatosis type I: Genetics and clinical manifestations. *Semin Ophthalmol.* 2008;23(1):45–51.

Tasman W, Jaeger E. *The Wills Eye Hospital Atlas of Clinical Ophthalmology.* 2nd ed. Philadelphia, PA: Lippincott Williams & Wilkins; 2001:466.

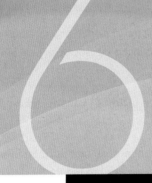

Misalignment of the Eyes

Leonard B. Nelson

Approach to the Problem

Misalignment of the eyes is one of the most common eye problems encountered in childhood, affecting approximately 4% of children younger than 6 years of age. This condition is usually referred to by the terms, strabismus or abnormal ocular alignment. Misalignment of the eyes may cause vision loss (amblyopia) and result in important and lifelong psychological effects. Misalignment of the eyes involves a number of clinical entities. Orthophoria is the condition of exact ocular balance. A convergent deviation, crossing, or turning in of the eyes is referred to as esotropia. Divergent deviation or turning outward of the eyes is referred to as exotropia. Hyperdeviation or hypodeviation, or hypotropia, refers to an upward or downward misalignment of the eyes, respectively. Misalignment of the eyes may be constant in all fields of gaze (comitant) or may change depending on where the child is looking (incomitant). Misalignments of the eyes prior to 3 months of age may not necessarily indicate an abnormality. However, if a misalignment of the eyes is present beyond 3 months of age, pediatricians must develop the clinical skill to detect the condition and refer the child for further evaluation and treatment. Early detection of a misalignment of the eyes is essential for restoring proper alignment and to prevent vision loss.

Key Points in the History

- When a parent informs a pediatrician of their concern about the possibility of a misalignment of the eyes of their child, there are a number of important questions to be asked:

  - Is there a family history of strabismus? Strabismus is commonly found in families.

  - How long have the eyes been misaligned? Different types of strabismus tend to occur at different ages. For example, congenital esotropia occurs by 6 months of age.

  - Any history of significant head trauma? Injury to the brain can result in a nerve palsy.

  - In what direction do the eyes appear to deviate? It is important for the parents to note the direction of the strabismus to determine whether it is consistent with the findings of the health care provider.

- Is the deviation noted intermittently or constantly? Different strabismus conditions may present as a manifest deviation as with congenital esotropia, or as an intermittent deviation as with intermittent exotropia.

- Does the child commonly close one eye when focusing? Closing one eye may indicate intermittent diplopia, or double vision.

- Does the child tilt his/her head or assume an abnormal face turn? Strabismus may be incomitant, forcing a child to turn or tilt his/her head to reduce the deviation.

- Do the eyes appear to move together in all directions of gaze? Asymmetric eye movements may indicate a nerve palsy or a strabismus disorder, such as Brown syndrome.

- Acute onset of a misalignment of the eyes may indicate a more ominous concern such as an intracranial abnormality.

- A variable misalignment of the eyes associated with intermittent ptosis may suggest myasthenia gravis.

Key Points in the Physical Examination

- If there is a concern that a child has a misalignment of the eyes, there are a number of methods to evaluate for strabismus:

  - Observation of the child is an important first step.

  - Corneal light (also known as Hirschberg) reflex is a rapid test, and the most easily performed diagnostic test for strabismus. This test is performed by projecting a light source onto the corneas of both eyes simultaneously as the child looks directly at the light. Comparison should be made of the placement of the corneal light reflex in each eye. The light reflex should be symmetrical in each eye. If not, strabismus is present.

  - Cover tests for a misalignment make up a more accurate and detailed method, but requires a child's attention and cooperation and reasonably good vision in both eyes.

  - In the cover–uncover test, a child looks at an object at a distance and then at near fixation. As the child looks at an object, the examiner covers one eye and observes for movement of the uncovered eye. If no movement occurs, there is no apparent misalignment of that eye. After one eye is tested, the same procedure is performed on the other eye.

  - In the alternate cover test, the examiner rapidly covers and uncovers each eye. If the child has a misalignment of the eyes, the eye rapidly moves as the cover is shifted to the other eye.

- By approximately 6 weeks to 2 months of age, children can usually follow objects in order to evaluate whether there are any abnormalities in their eye movements. Each eye should move symmetrically with the other eye. Any asymmetry in the eye movements may indicate a muscle weakness.

- Prior to age 3, evaluating visual acuity may be difficult because of poor cooperation and ability of the child to communicate. Therefore, covering each eye and observing the child's behavior in response is important. If a child objects asymmetrically to this technique, it may indicate that the uncovered eye has less than normal vision. If a deviation is constant and the child fixates more with one eye than with the other, the nonfixating eye may have less than normal vision (amblyopia).

- Amblyopia, or decreased vision in one eye, is an asymptomatic condition and is commonly found in children with strabismus, especially when the deviation is constant. Therefore, it is imperative to measure the vision in children with a misalignment of the eyes as soon as possible. Most children of age 3 and over can cooperate for a more formal vision testing. Children by age 3 can be tested with Allen card symbols. By age 5, children can usually be tested with letters, which is a better method to detect for differences in the vision between the two eyes.

PHOTOGRAPHS OF SELECTED DIAGNOSES

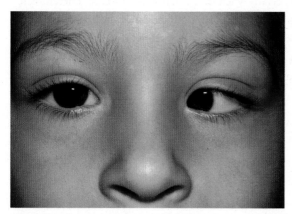

Figure 16-1 **Esotropia.** (Courtesy of Dean John Bonsall, MD, MS, FACS.)

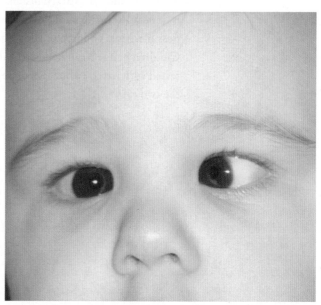

Figure 16-2 **Esotropia.** Large and constant turning in of the eyes. (Courtesy of Leonard B. Nelson, MD.)

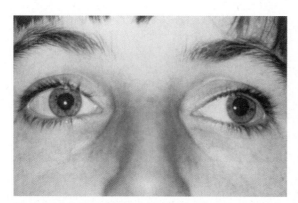

Figure 16-3 **Exotropia.** (Used with permission Wright KW. *Pediatric Ophthalmology for Pediatricians.* Baltimore, MD: Williams and Wilkins; 1999:41.)

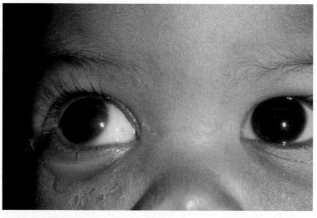

Figure 16-4 **Exotropia.** Large divergent deviation of the right eye. (Courtesy of Leonard B. Nelson, MD.)

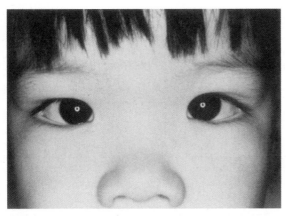

Figure 16-5 Pseudostrabismus. (Used with permission from Wright KW. *Pediatric Ophthalmology for Pediatricians*. Baltimore, MD: Williams and Wilkins; 1999:49.)

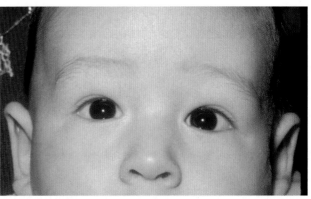

Figure 16-6 Pseudostrabismus. Apparent crossing of the eyes due to the wide nasal bridge and epicanthal folds. (Courtesy of Leonard B. Nelson, MD.)

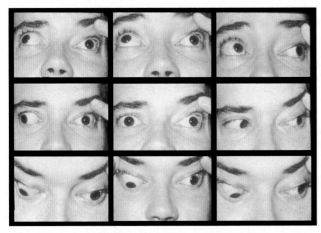

Figure 16-7 Left third cranial nerve palsy. Note the inability to elevate, depress, or move the left eye toward the nose. (Courtesy of Leonard B. Nelson, MD.)

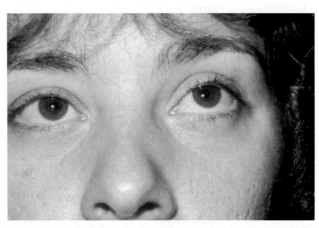

Figure 16-8 Left fourth cranial nerve palsy. Note the left hypertropia. (Courtesy of Leonard B. Nelson, MD.)

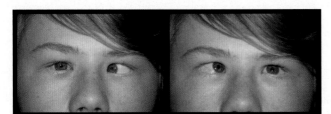

Figure 16-9 Bilateral sixth nerve palsy. Inability to abduct or turn either eye to the side. (Courtesy of Leonard B. Nelson, MD.)

DIFFERENTIAL DIAGNOSIS

DIAGNOSIS	ICD-10	DISTINGUISING CHARACTERISTICS	DISTRIBUTION	DURATION/ CHRONICITY
Infantile Strabismus	H50.00 Unspecified esotropia	Onset <6 months of age	Monocular/ binocular	May be present at birth
Pseudostrabismus	H50.00 Unspecified esotropia	Appearance of eyes deviating inward due to wide nasal bridge	N/A	Present until nose narrows with facial development
Accommodative Esotropia	H50.43	Age >2 months Typically 1–5 years of age Inward turning of one eye when focusing on a near object	Monocular	Chronic
Sensory Esotropia/ Exotropia	H50.00 Unspecified esotropia H50.10 Unspecified exotropia	<2 years: esotropia >2 years: exotropia	Monocular	Chronic
Intermittent Exotropia	H50.33 Intermittent monocular exotropia H50.34 Intermittent alternating exotropia	Ages 2–8 years Exotropia when the child is tired	Monocular/binocular	Chronic
Convergence Insufficiency	H51.11	Intermittent exotropia with near vision, but aligned with distance vision	Monocular/binocular	Chronic
Third Cranial Nerve Palsy	H49.00	Eye does not move up or down and is exotropic.	Monocular	Chronic
Fourth Cranial Nerve Palsy	H49.10	Vertical deviation of eye due to paralysis of superior oblique muscle	Monocular	Chronic
Sixth Cranial Nerve Palsy	H49.20	Inability to abduct affected eye Esotropia	Monocular	Chronic
Duane Syndrome	H50.81	Congenital absence of cranial nerve VI with aberrant innervation of lateral rectus muscle by cranial nerve III	Monocular/binocular	Chronic

ASSOCIATED FINDINGS	COMPLICATIONS	PREDISPOSING FACTORS	TREATMENT GUIDELINES
Vertical strabismus Latent nystagmus when one eye is covered	Visual loss Lack of binocular fusion	N/A	Surgical weakening of bilateral medial rectus muscles between 6 months and 2 years of age Eyeglasses are prescribed if there is significant farsightedness.
Centered corneal light reflex Negative cover–uncover test Asian descent	N/A	N/A	Reassurance
Farsightedness	Amblyopia	Farsightedness	Eyeglasses to treat accommodative error Sometimes miotic drops are used. Surgical correction may be needed if eyes are still misaligned with eyeglasses.
Blindness in one eye	N/A	Monocular blindness	Surgical correction of the muscles of the blind eye
Covering one eye causes it to become exotropic.	Significant amblyopia is rare.	Fatigue	Surgical correction if the deviation is not controlled
Reading fatigue	Diplopia when reading	Ocular muscle fatigue	Eye exercises to strengthen extraocular muscles
Ptosis Dilated, unresponsive pupil	Amblyopia	Congenital Closed head injury Migraine	Surgical correction
Compensatory head tilt to the strong side Deviation worsens with head tilt to the weak side Subtle facial asymmetry	Amblyopia Chronic head tilt	Congenital Closed head injury	Surgical correction to reduce head tilt
Diplopia	Amblyopia	Congenital Closed head injury Infratentorial neoplasms Postviral infection Following lumbar puncture	Varies depending on underlying condition
Head turn to keep eyes aligned Narrowing of the fissure (affected eye) with adduction Widening of the fissure with abduction	Amblyopia	Congenital	Surgical correction to reduce head turn

Other Diagnoses to Consider

- Children with cerebral palsy, developmental delay, hydrocephalus, or any other abnormality of the brain may develop strabismus.

- Children who are born premature, especially of a very low birth weight, may develop strabismus.

- Brown syndrome (also known as superior oblique tendon sheath syndrome)

- Hydrocephalus

- Intracranial mass

- Möbius syndrome (palsies of the cranial nerves VI and VII; limb and craniofacial anomalies)

- Myasthenia gravis

When to Consider Further Evaluation or Treatment

- Regardless of whether a misalignment is detected by an examiner, if the parents state that they notice a misalignment that does not resolve by or presents after 3 months of age, the child should be referred to an ophthalmologist.

- If a misalignment of the eyes is detected by any of the above tests for strabismus, the child should be referred to an ophthalmologist.

- An abnormal face turn or head tilt that cannot be accounted for by a structural abnormality of the neck should be referred to an ophthalmologist.

- If a child is noted to consistently close one eye, the child should be referred to an ophthalmologist.

SUGGESTED READINGS

Aronson S, Bridge C, Brunner RT, et al, eds. *Preschool Vision Screening for Healthcare Professionals*. Chicago, IL: Prevent Blindness America; 2005.

Committee on Practice and Ambulatory Medicine, Section on Ophthalmology. American Association of Certified Orthoptists, American Association for Pediatric Ophthalmology and Strabismus, American Academy of Ophthalmology. Eye examination in infants, children, and young adults by pediatricians. *Pediatrics*. 2003;111(4 Pt 1):902–907.

Nelson LB, Olitsky SE. *Harley's Pediatric Ophthalmology*. 6th ed. Philadelphia, PA: Lippincott Williams & Wilkins; 2013.

Olitsky SE, Nelson LB. *Pediatric Clinical Ophthalmology*. London, UK: Manson Publishing; 2012.

EARS

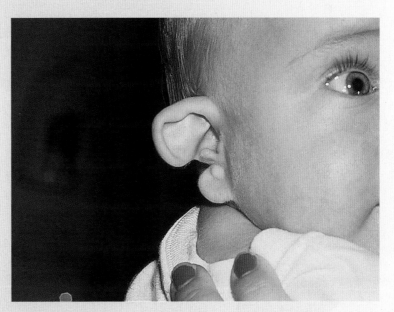

(Courtesy of Steven D. Handler, MD, MBE.)

Abnormalities in Ear Shape and Position

Charles A. Pohl

Approach to the Problem

Normally, there is a wide variation of shapes, sizes, and positions of ears in children. Most auricular growth (85%) is completed by 3 years of age, cartilaginous formation by 5 to 6 years, and ear width and its distance from the scalp by 10 years. Abnormalities in ear shape or position may occur as isolated findings or as part of a complex of congenital anomalies. Congenital malformations of the external ear, which occur in 1:10,000 to 1:20,000 live births, include problems with ear size (e.g., micro-ear), position (e.g., posteriorly rotated, low-set ears), maldevelopment (e.g., anotia, microtia, cleft earlobe, lobular attachment), and protrusion (e.g., prominent, lopped, cupped).

Malformed or underdeveloped auricles are frequently seen with genetic problems such as Beckwith–Wiedemann syndrome (creased lobes), CHARGE association (lopped or cupped ears), facio-auriculo-vertebral spectrum (Goldenhar syndrome; microtia), Levy–Hollister (cupped ears), or Trisomy 21 (small ears). Low-set ears commonly occur in syndromes such as Noonan, Smith–Lemli–Opitz, Treacher Collins, and Trisomy 18. Several studies have found an association between renal anomalies and various ear abnormalities. Although the underlying etiology is unclear, the anomalies usually are not found as isolated findings, but rather as components of more complex congenital syndromes, such as Beckwith–Wiedemann or Trisomy 18.

When inspecting the external ear, it is important to evaluate its position, size, shape, and symmetry compared with the other ear. The protrusion angle of the ear should not exceed 15 degrees in children. Fifteen percent of the auricle (the superior attachment of the pinna) should be above the horizontal line (an imaginary line drawn from the inner canthus through the outer canthus). The angle between the vertical axis (the line perpendicular to the horizontal line) and the longitudinal axis of the ear (superior aspect of the outer helix to the inferior border of the earlobe) is normally between 10 and 30 degrees. In addition, the length of an ear can be roughly estimated by measuring the distance between the arch of the eyebrow and the base of the ala nasi.

- Because hearing impairment is associated with microtia, lopped, or cupped ears, and with meatal atresia, it is essential to ask about hearing and language development.

- Underlying renal anomalies should be considered when children with ear abnormalities have a history of deafness or a maternal history of gestational diabetes.

- Children with microtia often have hearing loss on the side of their normal-appearing auricle.

- Familial inheritance patterns are seen with abnormal earlobe attachments and cupped ears; therefore, asking about a family history of ear abnormalities may be helpful.

- Children with posteriorly rotated, low-set ears should be inspected carefully for other congenital abnormalities.

- When a child has protruding ears, normal auricular architecture distinguishes prominent ears from lopped or cupped ears.

- Micro-ears, unlike maldeveloped auricles such as microtia, are small but normally formed.

- Marked skull molding can make normal auricles appear protruded.

- Abnormal facial features, including small chin, midfacial or nose hypoplasia, and highly arched eyebrows, can give the false impression of low-set, posteriorly rotated ears.

- Normally developed helices distinguish intrauterine compression abnormalities from the array of helix deformities. Also, intrauterine positioning effects do not generally result in symmetric abnormalities.

- Evaluation for renal anomalies should be considered when a patient with an auricular abnormality has other dysmorphic features, including facial asymmetry, choanal atresia, micrognathia, colobomas of the eye, branchial cysts, cardiac abnormalities, imperforate anus, and/or distal limb abnormalities.

PHOTOGRAPHS OF SELECTED DIAGNOSES

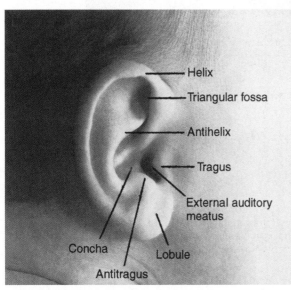

Figure 17-1 Normal anatomy of external ear. (Used with permission from Fletcher MA, ed. *Physical Diagnosis in Neonatology.* Philadelphia, PA: Lippincott–Raven Publishers; 1998:285.)

Labels: Helix, Triangular fossa, Antihelix, Tragus, External auditory meatus, Lobule, Antitragus, Concha

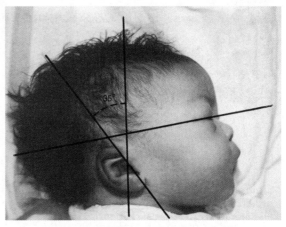

Figure 17-2 Posteriorly rotated, low-set ears. (Used with permission from Fletcher MA, ed. *Physical Diagnosis in Neonatology.* Philadelphia, PA: Lippincott–Raven Publishers; 1998:287.)

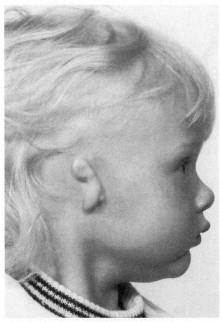

Figure 17-3 Microtia. (Used with permission from Cotton RT, Myer CM III, eds. *Practical Pediatric Otolaryngology.* Philadelphia, PA: Lippincott–Raven Publishers; 1999:345.)

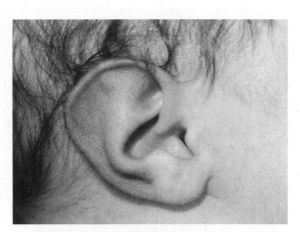

Figure 17-4 Helix deformity. (Used with permission from Fletcher MA, ed. *Physical Diagnosis in Neonatology.* Philadelphia, PA: Lippincott–Raven Publishers; 1998:288.)

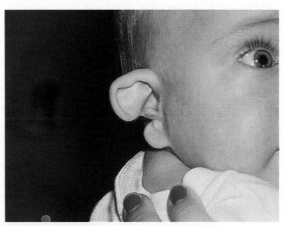

Figure 17-5 Cleft ear. (Courtesy of Steven D. Handler, MD, MBE.)

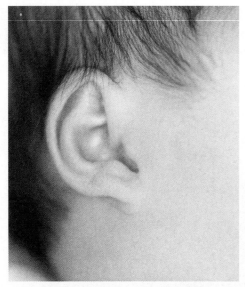

Figure 17-6 Adherent lobule/lobular attachment. (Used with permission from Fletcher MA, ed. *Physical Diagnosis in Neonatology*. Philadelphia, PA: Lippincott–Raven Publishers; 1998:289.)

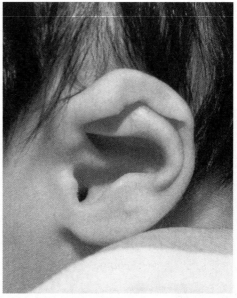

Figure 17-7 Lopped ear. (Used with permission from Fletcher MA, ed. *Physical Diagnosis in Neonatology*. Philadelphia, PA: Lippincott–Raven Publishers; 1998:297.)

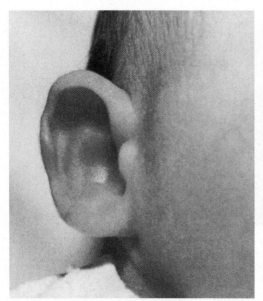

Figure 17-8 Cupped ear. (Used with permission from Fletcher MA, ed. *Physical Diagnosis in Neonatology*. Philadelphia, PA: Lippincott–Raven Publishers; 1998:298.)

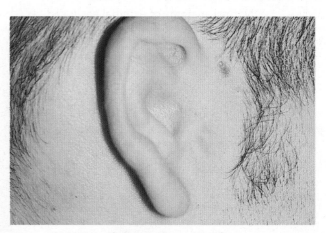

Figure 17-9 Meatal atresia. (Courtesy of Steven D. Handler, MD, MBE.)

DIFFERENTIAL DIAGNOSIS

CATEGORY	DIAGNOSIS	ICD-9	DISTINGUISHING CHARACTERISTICS	ASSOCIATED FINDINGS	OTHER FEATURES	TREATMENT GUIDELINES
Ear Size	Micro-ear	Q17.9 (congenital malformation of ear, unspecified)	Normal auricular architecture, but smaller size	Usually none	N/A	Cosmetic reconstructive surgery if severe
Ear Position	Posteriorly rotated, low-set ears	Q17.4 (misplaced ears)	External ear located inferior to normal location and rotated posteriorly	Isolated or component of complex syndrome, often involving the renal system	N/A	N/A
Maldeveloped Auricles	Microtia	Q17.2 (congenital microtia)	Dysplastic or disorganized external ear Variable presentation—from a small deformed auricular appendage to gross hypoplasia with a blind or absent external canal	Hearing loss (even in normal appearing ear) Other auditory malformations common (e.g., external auditory meatus, middle ear abnormality, ossicular abnormality) Other malformations (e.g., cardiac or renal anomalies)	1.7/10,000 live births 2:1 male-to-female ratio Autosomal dominant or recessive Risk with diabetic mothers, high altitudes	Cosmetic reconstructive surgery if severe Hearing augmentation
	Helix deformity	Q17.9 (congenital malformation of ear, unspecified)	Partial abnormality of auricle	Usually isolated	N/A	Cosmetic reconstructive surgery if severe
	Cleft ear (bifid lobule)	Q17.3 (other misshapen ear)	Isolated maldevelopment of earlobe	N/A	N/A	Cosmetic reconstructive surgery if severe
	Adherent lobule/lobular attachment	Q17.3 (other misshapen ear)	Earlobe attached anteriorly	Usually isolated	Familial	N/A
Protrusion	Prominent	Q17.5	Helix of ear is normally shaped and attached to the skull, but protrudes forward	N/A	N/A	Cosmetic reconstructive surgery if severe
	Lopped ear	Q17.3 (other misshapen ear)	Ear's helix and scapula fold downward because of inadequate development of antihelix; absence of antihelical fold	Hearing loss Similar to microtia Associated with anencephaly, microencephaly, severe congenital neuromotor deficiency; ossicular malformation	N/A	Cosmetic reconstructive surgery if severe
	Cupped ear	Q17.3 (other misshapen ear)	Ear malformation causes anterior protrusion of pinna and an exaggerated concave concha	Similar to lopped ear	Familial or sporadic	Cosmetic reconstructive surgery if severe
Maldevelopment of Ear Canal	Congenital absence, atresia and stricture of auditory canal	Q16.1	Atresia of auditory canal with or without pinna abnormality	Microtia Hearing impairment Craniofacial abnormality	1.5/20,000 live births Sporadic, autosomal dominant or recessive, chromosomal syndrome (e.g., Goldenhar syndrome)	Cosmetic reconstructive surgery if severe Early bone surgery if bilateral hearing impairment

SECTION 5 • EARS

Other
Diagnoses
to Consider

- Intrauterine compression, such as folded helix

- Marked skull molding (appears "protruded")

- Craniofacial disproportion forms such as severe microcephaly (ear appears large)

- Appearance of "low-set" or "posteriorly rotated" ears when abnormal facial features are present, such as a small chin, midface hypoplasia, or highly arched eyebrows

- Epidermal nevus on ear

- Arteriovenous malformation

When to
Consider
Further
Evaluation
or Treatment

- Malformed or underdeveloped auricles, as well as low-set ears, are often associated with more complex congenital syndromes or part of genetic disorders. Maldeveloped ears should be evaluated by otolaryngology and/or plastic surgery, particularly when considering cosmetic, reconstructive surgery.

- Closely monitor hearing, with periodic hearing evaluation, and language development in children with microtia, lopped, and cupped ears, as well as meatal atresia.

- Renal anomalies, often diagnosed by renal ultrasound, should be considered if a child with an ear abnormality has a history of deafness, a maternal history of gestational diabetes, or other dysmorphic features.

SUGGESTED READINGS

Bellucci RJ. Congenital aural malformation: Diagnosis and treatment. *Otolaryngol Clin North Am.* 1981;14:95–124.
Bordley JE, Brookhouser PE, Tucker GK, eds. *Ear, Nose and Throat Disorders in Children.* New York, NY: Raven Press; 1986.
Cotton RT, Myer CM III, eds. *Practical Pediatric Otolaryngology.* Philadelphia, PA: Lippincott–Raven Publishers; 1999.
Fletcher MA, ed. *Physical Diagnosis in Neonatology.* Philadelphia, PA: Lippincott–Raven Publishers; 1998.
Jones KL. *Smith's Recognizable Patterns of Human Malformation.* 7th ed. Philadelphia, PA: Saunders; 2013.
Wang RY, Earl DL, Ruder RO, et al. Syndromic ear anomalies and renal ultrasounds. *Pediatrics.* 2001;108(2):E32.

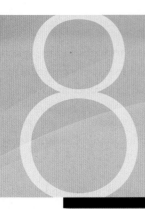

Ear Swelling

Kathleen Cronan

Approach to the Problem

Swelling of the external ear may be a concerning symptom to parents. Most causes of ear swelling are benign. Insect bites, for example, are a common cause of ear swelling in pediatric patients. However, the swelling seen with insect bites and other benign entities may mimic other diseases, such as cellulitis, perichondritis, and mastoiditis, all of which require immediate attention. Otitis externa can become diffuse and cause external ear swelling with an appearance similar to cellulitis. Blunt trauma to the ear results in swelling and discoloration of the auricle, pinna, or both. Mastoiditis, an acute bacterial infection, causes swelling and erythema of the pinna and posterior auricular swelling and tenderness.

Key Points in the History

- Pruritus, associated with swelling and erythema, is the typical presentation of an insect bite to the ear.

- A previous history of ear piercing or laceration to the ear lobe should raise the suspicion for a keloid. Patients with keloids will often have a history of keloids on other parts of their body.

- Recent ear pain with or without drainage in conjunction with posterior auricular swelling, fever, or both may indicate mastoiditis.

- The duration of symptoms often helps to distinguish an insect bite from cellulitis. Swelling and erythema resulting from an insect bite occur suddenly, whereas the swelling, tenderness, and redness of cellulitis may gradually develop.

- A history of active or recent, localized acute otitis externa may result in cellulitis of the auricle or diffuse otitis externa.

- A history of paroxysmal ear burning, redness, and swelling may indicate otomelalgia (red ear syndrome).

- Trauma, which may present as an auricular hematoma, and cellulitis typically present as swelling of the pinna and auricle, whereas mastoiditis presents as swelling and redness of the posterior auricular (e.g., in the area of the mastoid) and auricular areas.

- Forward displacement of the pinna usually indicates mastoiditis, although diffuse otitis externa or a posterior auricular insect bite may cause ear displacement when significant associated swelling is present.

- A rubbery, fleshy mass that extends beyond the wound margins indicates keloid formation.

- Erythema, swelling, warmth, and tenderness of the auricle usually indicate cellulitis. If there is no tenderness in association with the swelling and redness, an insect bite is more likely than cellulitis.

- Pain elicited with traction on the pinna and/or pressure on the tragus is associated with otitis externa.

- A bluish discoloration of the auricle accompanied by swelling suggests trauma. Petechial lesions on top of or inside the pinna are highly suspicious for an intentional injury that may be the result of pinching and pulling the pinna as seen with boxing or child physical abuse.

- Erythema and tenderness of the overlying skin and perichondrium suggest perichondritis.

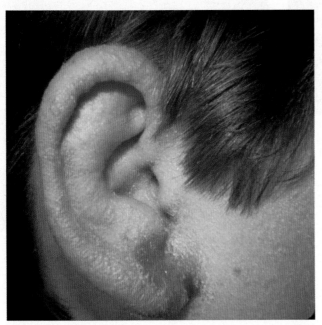

Figure 18-1 **Cellulitis.** Note the erythema and swelling. (Courtesy of Kathleen Cronan, MD.)

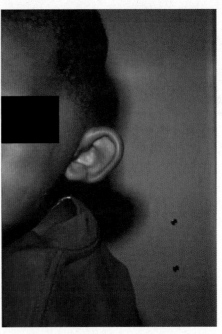

Figure 18-2 **Insect bite.** Ear protrusion and swelling in a healthy child with a papule on the posterior ear demonstrating an insect bite to the ear. (Courtesy of Kathleen Cronan, MD.)

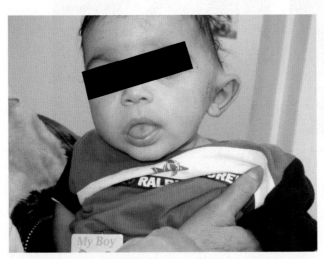

Figure 18-3 **Mastoiditis.** A protruding ear with evidence of acute otitis media, indicating mastoiditis. Frontal view. (Courtesy of Paul S. Matz, MD.)

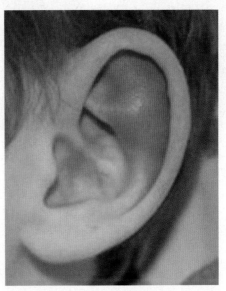

Figure 18-4 **Auricular hematoma.** This resulted from a direct blow to the ear. (Courtesy of Kathleen Cronan, MD.)

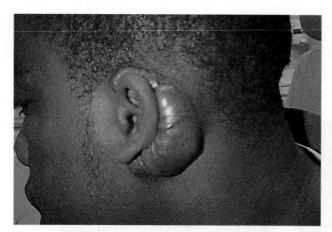

Figure 18-5 Keloid. Rubbery mass at the site of ear piercing is compatible with a keloid. (Courtesy of Steven P. Cook, MD.)

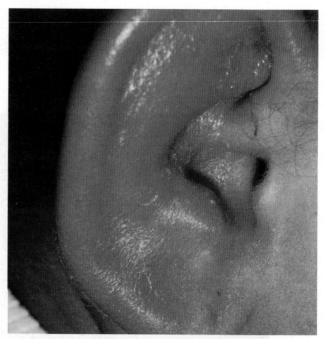

Figure 18-6 Perichondritis. Erythema and swelling of the pinna are consistent with perichondritis. (Used with permission from Handler SD, Myer CM. *Atlas of Ear, Nose and Throat Disorders in Children.* Ontario: BC Decker; 1998:12.)

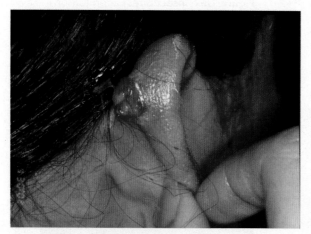

Figure 18-7 Infected ear-piercing site. Pustule with drainage at ear-piercing site, indicating infection. (Courtesy of Ellen Deutsch, MD.)

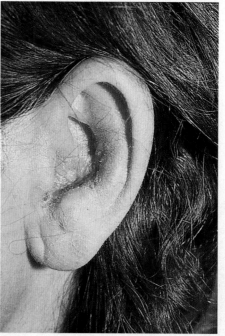

Figure 18-8 Ramsay Hunt syndrome. Vesicles in external auditory canal demonstrating Ramsay Hunt syndrome. (Courtesy of Steven D. Handler, MD, MBE.)

DIFFERENTIAL DIAGNOSIS

DIAGNOSIS	ICD-10 CODE	DISTINGUISHING CHARACTERISTICS	DISTRIBUTION	ASSOCIATED FINDINGS	PREDISPOSING FACTORS	TREATMENT GUIDELINES
Cellulitis	H60.10	Erythema Warmth Tenderness Originating from a wound Edema	Pinna Earlobe Preauricular and postauricular spaces	Fever Chills Malaise Red streaking Wound	Insect bites Laceration Earring related Ear piercing	Oral antibiotics; IV antibiotics if infection is spreading or no response to oral antibiotics If there is concurrent acute otitis externa, antibiotic drops are required.
Diffuse Otitis Externa	H60	Swelling Erythema Warmth Pain with manipulation of the pinna and pressure on the tragus Drainage from external auditory canal	External auditory canal Auricle Posterior auricular area Unilateral	Forward displacement of auricle Fever Thick otorrhea Pre- or postauricular lymphadenopathy	Prolonged moisture of ear canal (swimming) Excoriation of external auditory canal Foreign body Hearing aid use	Antibiotic ear drops If moderate to severe: aural lavage
Otomelalgia (Red Ear Syndrome)	H93.8X9	Painful Erythema Swelling Burning Unilateral Episodic	Entire ear, including earlobe	Migraine type headache Irritation of third cervical root Temporomandibular joint dysfunction Thalamic syndrome	Migraine headache	Medications used for migraine headaches Application of cool compresses
Insect Bite	S00.469	Erythema Swelling of sudden onset Nontender Papule or punctum at site of bite Pruritus	Pinna Posterior auricular space	Other papules on skin surface	Insect bite Sting	Oral antihistamines Cold packs
Mastoiditis	H70	Edema and erythema of pinna and skin overlying mastoid process Tenderness of mastoid process Displacement of pinna upward and outward in children >2 years	Postauricular area Mastoid periosteum Pinna	Acute otitis media Purulent otorrhea Fever Toxicity	Acute otitis media	Urgent evaluation IV antibiotics Drainage of abscess Referral to otolaryngology Myringotomy
Trauma	S00.439	Discoloration with ecchymoses Hematoma between the perichondrium and the cartilage Pallor of area	Pinna Earlobe Auricle	Hemotympanum Perforated tympanic membrane	Direct blow to the ear	Surgical evaluation for possible hematoma drainage If intentional injury from child physical abuse suspected, contact the local department of child protective services.
Keloid	L91.0	Flesh colored mass May be tender and pruritic initially Rubbery Extends beyond margins of wound	Ear lobe Site of wound or ear piercings	Other sites of keloid formation	Pierced ear Ear laceration Insect bites Burn Race/ethnicity of African descent	Intralesional steroid injections Surgical excision by plastic surgery, followed by steroid injections Topical silicon gel sheeting for several hours per day for several weeks
Perichondritis	H61.019 (acute pinna) H61.029 (chronic, of pinna)	Erythema Tenderness Swelling	Skin and perichondrium of pinna Auricular cartilage Site of wound	Puncture from earring Laceration Nodule Fever, chills Nausea	Trauma Ear piercing through the cartilage Laceration through cartilage	IV antibiotics Surgical drainage if abscess present Removal of ear jewelry

Other Diagnoses to Consider

- Malignant otitis externa

- Chilblains (pernio)

- Xanthomatosis

- Relapsing polychondritis

- Henoch–Schönlein purpura involving the ear lobe and pinna

- Ramsay Hunt syndrome or herpes zoster oticus

When to Consider Further Evaluation or Treatment

- Medical evaluation should be sought if ear swelling is accompanied by fever or ill appearance.

- Suspected cellulitis requires oral antibiotic treatment.

- Swelling from insect bites usually resolves with antihistamines and local treatment, such as ice or cold compresses.

- Mastoiditis requires urgent evaluation by an otolaryngologist.

- If the external ear is pale or ecchymotic following trauma and there is suspicion for an underlying hematoma, surgical evaluation is required to determine the need for emergent evacuation of the hematoma.

- Keloids may improve after monthly, intralesional injection of triamcinolone suspension by a dermatologist or plastic surgeon.

- Perichondritis requires systemic antibiotics and removal of all ear jewelry. Cartilage is susceptible to rapid destruction by bacterial infection; therefore, prompt treatment is essential.

- Otomelalgia usually resolves with the application of cool compresses and in some cases migraine headache medications.

SUGGESTED READINGS

Arnett AM. Pain-earache. In: Fleisher GR, Ludwig S, Henretig FM, eds. *Textbook of Pediatric Emergency Medicine.* 6th ed. Philadelphia, PA: Lippincott Williams & Wilkins; 2010:455–460.

Handler SD, Myer CM. *Atlas of Ear, Nose and Throat Disorders in Children.* Ontario: BC Decker, Inc.; 1998:12.

Kliegman R, Behrman RE, Jenson HB, et al. *Nelson's Textbook of Pediatrics.* 19th ed. Philadelphia, PA: Elsevier Saunders; 2011:2630–2631.

Long S. *Principles and Practice of Pediatric Infectious Disease.* 4th ed. Philadelphia, PA: Elsevier Saunders; 2012:220–222.

Paller A, Mancini A. Vascular disorders of infancy and childhood. In: *Hurwitz Clinical Pediatric Dermatology: A Textbook of Skin Disorders of Childhood and Adolescence.* 4th ed. Philadelphia, PA: Elsevier Saunders; 2011:295.

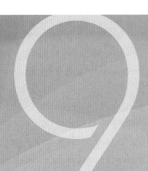

Ear Pits and Tags

Leora N. Mogilner and Risa L. Yavorsky

Approach to the Problem

Preauricular pits, sinuses, and tags are not unusual in the pediatric population and are often an incidental physical exam finding. Ear tags are flesh-colored appendages, and ear pits are small indentations, both most commonly located anterior and adjacent to the external ear. An ear pit may be the outermost sign of a sinus tract, which can be of variable length and may ultimately lead to the formation of a subcutaneous cyst. The prevalence of preauricular anomalies varies depending upon geographic location, ranging from 0.3% to 5% of the population, with the highest incidence in some areas of Asia and Africa. They may be sporadic or inherited, and bilateral findings are more commonly of the inherited type. When other craniofacial or physical anomalies are present, it is crucial to evaluate for genetic syndromes in which ear malformations are common, such as Treacher–Collins, Goldenhar, or Branchio-Oto-Renal (BOR) syndromes (see "Other Diagnoses to Consider" for complete list).

An isolated, asymptomatic preauricular pit, sinus, or tag requires no intervention. In contrast, a preauricular sinus that develops erythema, pain, swelling, or discharge due to acute infection should be treated with appropriate antibiotics, and recurrent or persistent infection requires surgical excision. While preauricular anomalies are generally benign conditions, a potential association with hearing loss and renal abnormalities exists. A number of studies show that children with preauricular anomalies may be at increased risk of hearing loss, particularly those with preauricular pits and tags as part of a syndrome. The evidence is inconclusive regarding the increased risk of renal anomalies in children with isolated preauricular sinuses, pits, and tags in the absence of a syndrome. Current guidelines suggest screening with renal ultrasound for children with preauricular anomalies only if they are associated with other malformations or dysmorphic features, a family history of deafness or auricular or renal malformations, or a maternal history of gestational diabetes.

151

- Preauricular pits and sinuses are generally asymptomatic but if infected, may present with swelling, pain, erythema, and discharge. A history of recurrent infection may warrant surgical intervention.

- Preauricular anomalies are often inherited, so family history is important to obtain. When inherited, the pattern is of incomplete autosomal dominance with reduced penetrance and variable expression. Bilateral preauricular pits and sinuses are more likely to be inherited than unilateral ones.

- While most ear pits and tags are incidental findings, they may be associated with genetic syndromes, so it is important to inquire about a history of other physical anomalies.

- Family and personal history of hearing loss must be obtained as preauricular pits and sinuses may be associated with a higher incidence of hearing impairment.

- Ear pits are small indentations located adjacent to the external ear, most often anterior to the helix, but may occur along the posterior margin of the helix, tragus, or ear lobe.

- A preauricular indentation may be the outermost sign of a sinus tract, which may branch or follow a tortuous route, and may ultimately lead to the formation of a cyst.

- Ear tags are flesh-colored appendages that may consist of skin, subcutaneous fat, and/or cartilage and are often located anterior to the tragus.

- Preauricular pits or sinuses may be unilateral, but 25% to 50% are bilateral. When unilateral, they are more commonly found on the right side.

- Since ear pits and tags may be associated with congenital anomalies, a close examination for other physical malformations is warranted.

  - BOR syndrome consists of preauricular pits, structural defects of the outer, middle, and inner ear associated with hearing loss, branchial cleft cysts or sinuses, and renal anomalies.

  - Oculo-auriculo-vertebral spectrum, which includes Hemifacial Microsomia and Goldenhar syndrome, consists of preauricular tags, hypoplasia of one side of the face, cervical vertebral malformations, and other findings.

- Erythema, tenderness, edema, or discharge at the site of a preauricular pit or sinus may indicate infection.

- A branchial cleft cyst/sinus/fistula, which may present as an opening anywhere from the external auditory canal to the angle of the mandible, must be differentiated from a preauricular pit or sinus.

PHOTOGRAPHS OF SELECTED DIAGNOSES

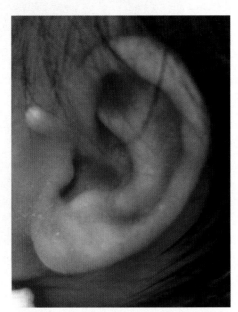

Figure 19-1 Preauricular tag in an infant. (Courtesy of Risa Yavorsky, MD.)

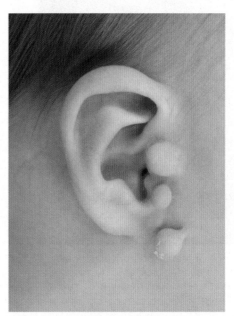

Figure 19-2 Multiple preauricular tags in a child with oculoauriculovertebral spectrum disorder. (Courtesy of David Tunkel, MD.)

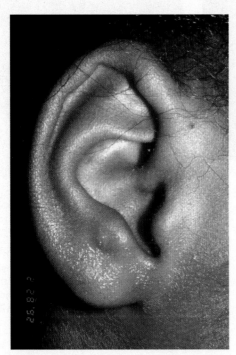

Figure 19-3 Preauricular pit. Note how the hairline can obscure visualization. (Courtesy of David Tunkel, MD.)

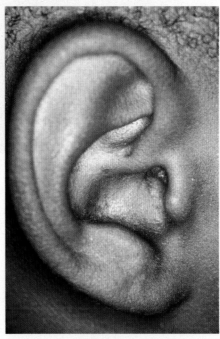

Figure 19-4 Auricular sinus on the inferior crus of the pinna. (Courtesy of David Tunkel, MD.)

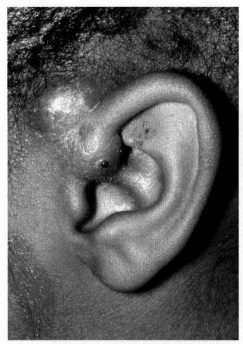

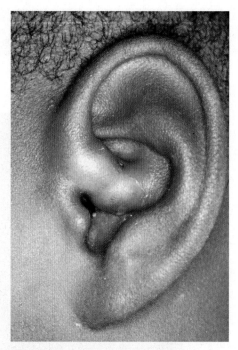

Figure 19-5 Infected preauricular sinus.
The swelling nearly obscures identification of
the offending sinus tract opening. (Courtesy
of David Tunkel, MD.)

**Figure 19-6 Infected auricular pit on
the inferior crus.** Note erythema and
edema. (Courtesy of David Tunkel, MD.)

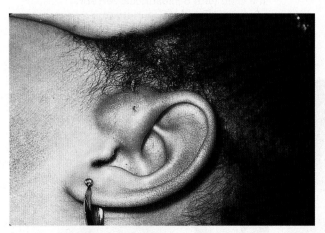

Figure 19-7 Preauricular abscess. (Courtesy of
Steven D. Handler, MD, MBE.)

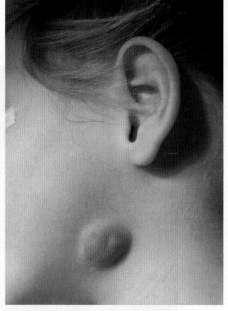

Figure 19-8 First branchial cleft sinus.
This lesion must be considered in the differential diagnosis of a preauricular pit or
sinus. (Courtesy of David Tunkel, MD.)

DIFFERENTIAL DIAGNOSIS

DIAGNOSIS	ICD-10 CODE	DISTINGUISHING CHARACTERISTICS	DISTRIBUTION	ASSOCIATED FINDINGS	COMPLICATIONS	TREATMENT GUIDELINES
Preauricular Tag	Q17.0	A flesh-colored appendage that may consist of skin, subcutaneous fat, and/or cartilage	Most often located anterior to the tragus	May be associated with other craniofacial or physical anomalies, especially when part of a genetic syndrome Increased risk of hearing impairment	Cosmetic concerns	An isolated, asymptomatic preauricular tag requires no intervention Surgical removal may be considered for cosmetic reasons
Preauricular/ Auricular Pit	Q17.9 Congenital malformation of the ear, unspecified	A small indentation adjacent to or on the external ear	Usually located anterior to the ascending limb of the helix, but may occur along the posterior superior margin of the helix, tragus, or earlobe	May be associated with other craniofacial or physical anomalies, especially when part of a genetic syndrome Increased risk of hearing impairment compared to the general population	Infection, particularly in older children who pick at the lesion	An isolated, asymptomatic preauricular pit requires no intervention Surgical removal in the case of recurrent or persistent infection
Preauricular or Auricular Sinus/Cyst	Q18.1	A small opening in the external ear leading to a track which may branch or follow a tortuous route, and may ultimately form a subcutaneous epithelial-lined cyst	Usually located anterior to the ascending limb of the helix, but may occur along the posterior superior margin of the helix, tragus, or earlobe	May be associated with other craniofacial or physical anomalies, especially when part of a genetic syndrome Increased risk of hearing impairment compared to the general population	Infection	An isolated, asymptomatic preauricular sinus requires no intervention Surgical removal in the case of recurrent or persistent drainage or infection
Preauricular Pit/Sinus Infection	L03.90 (cellulitis, unspecified site)	Erythema, tenderness, and edema surrounding the pit/sinus, often accompanied by discharge of purulent or squamous debris	N/A	Erythema, tenderness, warmth, edema, and/or discharge	Recurrent or persistent infection Scarring	Antibiotic treatment, followed by surgical excision in the case of recurrent or persistent infection
First Branchial Cleft Sinus/ Fistula/Cyst	Q18.0	Type I: A duplication anomaly of the external auditory canal, derived from ectoderm, and usually presenting as a preauricular cystic mass Type II: Usually presents as a fistula or mass at the angle of the mandible, derived from both ectoderm and mesoderm	Type I: Usually a sinus tract anterior and medial to the external auditory canal, in close proximity to the parotid gland and facial nerve Type II: Usually located at the angle of the mandible; may communicate with the external auditory canal, passing through the parotid gland and running alongside the facial nerve	In unusual cases, may coexist with aural atresia or stenosis May be associated with other craniofacial or physical anomalies, especially when part of a genetic syndrome	Infection or abscess formation Impingement on the facial nerve or postoperative facial nerve damage	Referral to ENT and/or plastic surgery Complete surgical excision with imaging in order to determine relationship to facial nerve In case of an abscess, emergency incision and/or drainage prior to surgical excision

- Body piercing

- Ear trauma

- Genetic syndromes with associated ear anomalies:

  - Beckwith–Wiedemann syndrome

  - BOR syndrome and other less common variants

  - CHARGE association

  - Diabetic embryopathy

  - Ectodermal dysplasia

  - Oculo-auriculo-vertebral spectrum (including Goldenhar syndrome and Hemifacial Microsomia)

  - Treacher–Collins syndrome

  - Trisomy 22 (mosaicism or complete)

  - Waardenburg syndrome

  - Wolf–Hirschhorn syndrome

- An isolated, asymptomatic preauricular sinus, pit, or tag requires no intervention.

- Preauricular tags may be removed for cosmetic reasons. If small and associated with a thin stalk, they are often tied off shortly after birth for this purpose. Removal of larger ear tags should be performed by an otolaryngologist or plastic surgeon for optimal cosmetic results and to avoid complications.

- Acute infection of a preauricular pit or sinus should be treated with antibiotics covering for staphylococcus, and less frequently proteus, streptococcus, or peptococcus.

- Recurrent or persistent infection requires surgical excision of the sinus, its tract, and the cartilage at the root of the helix. Incomplete excision can lead to recurrence of the preauricular sinus. For optimal outcomes, excision should be performed by an otolaryngologist.

- Screening with renal ultrasound is recommended if the preauricular anomaly is associated with another malformation or dysmorphic feature, a maternal history of gestational diabetes, or a family history of deafness and auricular or renal malformations.

- When other craniofacial or physical anomalies are present, it is crucial to evaluate for more complex genetic syndromes associated with ear malformations.

- In the case of a first branchial cleft cyst/sinus/fistula, due to the proximity to the facial nerve and the parotid gland, imaging and referral to otolaryngology or plastic surgery are required for further management.

SUGGESTED READINGS

Firat Y, Sireci S, Yakinci C, et al. Isolated preauricular pits and tags: Is it necessary to investigate renal abnormalities and hearing impairment? *Eur Arch Otorhinolaryngol.* 2008;265:1057–1060.

Gan EC, Anicete R, Tan H, et al. Preauricular sinuses in the pediatric population: Techniques and recurrence rates. *Int J Pediatr Otorhinolaryngol.* 2013;77:372–378.

Huang XY, Tay GS, Wansaicheong GK, et al. Preauricular sinus. *Arch Otolaryngol Head Neck Surg.* 2007;133:65–68.

McArdle AJ, Shroff R. Is ultrasonography required to rule out congenital anomalies of the kidneys and urinary tract in babies with isolated preauricular tags or sinuses? *Arch Dis Child.* 2013;98:84–87.

Roth DA, Hildesheimer M, Bardenstein S, et al. Preauricular skin tags and ear pits are associated with permanent hearing impairment in newborns. *Pediatrics.* 2008;122:e884–e890.

Scheinfeld NS, Silverberg NB, Weinberg JM, et al. The preauricular sinus: A review of its clinical presentation, treatment and associations. *Pediatr Dermatol.* 2004;21(3):191–196.

Tan T, Constantinides H, Mitchell TE. The preauricular sinus: A review of its aetiology, clinical presentation and management. *Int J Pediatr Otorhinolaryngol.* 2005;69:1469–1474.

Ear Canal Findings

Lee R. Atkinson-McEvoy and Esther K. Chung

20

Approach to the Problem

Physicians caring for children frequently see patients who have complaints about the ear, including pain, itching, drainage, and decreased hearing. Often, the initial concern is focused on middle ear abnormalities, but external auditory canal (EAC) abnormalities may cause complaints that are similar to those caused by middle ear pathology. Common diseases of the EAC include otitis externa (affecting up to 10% of the population), impacted cerumen, trauma, and foreign bodies in the ear.

There are many variations in cerumen, and canal size and shape. Flaky, dry cerumen may be found in East Asian patients. In some cases, as in Down syndrome, the canals may be narrowed, making it difficult for the examiner to evaluate the tympanic membrane on routine otoscopy.

Key Points in the History

- School-aged children may be exceptionally precise in their description of pain. Therefore, it is important to ask them to describe what they are feeling. Often, when parents report pain, the child instead reports ringing or fullness. For example, one child with water in his ear reported, "It sounds like I am under water."

- The use of cotton swabs or other objects to clean the ear may result in trauma to the EAC and tympanic membrane, and retained pieces of cotton may cause irritation and/or subsequent inflammation.

- The placement of a foreign body in the ear may lead to trauma and most often presents with pain. If the foreign body is not promptly removed, the EAC may become infected.

- Tinnitus and bleeding, in addition to pain, may be symptoms that occur from trauma to the external ear canal.

- Decreased hearing often occurs with cerumen impaction, fluid in the external canal, or otitis externa, but it may also be seen in trauma, particularly when perforation of the tympanic membrane exists.

- Drainage from the EAC may occur in acute otitis media with perforation, otitis externa, and external fluid in the canal (residual from swimming or bathing).

- The drainage seen with acute otitis media with perforation is often described as brownish and sticky, but at other times may be whitish and creamy.

- Pseudomonal and fungal infections should be considered in children with chronic symptoms of otitis externa.

- History of frequent swimming or submersion of ears while in the bathtub is suggestive of otitis externa (also known as *swimmer's ear*). Water from the pool or tub is believed to cause alterations in the normal flora of the EAC.

- Patients with eczema, seborrhea, or psoriasis may have the involvement of the epidermis of the EAC and may complain of pruritus.

- The use of medication or topical substances to the ear may result in an eczematous dermatitis.

- Earrings, particularly those made of alloy metals, may cause inflammation at the earring site and an eczematous dermatitis of the surrounding tissues.

- Pain preceding development of a vesicular rash suggests varicella zoster virus infection, which when associated with an acute facial neuropathy is known as Ramsay Hunt syndrome.

Key Points in the Physical Examination

- It is important to note that there may be variations in the amount, color, and consistency of cerumen.

- If blood is present, suspect trauma and carefully inspect the tympanic membrane for perforation or other injury.

- Pain elicited from pressure on the tragus and/or outward traction on the pinna is suggestive of otitis externa.

- Edema and inflammation of the ear canal are typically seen with otitis externa.

- When a significant amount of discharge is present, it may be difficult to differentiate acute otitis media with perforation from otitis externa.

- Greasy scales, dry or flaky skin, excoriation, and crusting of the external ear canal and pinna may be seen with eczematous or psoriatic dermatitis and seborrhea.

- Pustules on the outer portion of the EAC suggest furunculosis.

- Vesicular lesions suggest reactivation of varicella zoster or herpes simplex virus.

PHOTOGRAPHS OF SELECTED DIAGNOSES

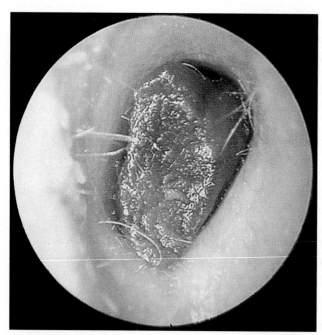

Figure 20-1 **Cerumen impaction of the ear canal.** (From Weber JR. *Nurses' Handbook of Health Assessment.* 7th ed. Philadelphia, PA: Lippincott Williams & Wilkins; 2009.)

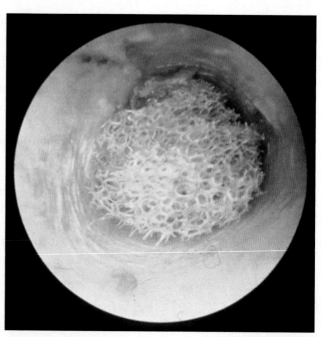

Figure 20-2 **Foreign body in ear canal.** (Courtesy of Welch Allyn, Inc. Skaneatleles Falls, NY.)

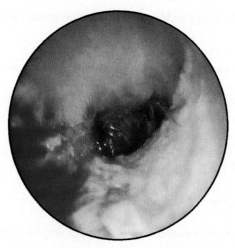

Figure 20-3 **Cockroach in external canal.** Note the visible body and legs from the cockroach. There is also surrounding edema and hyperemia. (Courtesy of Ellen Deutsch, MD.)

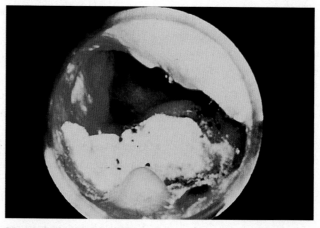

Figure 20-4 **Acute otitis externa.** Note that the EAC is edematous with narrowing. There is also discharge present. (Courtesy of Steven D. Handler, MD, MBE.)

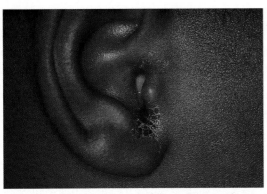

Figure 20-5 Otorrhea associated with a cholesteatoma. Note the white-colored discharge visible at the os of the EAC, as well as crust on the antitragus. (Courtesy of Ellen Deutsch, MD.)

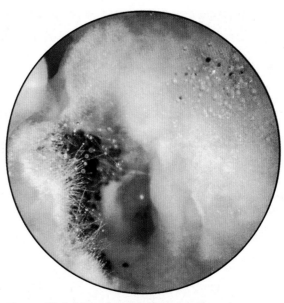

Figure 20-6 Mycotic otitis externa. Fungal overgrowth produces a moist appearing, whitish plaque. (Used with permission from Handler SD, Myer CM. *Atlas of Ear, Nose and Throat Disorders in Children.* Hamilton: BC Decker; 1998:24.)

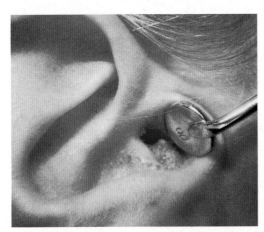

Figure 20-7 Furuncle of the EAC. Note the large erythematous papule with a pustular tip. (Used with permission from Handler SD, Myer CM. *Atlas of Ear, Nose and Throat Disorders in Children.* Hamilton: BC Decker; 1998:24.)

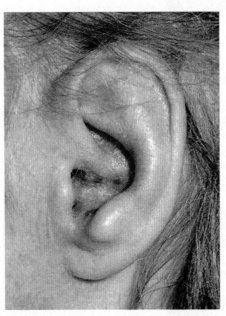

Figure 20-8 Ramsay Hunt syndrome. Vesicles in the external ear canal in a case of geniculate herpes. (From Campbell WW. *DeJong's The Neurologic Examination.* 7th ed. Philadelphia, PA: Lippincott Williams & Wilkins; 2012.)

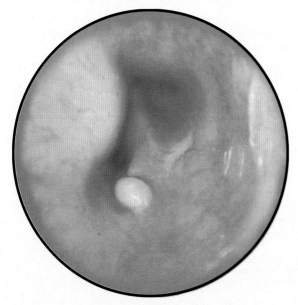

Figure 20-9 External auditory canal exostoses. Note the nontender nodular swellings covered by normal skin deep in the ear canal. (From Bickley LS, Szilagyi P. *Bates' Guide to Physical Examination and History Taking.* 8th ed. Philadelphia, PA: Lippincott Williams & Wilkins; 2003.)

DIFFERENTIAL DIAGNOSIS

DIAGNOSIS	ICD-10	DISTINGUISHING CHARACTERISTICS	DISTRIBUTION	DURATION/ CHRONICITY
Foreign Bodies in EAC	T16	Foreign bodies—most commonly seen in younger children Common foreign bodies include beads, paper, toys, and pebbles. Other foreign bodies found in the EAC include button batteries, insects, and food matter.	N/A	May present acutely or chronically
Trauma/Superficial Injury to EAC	S09.9	Bleeding or pain of the ear	N/A	Acute onset of symptoms
Acute Otitis Media with Perforation	H66.0 Acute otitis media H72.9 Perforation of tympanic membrane	Mucoid, whitish, grayish or brownish discharge in canal Canal walls, when visualized, are not irritated or red.	N/A	Acute
Acute Otitis Externa	H60.3 Acute infectious otitis externa H60.5 Noninfective acute otitis externa	Tenderness with pressure on the tragus and outward traction on the pinna	N/A	Acute or chronic
Seborrheic Otitis Externa	H60.5	Greasy appearing scales that may involve the auricle	N/A	Often chronic
Eczematous Otitis Externa	H60.5	Dry, flaky skin that may be pruritic	N/A	Often chronic
Psoriatic Otitis Externa	H60.5	Dry scaly plaques with a silvery quality	N/A	Often chronic
Chronic Mycotic Otitis Externa	H60.3	Intense itching, but usually painless Moist-appearing, white-colored plaque	N/A	Often chronic
Furunculosis	H60.0	Erythematous pustules in the anterior portion of the external ear canal	N/A	Acute or recurrent
Ramsay Hunt Syndrome	B02.2	Pain deep in the ear Pain precedes onset of rash Vesicular rash of ear and/or mouth in up to 80% Rash may occur in the following locations: tongue, soft palate, external ear canal, and pinna	VZV infection of the head and neck that involves the facial nerve, often the seventh cranial nerve (CN VII)	Self-limited

ASSOCIATED FINDINGS	COMPLICATIONS	PREDISPOSING FACTORS	TREATMENT GUIDELINES
Acute setting—possibly pain or decreased hearing Chronic setting—foul odor or discharge	Hearing loss Infection	Cleaning ears with cotton swabs Young age, particularly in the toddler years for most foreign bodies School-aged children more likely with button battery insertions	Removal of foreign body relieves symptoms. Can be removed directly with forceps, cerumen loop, or suction catheter, or with irrigation Acetone will dissolve a styrofoam foreign body. If inflammation of the EAC is present, combination of antibiotic and steroid topical treatments can be used.
Bloody discharge Decreased hearing whenever the tympanic membrane is affected	Hearing loss	Foreign body in ear Aggressive cleaning with an object of EAC	Careful exploration to evaluate for presence of concomitant perforation of the tympanic membrane. Combination of antibiotic and steroid topical treatment can be used to treat symptoms of inflammation of EAC in the absence of perforated tympanic membrane. If the tympanic membrane is perforated, refer to otolaryngologist.
May be associated with systemic symptoms, such as fever	Hearing loss Speech delays if recurrent	Associated with preceding upper respiratory tract infection	Treatment with topical antibiotics or systemic antibiotics, if warranted based on age and severity of infection
Edema of the external ear canal with seropurulent discharge or whitish to grayish exudate Generally no fever	Rarely, acute otitis media from invasion through the tympanic membrane Cellulitis	Trauma to external ear canal or exposure to water Wearing ear plugs, hearing aids, or headphones	Combination of antibiotic and steroid topical treatment can be used to treat symptoms of inflammation of EAC. For swimmers, prophylactic use of earplugs can help prevent otitis externa. Also installation of one teaspoon of a solution of equal parts of white vinegar and rubbing alcohol can prevent bacterial and fungal overgrowth.
Patient may have seborrheic dermatitis in other areas, especially the scalp	Scarring and narrowing of external ear canal	Family history of seborrheic dermatitis	Treatment with topical steroids can eliminate symptoms.
History of diffuse eczema	Scarring and narrowing of external ear canal	Use of topical medications or exposure to metals (earrings) or cosmetics	Treatment with emollients and topical steroids can eliminate symptoms.
History of psoriasis	Scarring and narrowing of external ear canal	History of psoriasis	Treatment with topical steroids can eliminate symptoms.
May form an exudate that may have a musty odor	Untreated infections can lead to bacterial superinfection.	Recurrent or chronic otitis externa	Treatment with topical antifungal agents can eliminate symptoms. In patients who are immunocompromised, systemic treatment may be warranted.
Point tenderness at the site of the furuncle	Scarring and narrowing of external ear canal	Infection of hair follicle	Heat, analgesics, and oral antistaphylococcal antibiotics are mainstays of treatment.
Tinnitus, hearing loss, nausea, vomiting, vertigo, fever, and nystagmus Peripheral facial nerve paralysis on ipsilateral side	Permanent facial nerve paralysis in >50%	Latent infection of varicella zoster virus Rare in children <6 years	Treatment includes medication to decrease inflammation and viral replication. It consists of systemic steroids, oral acyclovir and pain medication.

SECTION 5 • EARS

Other Diagnoses to Consider

- Osteomyelitis

- Acne

- Cholesteatoma

- EAC exostosis

- Malignant otitis externa

When to Consider Further Evaluation or Treatment

- In immunocompromised patients, consider parenteral treatment for EAC infections, and consider less common organisms as possible etiologic agents.

- If penetrating injury is suspected, consider imaging and consultation with subspecialists from trauma surgery, neurosurgery, and/or otolaryngology to evaluate for further injury.

- If acute otitis media with perforation is suspected, treat with oral antibiotics, and consider the use of topical antibiotic drops to the EAC.

- If symptoms do not improve within 48 to 72 hours of initiating treatment, consider other etiologies and referral to an otolaryngologist.

- Permanent facial nerve paralysis may be seen with reactivated varicella zoster virus in Ramsay Hunt syndrome. Early treatment with steroids and oral acyclovir and referral to an otolaryngologist should be considered.

SUGGESTED READINGS

Ely JW, Hansen MR, Clark EC. Diagnosis of ear pain. *Am Fam Physician.* 2008;77(5):621–628.

Handler SD, Myer CM. *Atlas of Ear, Nose, and Throat Disorders in Children.* Hamilton: BC Decker; 1998:22–27.

Kaushik V, Malik T, Saeed SR. Interventions for acute otitis externa. *Cochr Database Syst Rev.* 2010;(1):CD004740. doi:10.1002/14651858.CD004740.pub2.

Miravalle AA. Ramsay Hunt Syndrome. http://emedicine.medscape.com/article/1166804-overview. Accessed November 11, 2013.

Osguthorpe JD, Nielsen DR. Otitis externa: Review and clinical update. *Am Fam Physician.* 2006;74(9):1510–1516.

Sharpe SJ, Rochette LM, Smith GA. Pediatric battery-related emergency department visits in the United States, 1990–2009. *Pediatrics.* 2012;129:1111–1117.

Stoner MJ, Dulaurier M. Pediatric ENT emergencies. *Emer Med Clin N Am.* 2013;31:795–808.

Sweeney CJ, Gilden DH. Ramsay Hunt syndrome. *J Neurol Neurosurg Psychiatr.* 2001;71:149–154.

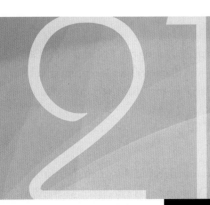

Tympanic Membrane Abnormalities

Charles A. Pohl

Approach to the Problem

Acute otitis media (AOM) is one of the most common diagnoses and reasons for antibiotic prescriptions in children. With more than 5 million cases diagnosed annually, it is associated with individual discomfort, family disruption, financial costs, serious sequelae, and antimicrobial resistance. For these reasons, it is important to make the correct diagnosis when evaluating the tympanic membrane (TM).

Pneumatic otoscopy allows the visualization of TM characteristics: color, contour (normal, retracted, full, bulging), position, and mobility. A normal TM is described as translucent, pearly gray, and mobile. A light reflex and boney landmarks, such as the arm of the malleus, are generally easily viewed. The examination requires that the child be restrained or held still and have patent and clear ear canal. Also, a pneumatic otoscope with a good seal and light source must be available.

Key Points in the History

- Acute onset, hyperpyrexia, and otalgia are features of AOM and not otitis media with effusion (OME).

- Concomitant or recent upper respiratory tract infections or allergies are commonly seen with AOM and OME.

- Hearing loss is a nonspecific finding that may be caused by middle ear (ME) fluid (AOM, OME), as well as by structural damage of the TM or ossicles (severe tympanosclerosis, TM perforation, or cholesteatoma).

- Refer children to a pediatric otolaryngologist whenever TM perforation is accompanied by hearing loss or vertigo, or when ME fluid is chronic and associated with hearing loss and/or speech delay.

- Suspect cholesteatoma if persistent middle ear effusion (MEE) or hearing impairment, greasy and/or whitish mass, or no clinical response is present when treating another suspected TM problem.

- When a cholesteatoma is associated with ataxia or headaches, neuroimaging should be considered to evaluate for the presence of a brain abscess.

- One must immobilize the head carefully and firmly when evaluating the TM and ear canal, while using a snug-fitting ear speculum. The small (2.5-mm diameter) ear speculum should be used in infants and preschool children, whereas the large (4-mm diameter) ear speculum should be used in school-aged children and adolescents.

- The light reflex may be absent in some normal children.

- Mobility, assessed by pneumatic otoscopy, should be measured, especially when the history and/or physical examination suggest a problem. Poor TM mobility is associated with AOM, MEE, TM perforation, or TM structural damage as with tympanosclerosis.

- Mild TM erythema can occur in association with fever, crying, upper respiratory tract infections, or irritation from cerumen or foreign objects.

- AOM should have evidence of MEE and acute inflammation, including TM bulging or fullness, marked erythema, otorrhea, or yellow or cloudy fluid.

- Air bubbles and amber TM discoloration are associated with serous ME fluid or OME.

- Blood in the ME causes a bluish, deep red, or brown ("chocolate") appearance of the TM.

- Chalky white plaques on the TM (tympanosclerosis) are seen with healed inflammation.

- TM mobility is absent or decreased with TM perforation.

- Manipulation of the ear pinna to ensure proper visualization of TM varies with age. As in adults, the pinna should be lifted posterosuperiorly in older children. The pinna should be pulled horizontally backward in infants and younger children.

- Localized TM atelectasis, especially in the posterosuperior quadrant of the pars tensa, is seen with retraction pockets.

- Excessive localized mobility reflects a healed perforation or TM thinning.

- OME is evidenced by fluid bubbles and air–fluid levels or by at least two of the following TM changes: abnormal color including white, yellow, amber, or blue; opacification; decreased mobility.

PHOTOGRAPHS OF SELECTED DIAGNOSES

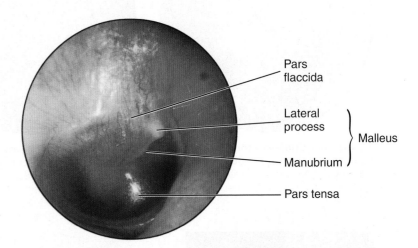

Figure 21-1 Normal tympanic membrane. (Photo used with permission from Handler SD, Myer CM. *Atlas of Ear, Nose and Throat Disorders in Children.* Ontario: BC Decker; 1998:28.)

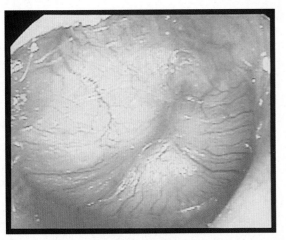

Figure 21-2 Acute otitis media. Typical acute otitis media with a red, distorted, bulging tympanic membrane in a highly symptomatic child. (Courtesy of Alejandro Hoberman, Children's Hospital of Pittsburgh, University of Pittsburgh.)

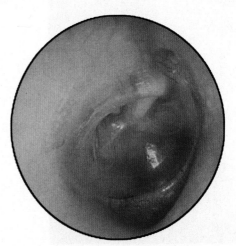

Figure 21-3 Otitis media with effusion. (Courtesy of Glenn Isaacson, MD.)

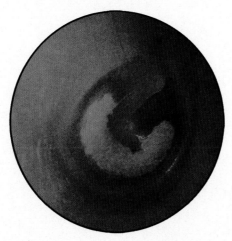

Figure 21-4 Tympanosclerosis. (Courtesy of Steven D. Handler, MD, MBE.)

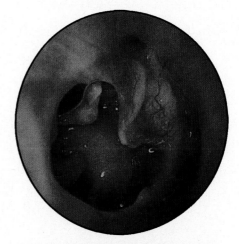

Figure 21-5 Tympanic membrane perforation. (Courtesy of Steven D. Handler, MD, MBE.)

SECTION 5 • EARS

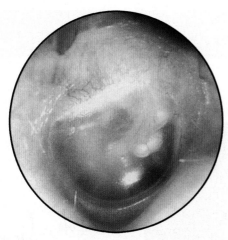

Figure 21-6 **Cholesteatoma.** (Used with permission from Handler SD, Myer CM. *Atlas of Ear, Nose and Throat Disorders in Children*. Ontario: BC Decker; 1998:30.)

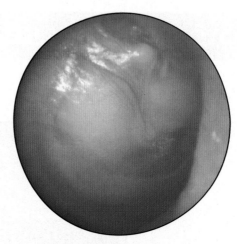

Figure 21-7 **Cholesteatoma.** Note the white, pearly lesion seen behind the TM in the anterior and posterior superior quadrants. (Courtesy of John A. Germiller, MD, PhD.)

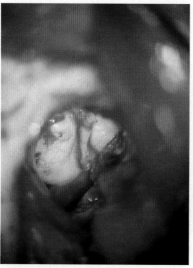

Figure 21-8 **Cholesteatoma.** Intraoperative view of the lesion that corresponds with the previous figure. (Courtesy of John A. Germiller, MD, PhD.)

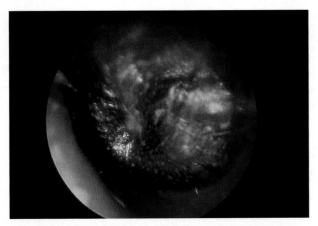

Figure 21-9 Hemotympanum. This hemotympanum was seen in association with a left temporal bone fracture. (Courtesy of Ellen Deutsch, MD.)

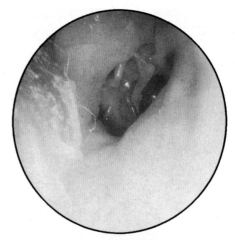

Figure 21-10 Atelectasis, severe. (Courtesy of Ellen Deutsch, MD.)

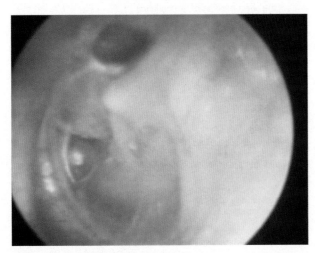

Figure 21-11 Retraction pocket. (Courtesy of Steven D. Handler, MD, MBE.)

DIFFERENTIAL DIAGNOSIS

DIAGNOSIS	ICD-10	DISTINGUISHING CHARACTERISTICS	ASSOCIATED FINDINGS
Acute Otitis Media	H66.4 Suppurative otitis media, unspecified	Most under the age of 2 years MEE and features of acute inflammation: otalgia, fullness or bulging TM, marked TM erythema, otorrhea, yellow or cloudy fluid Malleus may be obscured TM will have poor mobility Acute onset	Fever Otalgia Dizziness Unsteady gait
Otitis Media with Effusion	H65.00 Acute serous otitis media, unspecified ear	Absence of pain or fever Nonerythematous, nonmobile TM with serous or mucoid fluid Bubbles or air–fluid interface noted on otoscopy TM discoloration (white, yellow, or amber) TM atelectasis common (prominence of the short process of the malleus) Usually indolent course	Ear popping Feeling of fullness or pressure Hearing loss Vertigo
Tympanosclerosis (Myringosclerosis)	H74.09 Tympanosclerosis, unspecified ear	"Chalky white plaque" in fibrous layer of TM Reddish or yellowish, localized deposit early Poor mobility when severe	Conductive hearing loss when AOM is present Asymptomatic if small patch
TM Perforation	H72	Hole in TM Everted, ragged edges resulting from sudden pressure changes; bloody when resulting from direct TM trauma Anteroinferior quadrant when resulting from sudden pressure changes; posteriorly when resulting directly from trauma	Hearing loss Bleeding Pain Tinnitus
Cholesteatoma	H71.9 Unspecified cholesteatoma	Greasy, whitish mass of keratin debris	Dizziness Ataxia and headaches (suggests brain abscess) Hearing loss Chronic otorrhea
Hemotympanum	H74.8X9 Other specified disorders of ME and mastoid, unspecified ear	Extravasated blood or blood-stained fluid in ME space Bright red or dark red, blue, or brown ("chocolate" ear drum) TM	Hearing loss Pain Feeling of pressure or fullness
Atelectasis	H73.9 Unspecified disorder of the TM	Retracted and atrophic TM Golden-yellow serous effusion TM thinning and transparent over time (may resemble perforation)	Often asymptomatic Muffled sounds; feeling of pressure or fullness
Retraction Pockets	H73.9 Unspecified disorder of the TM	Localized atelectasis Usually on posterosuperior quadrants of pars tensa	Usually asymptomatic

COMPLICATIONS	PREDISPOSING FACTORS	TREATMENT GUIDELINES
Structural damage of TM or ear bones (ossicles) Hearing impairment Mastoiditis Facial paralysis Persistent perforation Intracranial infection (rare) Cholesteatoma formation	Upper respiratory tract infection Allergies Environmental tobacco smoke Daycare Pacifier use Absence of breastfeeding Family history	Antimicrobial therapy covering *Streptococcus pneumoniae*, nontypeable *Haemophilus influenzae*, and *Moraxella catarrhalis*
Hearing loss Speech/language delay TM atelectasis Developmental/learning impairment Cholesteatoma Usually spontaneously resolves (50–60% resolve 2 weeks after AOM treated, 80% after 4 weeks treatment, 90% after 8 weeks treatment)	Concomitant resolving AOM Allergies Upper respiratory tract infection	Supportive care Decongestants and steroids have not been shown to have long-term benefits.
Conductive hearing loss	Ear infections (severe AOM) Ventilation tube insertion	Supportive care
Marginal perforation less likely to heal than central ones and more likely to lead to cholesteatoma or intracranial infection Residual perforation Water entering ME Ear infections Ossicular damage (more likely when resulting from direct TM trauma)	Direct TM trauma (e.g., from cotton swab, hairpins) Ear trauma Sudden ear pressure changes in ear canal (e.g., gunfire or violent slap) AOM Chronic OME	Usually heals spontaneously Refer if vertigo, persistent hearing loss, or when perforation does not heal Surgical repair if persistent hearing loss
Bony structure erosion Hearing loss Facial nerve paralysis Intracranial process (e.g., brain abscess, meningitis)	Congenital Recurrent AOM Persistent MEE	Referral to otolaryngology Surgical resection
Usually resolves spontaneously Hearing loss TM perforation	Head injury Barotrauma (e.g., flying, diving) Basilar skull, including temporal bone, fracture Severe AOM ME surgery	Consider CT to rule out basilar skull fracture from accidental or nonaccidental trauma. Referral to otolaryngology Surgical evacuation if associated with significant pain or persistent hearing loss, vestibular symptoms, or facial nerve palsy
Fluctuating conductive hearing loss	Untreated OME (prolonged negative pressure)	Supportive care Refer if persistent hearing loss or persistent symptoms
Cholesteatoma Hearing loss	Atrophic TM from recurrent OM, atelectasis, chronic eustachian tube dysfunction Trauma	Supportive care Refer if you suspect a cholesteatoma or if persistent hearing loss

Other Diagnoses to Consider

- Bullous myringitis

- Improper technique (e.g., inadequate light resource, poor speculum seal)

- Cerumen

- Mastoiditis

- Trauma to temporal bone

- Foreign body in ear canal

- Bleeding disorder

- Glomus tympanicum or glomus jugulare tumor

- Otosclerosis (Schwartze sign)

When to Consider Further Evaluation or Treatment

- Consider antibiotic treatment when MEE is associated with acute inflammation, as evidenced by TM bulging or fullness, marked erythema, otorrhea, or yellow or cloudy fluid.

- Chronic MEE associated with hearing loss and/or speech delay should be referred to a pediatric otolaryngologist.

- Investigate for a cholesteatoma if MEE persists or AOM does not respond to antibiotic therapy.

- Suspect a brain abscess when a cholesteatoma is associated with ataxia or headaches.

- Consider an atypical or resistant organism in a child who is immunocompromised or has been exposed to frequent or recent antimicrobial therapy.

- Persistent TM perforation or TM perforation associated with hearing loss or vestibular symptoms (i.e., nausea, vomiting, nystagmus, ataxia, vertigo) should be referred to an otolaryngologist.

SUGGESTED READINGS

American Academy of Family Physicians, American Academy of Otolaryngology—Head and Neck Surgery, American Academy of Pediatrics Subcommittee on Otitis Media with Effusion. Otitis media with effusion. *Pediatrics.* 2004;113:1412–1429.

Bluestone CD, Klein JO, Definitions, terminology, and classification. In: Bluestone CD, Klein JO, eds. *Otitis Media in Infants and Children.* 4th ed. Hamilton: BC Decker, 2007:1–19.

Coker TR, Chan LS, Newberry SJ, et al. Diagnosis, microbial epidemiology, and antibiotic treatment of acute otitis media in children: A systematic review. *JAMA.* 2010;304:2161–2169.

Hoberman A, Paradise JL, Rockette HE, et al. Treatment of acute otitis media in children under 2 years of age. *N Engl J Med.* 2011;364:105–115.

Lieberthal AS, Carroll AE, Chonmaitree T, et al. The diagnosis and management of acute otitis media. *Pediatrics.* 2013;131:e964–e999.

Shaikh N, Hoberman A, Kaleida PH, et al. Otoscopic signs of otitis media. *Pediatr Infect Dis J.* 2011;30:822–826.

NOSE

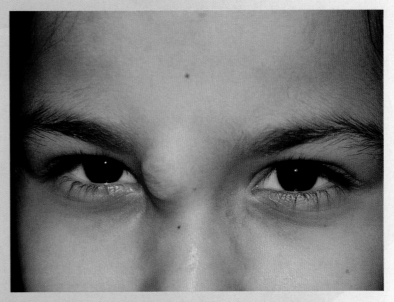

(Courtesy of E. Douglas Thompson, Jr, MD.)

SIX

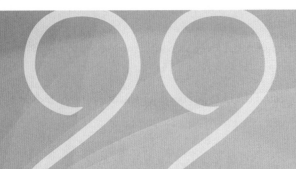

Nasal Bridge Swelling

E. Douglas Thompson, Jr

Approach to the Problem

Swelling of the nasal bridge is an uncommon problem that can present a diagnostic dilemma to the practitioner. Lesions resulting in swelling can be divided into congenital and acquired etiologies. Congenital lesions of the nose occur in 1 in 20,000 to 40,000 live births. The most common congenital lesions to consider in the differential diagnosis include hemangiomas, dacryocystoceles, dermoid cysts, gliomas, and encephaloceles. Teratomas, lymphangiomas, lipomas, and angiofibromas are less frequently encountered. Acquired lesions occur secondary to trauma or infection.

Key Points in the History

- Rapid growth of the lesion in the first weeks to months of life is suggestive of a hemangioma.

- Multiple cutaneous hemangiomas are associated with diffuse neonatal hemangiomatosis.

- Increased size when crying or straining raises the possibility of a connection to the central nervous system consistent with an encephalocele.

- Intermittent discharge of sebaceous material can occur with nasal dermoid cysts.

- Fever can be evidence of an infected congenital cystic lesion or meningitis complicating lesions that extend to the central nervous system.

- Anterior encephaloceles are associated with hydrocephalus, agenesis of the corpus callosum, and other brain malformations.

- A history of trauma may result in a nasal fracture or contusion.

- Reddish or bluish discoloration and telangiectasias are most consistent with hemangiomas, but may be seen in gliomas.

- Cystic lesions located on the lateral aspect of the nose just under the medial canthus indicate the presence of a dacryocystocele.

- Dermoid cysts are midline lesions.

- Hair protruding from a midline mass most likely represents a dermoid cyst.

- Compressible lesions suggest encephaloceles and hemangiomas.

- Transillumination may be evident in encephaloceles.

- A positive Furstenberg sign, represented by enlargement of the mass with compression of the jugular veins, makes the diagnosis of an encephalocele probable.

PHOTOGRAPHS OF SELECTED DIAGNOSES

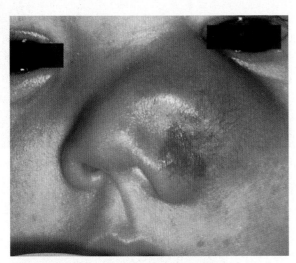

Figure 22-1 **Nasal hemangioma in a child 6 months of age.** Note the vascularity of this nasal mass. (Used with permission from Handler SD, Myer CM. *Atlas of Ear, Nose, and Throat Disorders in Children*. Ontario: BC Decker; 1998:55.)

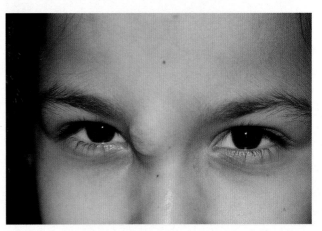

Figure 22-2 **Resolving hemangioma.** A compressible mass without obvious vascularity on the nasal bridge of a child. (Courtesy of E. Douglas Thompson, Jr, MD.)

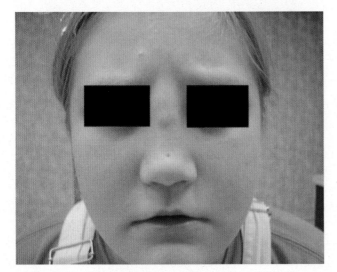

Figure 22-3 **Dermoid cyst.** A midline mass on the upper nasal bridge. (Courtesy of Kathleen Cronan, MD.)

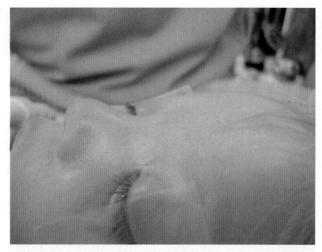

Figure 22-4 Dermoid cyst. Preoperative view. (Courtesy of John A. Germiller, MD, PhD.)

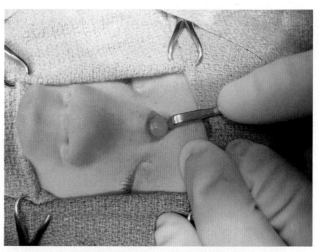

Figure 22-5 Dermoid cyst. Intraoperative view of a well-circumscribed dermoid cyst that corresponds with the previous figure. (Courtesy of John A. Germiller, MD, PhD.)

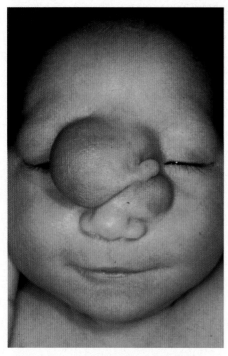

Figure 22-6 Nasal bridge encephalocele. Large nasal bridge mass in a neonate. (Courtesy of Joseph Piatt, MD.)

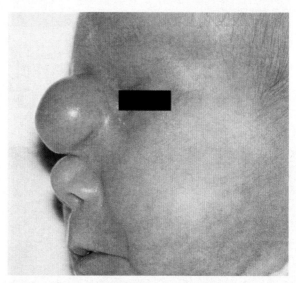

Figure 22-7 Large frontal encephalocele. A midline nasal protrusion in a newborn. (Used with permission from Handler SD, Myer CM. *Atlas of Ear, Nose, and Throat Disorders in Children*. Ontario: BC Decker; 1998:48.)

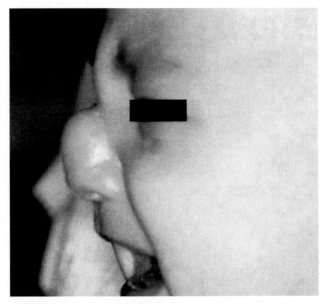

Figure 22-8 Large glioma under the nasal dorsum. Deformity of the nasal bridge in a newborn. (Used with permission from Handler SD, Myer CM. *Atlas of Ear, Nose, and Throat Disorders in Children.* Ontario: BC Decker; 1998:48.)

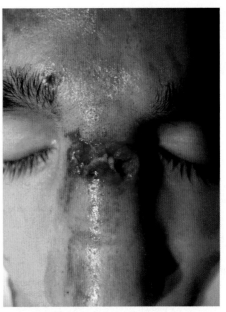

Figure 22-9 Nasal trauma from an assault. Note the swelling, ecchymosis, and laceration. (Courtesy of Brooke Burkey, MD.)

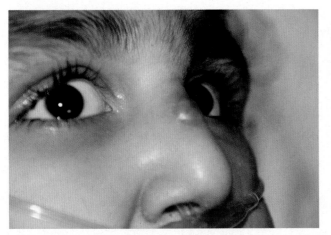

Figure 22-10 Hypertrophic scar. Nasal bridge scarring due to use of a continuous positive airway pressure machine. (Courtesy of E. Douglas Thompson, Jr, MD.)

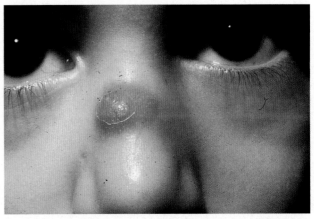

Figure 22-11 Nasal bridge abscess. Painful, erythematous lesion with purulent center on a child's nasal bridge. (Courtesy of the late Peter Sol, MD.)

SECTION 6 • NOSE

DIFFERENTIAL DIAGNOSIS

DIAGNOSIS	ICD-10	DISTINGUISHING CHARACTERISTICS	ASSOCIATED FINDINGS	DURATION/ CHRONICITY	COMPLICATIONS	TREATMENT GUIDELINES
Hemangioma	D18.0	Soft, compressible mass Red or blue discoloration	Multiple cutaneous lesions may be associated with visceral hemangiomas	Present in first 3 months of life Grow until 6 months of life Regress after 1 year of life 50% resolve by 5 years; 90% by 9 years	Bleeding Ulceration Scarring Airway obstruction Obstruction of visual axis Amblyopia	Observation only for most lesions Referral to dermatology and/or plastic surgery for beta blocker therapy, corticosteroids, laser therapy, or surgical excision when involving airway or when in periorbital region
Dacryocystocele	H04.6	Cystic mass Lateral aspect of nose below medial canthus of eye	Eye drainage and tearing	Present from birth 85% resolve by 9 months of age	Dacryocystitis Nasal obstruction	Digital massage May drain spontaneously Lacrimal duct probing under anesthesia by an ophthalmologist, if persistent
Dermoid Cyst	L72.0	Midline mass Variable presence of a pit Hair may protrude from mass	Intermittent drainage of sebaceous material Intracranial extension in 45%	Mean age at presentation 14–34 months Grow with age	Abscess Bony erosion CNS infection	Brain MRI to rule out intracranial extension Surgical resection
Glioma	Q30.8	Firm mass lateral to the midline that is unaffected by crying or straining Negative Furstenburg sign	Tearing Intracranial extension occurs in up to 15%–25%	Present at birth Demonstrates slow growth	Nasal obstruction	Brain MRI to rule out intracranial extension Surgical resection
Encephalocele	Q01.1	Compressible mass Demonstrates transillumination positive Furstenberg sign	CSF leak Cleft palate	Present from birth	Meningitis Brain abscess Nasal obstruction	Neurosurgical evaluation Brain MRI Surgical resection
Nasal Contusion or Fracture	S02.2	Swelling Deformity Ecchymosis Laceration Epistaxis	Trauma	Swelling and contusion resolve within weeks Deformity from healed fracture may worsen through adolescence	Nasal fracture Septal hematoma Septal abscess Nasal obstruction Facial asymmetry	Pain control Head CT if CSF leak suspected ENT referral for nasal deformity, septal hematoma or deviation, persistent or severe epistaxis

Other Diagnoses to Consider

- Diffuse neonatal hemangiomatosis

- PHACE syndrome (posterior fossa malformations, hemangiomas, arterial anomalies, cardiac defects, and eye abnormalities)

- Complex craniofacial anomalies

- Hypertrophic scar

When to Consider Further Evaluation or Treatment

- Nasal hemangiomas resulting in obstruction of the airway, impairment of vision, or significant cosmetic concerns should be referred to a pediatric dermatologist or plastic surgeon for treatment.

- Hemangiomas obscuring vision should be referred to a pediatric ophthalmologist for evaluation for amblyopia.

- Oral propranolol is the preferred treatment for hemangiomas. Propanolol is more effective with fewer adverse effects than traditional therapies such as surgical excision or systemic/intralesional corticosteroids.

- Laser therapy is a promising alternative therapy for some hemangiomas, but the evidence is more anecdotal.

- MRI of the head and neurosurgical referral are indicated if a dermoid cyst, glioma, or encephalocele is suspected.

- Nasal fractures with deformity, septal hematoma, septal deviation, or difficult to control epistaxis should be referred to an ENT specialist.

SUGGESTED READINGS

Chen TS, Eichenfield LF, Friedlander SF. Infantile hemangiomas: An update on pathogenesis and therapy. *Pediatrics.* 2013;131(1):99–108.
Dasgupta NR, Bentz ML. Nasal gliomas: Identification and differentiation from hemangiomas. *J Craniofac Surg.* 2003;14:736–738.
Lee WT, Koltai PJ. Nasal deformity in neonates and young children. *Pediatr Clin North Am.* 2003;50(2):459–467.
Mahapatra AK, Suri A. Anterior encephaloceles: A study of 92 cases. *Pediatr Neurosurg.* 2002;36(3):113–118.
Wong RK, VanderVeen DK. Presentation and management of congenital dacryocystocele. *Pediatrics.* 2008;122(5):e1108–e1112.
Wright RJ, Murakami CS, Ambro BT. Pediatric nasal injuries and management. *Facial Plast Surg.* 2011;27(5):483–490.
Zapata S, Kearns DB. Nasal dermoids. *Curr Opin Otolaryngol Head Neck Surg.* 2006;14(6):406–411.

SECTION 6 • NOSE

Nasal Swelling, Discharge, and Crusting

Shareen F. Kelly

Investigating the causes of nasal swelling and discharge involves acquiring a careful history that includes the duration and timing of symptoms, the environment in which the symptoms occurred, whether anything has relieved the symptoms, and to what extent the problem has disrupted the child's daily functioning. Radiological studies may be useful in select cases. Noting the age of the patient is important because the sinus and nasopharyngeal complex changes with growth, and potential infectious causes of rhinorrhea vary with age.

- Rhinorrhea accompanying viral infections may be associated with fever, cough, and/or lymphadenopathy.

- Most rhinorrhea from viral upper respiratory tract infections resolves in 6 to 10 days.

- Prolonged purulent rhinorrhea (>10 days) or acute symptoms including headache, facial pain, and/or fever are suggestive of bacterial rhinosinusitis.

- Increased cough while supine and halitosis are symptoms of bacterial rhinosinusitis.

- Seasonal allergic rhinitis is generally accompanied by sneezing and intense nasal pruritus, and is often associated with ocular pruritus.

- Children with allergic rhinitis often have family members with atopic diseases.

- Fits of sneezing that occur soon after rising from sleep and nasal symptoms in the presence of specific allergens, such as dust or animals, are characteristic of seasonal allergic rhinitis.

- Chronic use of decongestant nasal sprays can result in paradoxical nasal swelling and rebound congestion.

- Rhinorrhea in the setting of exposure to cold outdoor temperatures is suggestive of vasomotor rhinitis.

- Children with impetigo generally do not complain of pain at the affected site.

- Nasal drainage resulting from a foreign body, typically occurring in younger children, is usually acute, unilateral, and often associated with a foul odor.

- Recurrent nasal infections or persistent inflammation may contribute to the development of nasal polyps.

- Direct trauma to the nose may result in a septal hematoma, manifesting as pain and nasal congestion; occluding one nostril at a time after trauma should still allow child to breathe through the open nostril in the setting of septal hematoma.

Key Points in the Physical Examination

- Viral rhinorrhea may be of varied color, thickness, and amount.

- Tenderness over the facial bones and increased headache and/or facial pain on forward bending of the neck are signs of sinusitis.

- Foul-smelling breath and visible irritation of the posterior pharynx can be signs of postnasal drip and acute bacterial rhinosinusitis.

- Difficulty with nasal breathing in the absence of swollen turbinates is usually indicative of enlarged adenoids.

- Rhinorrhea from allergic rhinitis is generally thin, profuse, and clear.

- Examination of the nares in a child with allergic rhinitis usually reveals enlarged nasal turbinates with pale boggy mucosa and cobblestoning of the posterior pharynx.

- Children with allergic rhinitis often have associated Dennie–Morgan lines and allergic shiners.

- Nasal drainage from a foreign body is unilateral, thick, purulent, and sometimes bloody or foul smelling.

- Impetigo may occur as a single "honey-crusted" lesion of the nares. Because of autoinoculation, it often presents with multiple lesions in close proximity to the original lesion.

- Nasal polyps are painless, lucent-gray, yellow, or erythematous nasal masses that are most often solitary.

- A septal hematoma appears as a midline, tense, ecchymotic mass over the nasal septum.

PHOTOGRAPHS OF SELECTED DIAGNOSES

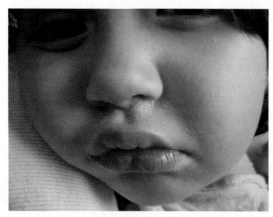

Figure 23-1 **Viral rhinorrhea.** Scant mucoid rhinorrhea in a child with an upper respiratory tract infection. (Courtesy of Paul S. Matz, MD.)

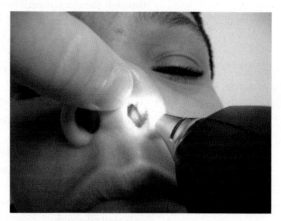

Figure 23-2 **Allergic rhinitis.** Pale boggy inferior turbinates are visible. (Courtesy of Paul S. Matz, MD.)

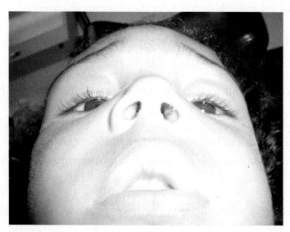

Figure 23-3 **Nasal discharge/crusting because of a foreign body.** This child had persistent unilateral, foul-smelling discharge until paper was removed from the left side by an otolaryngologist. (Courtesy of Paul S. Matz, MD.)

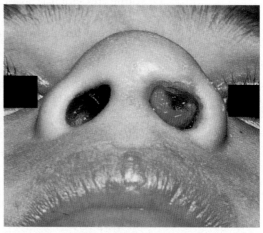

Figure 23-4 **Nasal polyp.** Erythematous mass visible in the left nare. (Used with permission from Handler SD, Myer CM. *Atlas of Ear, Nose and Throat Disorders in Children*. Ontario: BC Decker; 1998:59.)

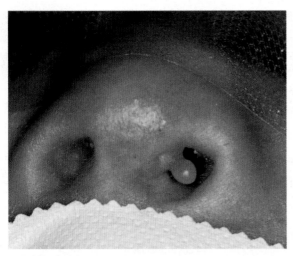

Figure 23-5 Skin tag at nasal vestibule. Small protuberant nodule at entrance to left nare. (Used with permission from Handler SD, Myer CM. *Atlas of Ear, Nose and Throat Disorders in Children.* Ontario: BC Decker; 1998:49.)

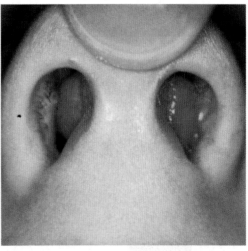

Figure 23-6 Bilateral septal hematoma. Bilateral erythematous masses arising from the nasal septum. (Used with permission from Handler SD, Myer CM. *Atlas of Ear, Nose and Throat Disorders in Children.* Ontario: BC Decker; 1998:52.)

DIFFERENTIAL DIAGNOSIS

DIAGNOSIS		ICD-10	DISTINGUISHING CHARACTERISTICS	DISTRIBUTION	DURATION/ CHRONICITY
Viral Rhinorrhea		J00	Thin and clear or thick white or yellow rhinorrhea	Any age More frequent in daycare attendees	Lasts 5–10 days Occurs most often in winter
Bacterial Rhinosinusitis		J01	Persistent (>10 days) purulent nasal discharge Facial pain, headaches, or fever	Any age More common in children with allergic rhinitis	Depends on treatment— days to months
Allergic Rhinitis		J30	Thin, profuse, watery rhinorrhea	Unusual in children less than 3 years Peak incidence in adolescence	Occurs more seasonally or upon exposure to allergens or irritants, such as smoke, animals, and dust
Impetigo		L01	Golden "honey-crusted" erythematous area	Any age but may be associated with children who pick their noses Usually near the nares but may be seen anywhere on the body	Easy to treat but contagious May recur if child is colonized with *Staphylococcus aureus*
Nasal Foreign Body		T17.1	Unilateral purulent nasal discharge	Most common in children of preschool age	N/A
Nasal Polyp		J33	Glistening gray, yellow, or erythematous mass in nares	Usually solitary Unusual in children less than 10 years	Long lasting unless removed
Septal Hematoma		J34.8 (Other specified disorders of nose and nasal sinuses)	Purple or dark fluctuant mass on mucosa of nasal septum	No age or gender predilection	Should be treated within 48 hours of occurrence to avoid necrosis

ASSOCIATED FINDINGS	COMPLICATIONS	PREDISPOSING FACTORS	TREATMENT GUIDELINES
Sore throat Cough Fever Enlarged cervical lymph nodes	Rhinosinusitis	Exposure to others with upper respiratory tract infections	Supportive treatment Nasal saline washes
Fever Headache Facial bone ache/pressure	Chronic sinusitis Periorbital cellulitis Orbital cellulitis Brain abscess	Allergic rhinitis Facial anomalies preventing sinus drainage	High-dose amoxicillin as first line
Associated with ocular symptoms of tearing and itchiness Often associated with atopic dermatitis	Headaches from sinus pressure Postnasal drip with or without halitosis	Allergens Familial predisposition with other allergic symptoms	Systemic antihistamines and/or nasal corticosteroids Environmental allergen elimination
May have skin lesions in other areas	Rarely, invasive infection with S. aureus Generally does not result in scarring	Nasal colonization with S. aureus Nose picking	Topical antibiotic cream if lesions are small and localized Oral antibiotics if lesions are widespread
Malodorous nasal discharge, sometimes bloody	Nasal septum erosion with retained foreign body	Behavior of child	Removal of foreign body
May be associated with epistaxis	Persistent nasal congestion and decreased ability to breathe through affected side	Recurrent infections and persistent inflammation Associated with cystic fibrosis	Decrease inflammation by use of nasal steroids Removal of polyps
Facial tenderness or contusions over other facial bones	Nasal septum erosion	Trauma	Prompt evacuation of hematoma

SECTION 6 • NOSE

Other Diagnoses to Consider

- Cerebrospinal fluid leak

- Rhinitis medicamentosa

- Vasomotor rhinorrhea

- Gustatory rhinitis

- Epistaxis

- Nasal glioma or encephalocele

- Craniofacial anomalies

- Nasopharyngitis from gastroesophageal reflux

- Choanal atresia

- Anterior nasal stenosis

- Cocaine use

When to Consider Further Evaluation or Treatment

- Recurrent or chronic sinusitis should prompt consideration and investigation of diagnoses, including cystic fibrosis, specific immunodeficiencies, and disorders of ciliary motility.

- Allergic rhinitis unresponsive to treatment may be secondary to enlarged adenoids or lack of allergen control in the child's environment.

- Impetiginous skin lesions near the nares that are painful or associated with fever must be considered as possibly representing invasive staphylococcal or streptococcal infections. Treatment for invasive disease warrants consideration of methicillin-resistant *S. aureus* (MRSA) when choosing antibiotic coverage.

- Nasal polyps in a child with growth failure, malabsorption, and/or frequent lower respiratory tract infections or inflammation should prompt a workup for cystic fibrosis.

- Nasal foreign body removal can be attempted in the pediatrician's office, but failure to accomplish removal necessitates prompt referral to the otolaryngologist.

- Diagnosis of septal hematoma necessitates referral to the otolaryngologist to prevent erosion through or perforation of the nasal septum.

SUGGESTED READINGS

Gargiulo KA, Spector ND. Stuffy nose. *Pediatr Rev.* 2010;31:320–324.

Mahr TA, Sheth K. Update on allergic rhinitis. *Pediatr Rev.* 2005;26:284–288.

Yellon RF, McBride TB, Davis HW. Otolaryngology. In: *Atlas of Pediatric Physical Diagnosis.* 5th ed. Philadelphia, PA: Mosby; 2007:818–866.

Wald ER, Applegate KE, Bordley C, et al.; American Academy of Pediatrics. Clinical practice guideline for the diagnosis and management of acute bacterial sinusitis in children aged 1 to 18 years. *Pediatrics.* 2013;132:e262–e280.

Wallace DV, Dykewicz MS, Bernstein DI, et al. The diagnosis and management of rhinitis: An updated practice parameter. *J Allergy Clin Immunol.* 2008;122(2):S1–S84.

Section 7

SEVEN

MOUTH

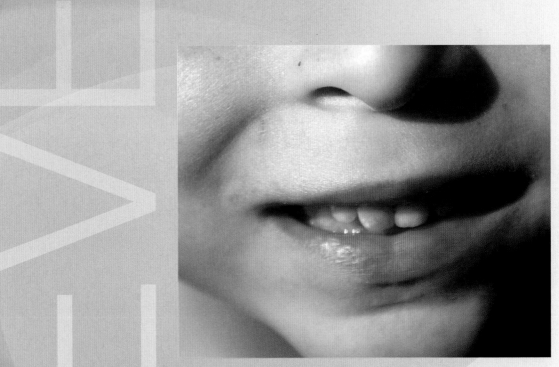

(Courtesy of Daniel R. Taylor, DO.)

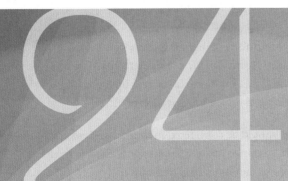

Mouth Sores and Patches

Elizabeth C. Maxwell and
Nancy D. Spector

Approach to the Problem

Mouth sores and patches are commonly found on careful oral examination of pediatric patients. Lesions may be asymptomatic or may lead to ulceration, pain, and decreased oral intake. Oral lesions may be categorized as anatomic, traumatic, or infectious. Many of these lesions are isolated to the oral cavity and mucosa, but certain systemic illnesses and conditions can present with oral sores or patches as part of a constellation of symptoms. Diagnosis is primarily clinical. Management is often limited to supportive care, including pain control and ensuring adequate hydration.

Key Points in the History

- Oral candidiasis is the most common oral fungal infection in infants and children, with *Candida albicans* being the most frequently identified species. When infections are persistent in children older than 6 months, the clinician should consider an underlying defect in the systemic immune system.

- Epstein pearls are asymptomatic and self-resolving, keratin-filled, epithelial-lined cysts that are extremely common in newborns.

- A sucking blister, also referred to as a sucking pad or callus, is a hyperkeratotic thickening at the closure line of the upper and lower lips caused by the mechanical effects of sucking, and may be white or pigmented. These lesions, found in newborns and young infants, usually disappear by 3 to 6 months of age.

- Traumatic oral lesions arise from mouthing objects in the period of infancy, and accidental biting or injury from objects placed in the oral cavity in older children. Pain is the predominant symptom, occurring 24 to 48 hours after the initial injury.

- Small gingival vesicles that progress into painful ulcerations following high fever, irritability, and malaise should prompt consideration of primary herpetic gingivostomatitis caused by herpes simplex virus (HSV) type 1 as a diagnosis.

- Herpangina also produces oral ulcerations and follows a prodrome that includes malaise, sore throat, and low-grade fever. It is caused by coxsackievirus group A, usually in the summer and early fall. The oral ulcerations are isolated in herpangina. When oral ulcerations occur in conjunction with palmar and plantar papulovesicles, hand, foot, and mouth disease should be strongly considered.

- Recurrent aphthous stomatitis (RAS) is the most common inflammatory ulcerative condition of the oral mucosa in patients in North America, with up to 20% of the population affected during childhood or early adulthood. Its cause is unknown. It is categorized into major and minor forms based on size and location of ulcers.

- Other viruses can cause enanthems, and should be considered in the diagnosis of oral lesions when prodromal symptoms are present. Examples include Koplik spots associated with measles, and ulcerations found in infectious mononucleosis and varicella.

Key Points in the Physical Examination

- Lesions of oral candidiasis include white or whitish-yellow plaques and erythema of the tongue, soft palate, or buccal mucosae. When plaques are scraped off, there is often underlying raw, erythematous mucosa, which may bleed. These mucosal changes may help the clinician differentiate the white plaques from milk residue seen on the tongue of infants.

- Epstein pearls, found in newborns, are white, nodular lesions typically found on the alveolar ridge or midline of the hard palate.

- Drooling and tenderness may be predominant features on physical examination when ulcerative lesions are present.

- Location of lesions can help differentiate between HSV gingivostomatitis and herpangina. HSV lesions are located in both the anterior and the posterior oropharynx, and lesions of herpangina are located predominantly in the posterior oropharynx, sparing the lips and gingiva.

- Both HSV and herpangina present with painful, small, grouped vesicles that eventually ulcerate. Gingival erythema, friability, and edema are commonly seen in HSV gingivostomatitis, but not in herpangina.

- RAS may produce ulcers of nonkeratinized mucosa (unattached gingiva) and keratinized surfaces. Lesions of major RAS are larger and can cause scarring.

- Koplik spots occur early in the course of measles, before other cutaneous signs, and are often missed.

PHOTOGRAPHS OF SELECTED DIAGNOSES

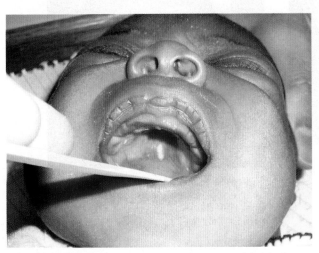

Figure 24-1 Epstein pearls. Whitish cysts visible on the midline palate of a neonate. (Courtesy of Paul S. Matz, MD.)

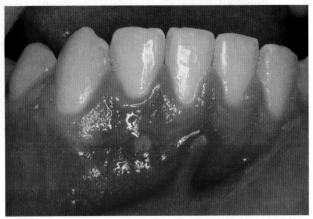

Figure 24-2 Aphthous stomatitis. This tender lesion is visible on the gingival mucosa. (Courtesy of T.P. Croll, DDS.)

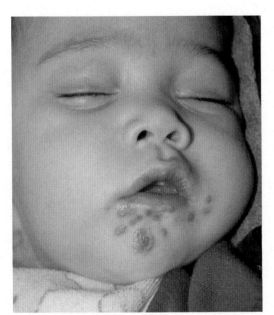

Figure 24-3 HSV stomatitis. An infant with extraoral HSV lesions. (Courtesy of George A. Datto, III, MD.)

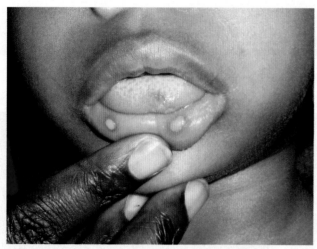

Figure 24-4 **HSV stomatitis.** Lesions are visible on the tongue and labial mucosa. (Courtesy of Paul S. Matz, MD.)

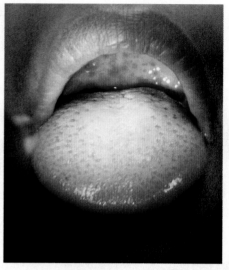

Figure 24-5 **Herpangina.** Posterior pharyngeal lesions distinguish this illness from HSV gingivostomatitis. (Courtesy of Paul S. Matz, MD.)

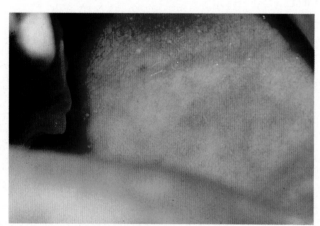

Figure 24-6 **Koplik spots.** Fine, white spots with red halos seen on the buccal mucosa. (Used with permission from The Wellcome Trust, National Medical Slide Bank, London, UK.)

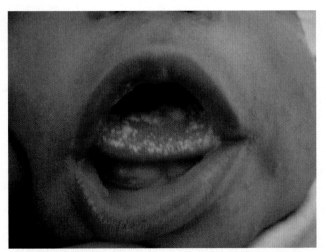

Figure 24-7 Oral thrush. An infant with numerous whitish tongue plaques. (Courtesy of Paul S. Matz, MD.)

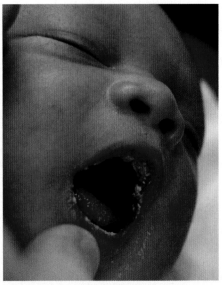

Figure 24-8 Oral thrush. Note the whitish plaques on the labial mucosa. (Courtesy of George A. Datto, III, MD.)

DIFFERENTIAL DIAGNOSIS

DIAGNOSIS		ICD-10	DISTINGUISHING CHARACTERISTICS	DISTRIBUTION
Thrush		B37.0	White/whitish-yellow plaques on erythematous base	Tongue, soft palate, buccal mucosae
Epstein Pearls		K09.8	Small, white papules or translucent cysts	Midline at junction of hard and soft palate Called Bohn nodules if located on alveolar ridges
Sucking Blister		K13.79	White or yellow hyperkeratotic thickening	At closure line of upper and lower lips Extending inward to involve mucosa
Traumatic Ulcer		K13.79	Yellow, pseudomembranous ulcer with erythematous border	Anywhere in oropharynx, commonly involving buccal mucosae
HSV Gingivostomatitis		B00.9	Small clustered vesicles Rupture into painful ulcerations	Anterior oropharynx: tongue, gingiva, buccal mucosae, lips
Herpangina		B08.5	Red macular lesions, evolve to cluster of fragile vesicles that rapidly ulcerate	Posterior oropharynx: soft palate, tonsillar pillars
Recurrent Aphthous Stomatitis		K12.0	One or more small oval or round, shallow, gray or tan ulcer with erythematous halo	Distribution is determined by type Nonkeratinized mucosa in minor RAS Keratinized mucosa in major RAS
Koplik Spots		B05.9	Small white lesions resembling grains of salt	Buccal mucosae

ASSOCIATED FINDINGS	COMPLICATIONS	PREDISPOSING FACTORS	TREATMENT GUIDELINES
Pain Dysphagia Poor feeding	Recurrence or persistence raises concern for immunosuppression	Infants Antibiotic use, immunocompromised Common oral flora in infants	Topical antifungal Discard or disinfect contaminated objects, such as pacifiers
None	None	None	No therapy as these are self-limited
None	None	Feeding and sucking in the neonatal period Breastfeeding	No therapy
None	Pain, decreased oral intake	Inadvertent self-inflicted trauma, often following anesthesia for dental procedure Use of microwaves to heat bottled milk	Topical or systemic analgesia
"Fire engine red," edematous, hemorrhagic gingiva Prodrome of high fever, irritability, malaise	Severe pain Decreased oral intake and dehydration Superinfection Recurrence	Contact with infected person shedding virus, usually HSV-1 Peak incidence: 2 years	Oral or IV hydration Topical and systemic analgesia Systemic antiviral therapy, if severe or immunocompromised
Prodrome of malaise, sore throat, low-grade fever	Pain Decreased oral intake leading to dehydration	Summer or early fall Exposure to coxsackievirus group A	Supportive care with topical or oral analgesia Lesions spontaneously resolve
Pain Recurrence	Scarring in major form	Unknown etiology Stress, trauma, food allergy, and vitamin deficiency are thought to play a role	Rinses containing steroid, antihistamine, analgesia may provide symptomatic relief. The role of vitamins is unclear at this time.
Fever, cough, coryza, conjunctivitis, morbilliform rash	None from lesions	Incomplete immunization Exposure to index case of measles	Supportive care for measles infection

SECTION 7 • MOUTH

Other Diagnoses to Consider

- Mucous cysts (mucoceles, ranulas)

- Hemangiomas

- Intraoral abscess

- Leukoplakia

- Erythema multiforme

When to Consider Further Evaluation or Treatment

- Atypical presentation or unexpected clinical course of a common superficial ulcerative lesion should prompt further workup to investigate underlying immunologic or rheumatologic conditions.

- Ulcerative lesions with granulation may require biopsy by a specialist to verify the diagnosis based on clinical suspicion.

- Dental evaluation is indicated if dental trauma is suspected as an underlying cause of a mouth sore or ulceration.

- Severe pain or dehydration may require systemic therapy and intravenous fluids and warrants inpatient management.

SUGGESTED READINGS

Gonsalves WC, Chi AC, Neville BW. Common oral lesions: Part I. Superficial mucosal lesions. *Am Fam Physician*. 2007;75(4):501–506.
Hebert AA, Del Carmen Lopez M. Oral lesions in pediatric patients. *Adv Dermatol*. 1997;12:169–194.
Krol DM, Keels MA. Oral conditions. *Pediatr Rev*. 2007;28:15.
Patel NJ, Sciubba JS. Oral lesions in young children. *Pediatr Clin N Am*. 2003;50:469–486.
Witman PM, Rogers RS. Pediatric oral medicine. *Dermatol Clin*. 2003;21:157–170.

Focal Gum Lesions

Blair J. Dickinson and Nancy D. Spector

Approach to the Problem

Oral lesions are very common in newborns, infants, and young children. As today's medical providers increasingly discuss oral health, parents may be particularly concerned when a focal lesion appears on their child's gum. Fortunately, most of these lesions are benign. Bohn nodules affect up to 85% of children, and natal teeth are present in one to two of 6,000 births. Many gum lesions resolve without intervention, and their presence does not have adverse effects. However, some untreated lesions, such as dental abscesses, may extend to involve adjacent tissue and result in the formation of fistulas, facial cellulitis, and even osteomyelitis. Meticulous oral hygiene is critical to prevent infectious lesions that result from untreated dental caries and poor oral hygiene.

Key Points in the History

- Natal teeth are present at birth, whereas neonatal teeth develop in the first month of life.

- Approximately 85% of natal and neonatal teeth are mandibular.

- Bohn nodules and alveolar cysts, often present at birth, generally do not interfere with feeding.

- Parents may confuse Bohn nodules with oral thrush.

- Eruption cysts are common in infants and children during the mixed-dentition stage, when primary and permanent teeth are present in the mouth.

- Eruption cysts tend to rupture spontaneously and are generally nontender.

- A deflection in the path of tooth eruption (e.g., crowding or overretention of primary teeth) may result in a mucogingival defect.

- Poor dental hygiene and dental caries are risk factors for dental abscesses.

- Children with dental abscesses may have a history of fever, mouth pain, or facial swelling.

- Children with a fistula between a dental abscess and the gum may report drainage, a funny or sour taste in their mouth, or both.

Key Points in the Physical Examination

- Natal and neonatal teeth are most commonly primary, but may be supernumerary.

- Natal teeth are erupted teeth present at the time of birth.

- Bohn nodules are smooth, translucent, pearly white cysts that range from approximately 1 to 3 mm in size.

- Bohn nodules may be isolated or clustered.

- Eruption cysts are usually found in the region of the incisors on the edge of the alveolar ridge where a tooth is erupting.

- Eruption cysts may feel rubbery, be nontender, and have a bluish hue.

- Alveolar cysts are visible along the alveolar ridges.

- A retrocuspid papilla, often bilateral, is a firm, round, pink to red 2- to 3-mm papule attached to the lingual gingiva adjacent to the mandibular canines.

- The presence of fever in association with a focal gum lesion should raise suspicion for a dental abscess.

- Dental abscesses may appear as erythema and swelling of the gum, often in the region of dental caries, and may be associated with purulent drainage.

- Dental abscesses may cause swelling of the overlying cheek.

- Dental abscesses may develop a fistula between the tooth apex and the oral cavity.

PHOTOGRAPHS OF SELECTED DIAGNOSES

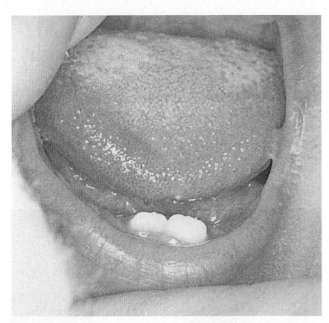

Figure 25-1 **Natal teeth.** Bilateral lower central incisors in a neonate (Used with permission from O'Doherty N. *Atlas of the Newborn*. Philadelphia, PA: JB Lippincott; 1979:51.)

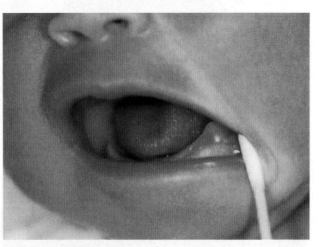

Figure 25-2 **Bohn nodule.** Pearly nodule on the gum of a neonate. (Used with permission from Fletcher MA. *Physical Diagnosis in Neonatology*. Philadelphia, PA: Lippincott–Raven Publishers; 1998:216.)

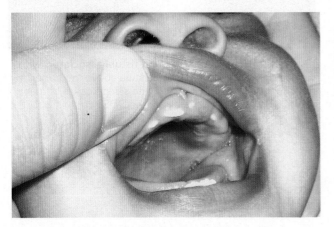

Figure 25-3 **Eruption cyst.** Swelling and blue discoloration are visible along the alveolar ridge shortly before the upper left central incisor erupted. (Courtesy of Paul S. Matz, MD.)

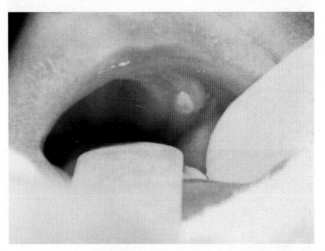

Figure 25-4 **Alveolar cyst.** Cyst on the alveolar ridge of a newborn. (Used with permission from Fletcher MA. *Physical Diagnosis in Neonatology*. Philadelphia, PA: Lippincott–Raven Publishers; 1998:216.)

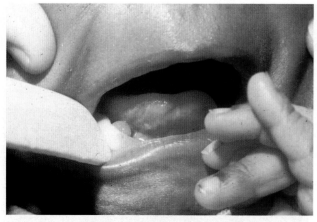

Figure 25-5 **Alveolar cyst.** Cyst on the alveolar ridge of a newborn. (Courtesy of the late Peter Sol, MD.)

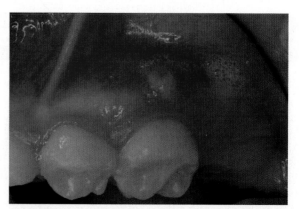

Figure 25-6 **Dentoalveolar abscess.** Swelling and erythema are present in this photo of an abscessed primary second molar. In this case, the permanent first molar came in too far anteriorly and destroyed the roots of the baby tooth. (Courtesy of Theodore P. Croll, DDS.)

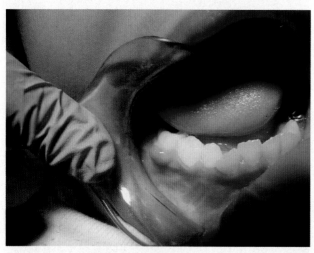

Figure 25-8 **Gingival abscess.** Erythematous mass on the lower gum, associated with dental caries. (Courtesy of Michael Lemper, DDS.)

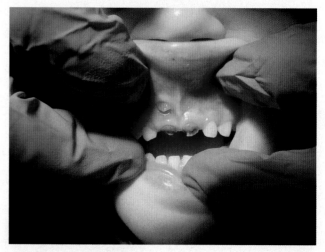

Figure 25-7 **Dental abscess and fistula associated with severe dental caries.** Note the fistula above the upper right central incisor, associated with severe caries of that tooth. (Courtesy of Michael Lemper, DDS.)

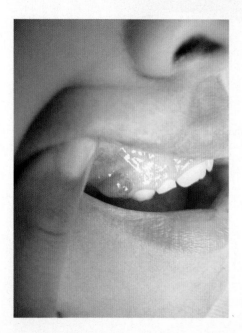

Figure 25-9 **Dental abscess with fistula to the gum.** Spongy mass on the gum associated with nearby caries. (Courtesy of Paul S. Matz, MD.)

DIFFERENTIAL DIAGNOSIS

DIAGNOSIS	ICD-10	DISTINGUISHING CHARACTERISTICS	DISTRIBUTION	DURATION/ CHRONICITY	ASSOCIATED FINDINGS	COMPLICATIONS	PREDISPOSING FACTORS	TREATMENT GUIDELINES
Natal or Neonatal Teeth	K00.6	Natal teeth present at birth Neonatal teeth present in first month of life	85% are mandibular 90% are primary teeth	Usually extracted	None	Aspiration Interference with feeding	N/A	Extract if hypermobile or if supernumerary
Bohn Nodule	K05.5	Occurs commonly in up to 85% of newborns Smooth, translucent, pearly white, keratin-filled, 1- to 3-mm cysts	Buccal or alveolar surface of the gums	Ruptures spontaneously in the first month of life	None	None	N/A	No intervention required
Eruption Cyst	K09.0	Common in infants and children during the mixed-dentition phase Dome-shaped, fluid-filled, rubbery cyst Bluish hue Ruptures spontaneously	On the edge of the alveolar ridge overlying erupting tooth Usually, in the region of the incisors Less often in the region of the permanent molars	Related to tooth eruption	Mixed dentition Tooth eruption Hematoma	May precede neonatal teeth Infrequently delays tooth eruption	Process of tooth eruption	No intervention required Resolves spontaneously as the tooth erupts through the lesion Consider uncovering tooth if symptomatic or there is delayed tooth eruption.
Alveolar (Gingival) Cyst	K09.0	Some report gingival cysts in up to 50% of newborns. Smooth, translucent, pearly white, keratin-filled, 1- to 3-mm cysts Single or multiple Discrete or clustered	Alveolar mucosa, most commonly on the maxillary mucosa	Ruptures spontaneously in first 3 months of life	None	None	N/A	No intervention required
Retrocuspid Papilla	K13.79	Fibroepithelial papule Firm, round, pink to red, 2–3 mm in diameter Usually bilateral More common in females	Attached to lingual gingiva adjacent to the mandibular canines	Decreases in size with age	None	None	N/A	No intervention required
Dental Abscess with Fistula to the Gum	K04.7 (No sinus), K04.6 (Sinus present)	Dental caries progress to involve the tooth pulp and cause an abscess. May progress to the development of a fistula to the gum Tooth and gum pain	Fistula between the tooth apex and the oral cavity	Takes months to develop Will not resolve without intervention	Dental caries Pain Discharge from the gum	Facial space infection Sepsis Primary tooth infection may disrupt normal development of the secondary tooth. Destruction of underlying bone	Dental caries, poor oral health	Refer to dentistry. Administer oral antibiotics

Other Diagnoses to Consider

- Oral lymphoepithelial cyst

- Hemangioma

- Pyogenic granuloma

- Irritation fibroma

- Peripheral giant cell granuloma

- Sialolithiasis congenital epulis (granular cell tumor of the alveolar ridge)

- Teratoma and dermoid cyst

- Alveolar lymphangioma

- Rhabdomyosarcoma

- Osteogenic sarcoma

- Fibrosarcoma

- Mucoepidermoid carcinoma

When to Consider Further Evaluation or Treatment

- Most focal gum lesions are benign, do not interfere with feeding, and do not require intervention. They generally rupture spontaneously.

- Natal or neonatal teeth should be extracted if supernumerary or if overly mobile, as they may lead to aspiration.

- For eruption cysts that do not resolve spontaneously, consider referral to dentistry in order to uncover the underlying tooth.

- The presence of a dental abscess requires referral to dentistry for debridement and the administration of oral antibiotics.

- Consider referral to dentistry for any painful, localized gum lesions.

- A focal gum lesion that continues to enlarge or is associated with systemic symptoms or signs warrants further evaluation for an oncologic or genetic process.

SUGGESTED READINGS

DaSilva CM, Ramos MM, de Carvalho Carrara CF. Oral characteristics of newborns. *J Dent Child.* 2008;75:4–6.

Flaitz CM. Differential diagnosis of oral lesions and developmental anomalies. In: Casamassimo PS, Fields HW, McTigue DJ, Nowak AJ, eds. *Pediatric Dentistry: Infancy Through Adolescence.* 5th ed. St. Louis, MO: Elsevier Saunders; 2013:11–53.

Markman L. Teething: Facts and fiction. *Pediatr Rev.* 2009;30:e59–e64.

Noffke CEE, Chabikuli NJ, Nzima N. Impaired tooth eruption: A review. *SADJ.* 2005;60:422–425.

Roback MG. Oral lesions. In: Fleisher GR, Ludwig S, eds. *Textbook of Pediatric Emergency Medicine.* 6th ed. Philadelphia, PA: Wolters Kluwer/Lippincott Williams & Wilkins Health; 2010:463–467.

Weber-Gasparoni K. Examination, diagnosis, and treatment planning of the infant and toddler. In: Casamassimo PS, Fields HW, McTigue DJ, Nowak AJ, eds. *Pediatric Dentistry: Infancy Through Adolescence.* 5th ed. St. Louis, MO: Elsevier Saunders; 2013:184–199.

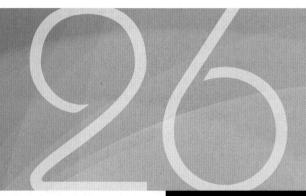

Discoloration of Teeth

Roy Benaroch

Approach to the Problem

Visible discoloration of the teeth can be caused by extrinsic factors, which stain the outside of the tooth. Alternatively, discoloration can be caused by intrinsic changes in the tooth, which are triggered during or after tooth development. Because the inner dentin of a tooth is darker than the white enamel covering a tooth, pits caused by thinning of the enamel can appear as dark areas. Problems with dental health such as trauma, genetics, exposures to chemicals and antibiotics, systemic diseases, malnutrition, or poor dental care can all contribute to discoloration.

Key Points in the History

- The risk of developing dental caries depends on multiple overlapping factors. Caries risk is influenced by family history, diet and feeding style, dental hygiene, and fluoride use. The highest caries risk is seen in children with complex medical needs, those from disadvantaged families, and in babies who bottle feed through the night. Dental caries risk assessment and counseling should be part of early childhood care.

- Children's vitamins, especially those containing iron, can lead to external tooth stains. External tooth staining can also be seen from cigarettes or other tobacco products, coffee, and red wine.

- Dental trauma can damage primary teeth and influence the development of preeruptive permanent teeth. Even mild trauma, depending on timing and location, can lead to significant changes in tooth appearance.

- Systemic fluoride given during tooth formation helps teeth develop strong enamel. Topical fluoride throughout life helps protect teeth by preventing and repairing damage to enamel. However, excessive fluoride exposure during tooth development can lead to fluorosis. Despite some cosmetic consequences, most degrees of fluorosis strengthen the teeth against caries. Common sources of fluoride exposure are from fluoridated municipal water, toothpastes and rinses (if swallowed), and from dental treatments. Fluoride exposure after tooth development, past age 8, will not cause fluorosis.

- Significant systemic illness can alter a tooth's appearance. Children with cystic fibrosis or renal insufficiency, for example, may have mottled teeth or hypoplastic enamel.

- Stains occur from tetracycline antibiotics, including doxycycline, when they are incorporated into a tooth during development. These antibiotics will not stain fully formed permanent teeth. Pregnant women, and children younger than 8 years old, should avoid tetracyclines.

Key Points in the Physical Examination

- Milk bottle caries causes the most damage to the upper teeth and is associated with staining, caries, and destruction of the primary teeth.

- Most fluorosis causes easily overlooked subtle discoloration, including tiny white spots or streaks. Moderate to severe fluorosis affects the appearance of all teeth.

- Staining from iron vitamin drops is dark brown or black. It will not come off with routine toothbrushing, but can be removed by a dentist.

- White, opaque spots or patches can be caused by early caries or from altered mineralization related to illness, malnutrition, or trauma. They may also be idiopathic. These spots are sometimes referred to by the technically incorrect terms of hypocalcification or demineralization.

- Discoloration affecting all teeth is most likely related to systemic illness or exposures, and warrants thorough evaluation.

- Tetracycline staining may be brown or gray, and may affect the entire tooth. The staining is intrinsic to the tooth and cannot be buffed off. The best cosmetic result may be reached by covering the tooth with a veneer.

PHOTOGRAPHS OF SELECTED DIAGNOSES

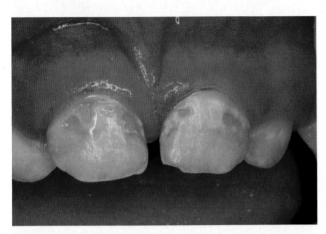

Figure 26-1 **Dental caries.** The upper incisors show significant caries and decalcification, along with gingivitis. (Courtesy of Theodore P. Croll, DDS.)

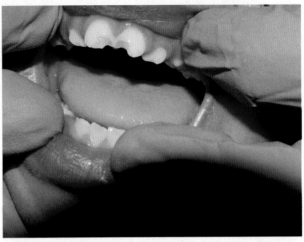

Figure 26-2 **Moderate milk bottle caries.** Brown discoloration and decay of the upper incisors. (Courtesy of Michael Lemper, DDS.)

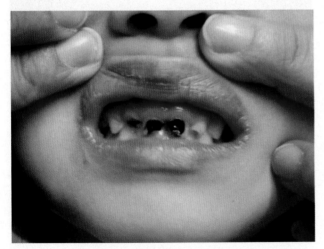

Figure 26-3 **Severe milk bottle caries.** Severe erosion of the upper incisors, associated with black staining. (Courtesy of Philip Siu, MD.)

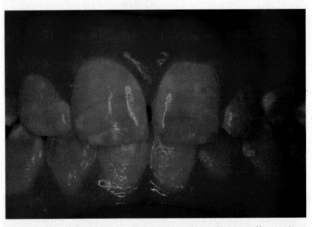

Figure 26-4 **Moderate fluorosis.** All teeth are affected by staining from excessive systemic fluoride during tooth formation. (Courtesy of Theodore P. Croll, DDS.)

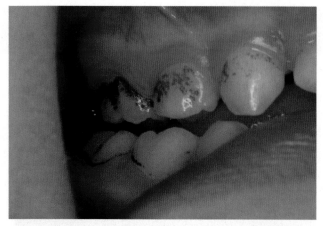

Figure 26-5 Iron staining. Iron solutions or multivitamin solutions that contain iron can stain teeth, as shown here most prominently near the gums. (Courtesy of Theodore P. Croll, DDS.)

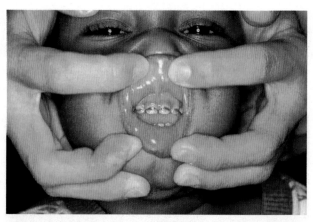

Figure 26-6 Tetracycline staining. Brown, band-like staining visible on all four maxillary incisors. (Courtesy of Jan Edwin Drutz, MD.)

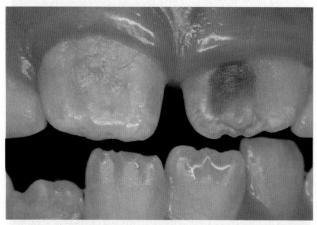

Figure 26-7 Enamel hypoplasia. Brown dentin is visible through hypoplastic enamel of the upper incisors, in this case probably related to trauma affecting the developing tooth. (Courtesy of Theodore P. Croll, DDS.)

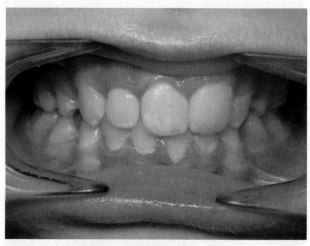

Figure 26-8 Hypocalcification. Caused by dysregulated mineralization that is often idiopathic, these white "chalk marks" are most prominent on the upper teeth. (Courtesy of Jason Kaplan, DDS, MS.)

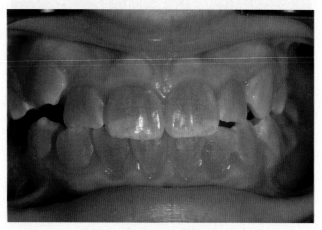

Figure 26-9 Dentinogenesis imperfecta. This genetic disorder of tooth development causes blue-gray or yellow-brown discoloration of all of the teeth. (Courtesy of Theodore P. Croll, DDS.)

DIFFERENTIAL DIAGNOSIS

DIAGNOSIS	ICD-10	DISTINGUISHING CHARACTERISTICS	DISTRIBUTION	DURATION/ CHRONICITY	ASSOCIATED FINDINGS	COMPLICATIONS	PREDISPOSING FACTORS	TREATMENT GUIDELINES
Caries	K02.9	Early: white spots Late: brown decay	Mostly on occlusal surfaces	Very mild caries can resolve without treatment	Halitosis, gingivitis, pain	Abscess, failure to thrive	High sugar diet; dry mouth; mouth breathing; poor dental hygiene; insufficient fluoride, genetic factors	Dental fillings; tooth extraction; reconstruction for permanent teeth
Milk Bottle Caries	K02.9	Decay and tooth erosion	Maxillary incisors	Seen after eruption after the use of bottles or sippy cups	Changes in oral occlusion; halitosis, gingivitis, pain	Abscess, failure to thrive, changes in maxillary shape and bite	Bottle feeding through the night	Appropriate feeding and dental hygiene; tooth extractions
Fluorosis	K00.3	Mild: easy to overlook Moderate: white chalk marks Severe: brown spots	All teeth	Teeth are permanently affected.	Extreme fluorosis can affect bone health	If severe, weakened enamel	Excessive ingested fluoride prior to age 8 years	Appropriate fluoride use
Iron Staining	K03.6	Dark black to brown spots or lines	Mostly lower incisors	Stains can be removed by dentist.	None	None	Iron-containing vitamins	Rinse mouth after administration of vitamins; stains can be removed by dentist
Enamel Hypoplasia	K00.4	Gray discoloration of entire tooth	Often caused by trauma; therefore, usually affects front teeth	Permanent; trauma to primary teeth may or may not affect permanent teeth	Adjacent gingival changes	Possible damage to permanent teeth from trauma	Trauma, malnutrition, serious illness	If severe, veneers or dental reconstruction
Abnormal Mineraliza-tion	K00.3	White spots	Most visible on incisors	Permanent	None	Cosmetic outcome	Trauma, malnutrition, serious illness, idiopathic	If severe, veneers or dental reconstruction
Tetracycline Staining	K00.8	Yellow-brown or gray coloring, in horizontal band or spots	All teeth	Permanent	None	Cosmetic outcome	Exposure to tetracycline-class antibiotics during pregnancy or in first 8 years of life	Best cosmetic result is from veneers

Other Diagnoses to Consider

- Rickets, parathyroid disorders, and other disorders of calcium and vitamin D metabolism

- Kidney failure

- Cystic fibrosis

- Ectodermal dysplasias

- Disorders of tooth development, including amelogenesis imperfecta and dentinogenesis imperfecta

When to Consider Further Evaluation or Treatment

- Even without staining, the American Dental Association and the American Academy of Pediatrics recommend children establish a dental home at age 12 months.

- Significant dental disease can contribute to malnutrition and a poor quality of life. Children, particularly those with multiple risk factors, may need early referral to prevent the progression of dental disease.

- Dental findings may be a clue to serious, systemic illness, especially when accompanied by other signs and symptoms. For instance, children with malabsorption syndromes may present with abdominal complaints and poor growth in addition to poorly mineralized or discolored teeth. Other illnesses can increase the risk of caries, including diabetes and Sjogren syndrome.

SUGGESTED READINGS

Croll T. *The ASDC Kid's Mouth Book*. Chicago, IL: The American Society of Dentistry for Children; 1999:144.
Norwood KW, Slayton RL. Oral health care for children with developmental disabilities. *Pediatrics*. 2013;131:614–619.
Schafer TE, Adair SM. Prevention of dental disease: The role of the pediatrician. *Pediatric Clin N A*. 2000;47:1021–1042.
Section on Pediatric Dentistry and Oral Health. Preventive oral health intervention for pediatricians. *Pediatrics*. 2008;122(6):1387–1394.

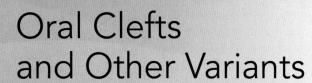

Oral Clefts and Other Variants

Darshita P. Bhatia and Nancy D. Spector

Approach to the Problem

Oral clefts are among the most common birth defects in children and the most common craniofacial abnormality. A failure of the medial and lateral nasal and maxillary processes to fuse results in a cleft lip, whereas a failure of the palatal shelves to join results in a cleft palate. A combination of genetic and environmental factors plays a role in the etiology of oral clefts. Males are twice as likely as females to present with both a cleft lip and a cleft palate. Females commonly have an isolated cleft palate. Asian and Native American populations have the highest frequency of oral clefts, whereas African Americans have the lowest frequency. Oral clefts can cause feeding problems in the newborn child that may be overcome by the use of special nipples and bottles. The first stage of surgical repair for cleft lip should take place by 3 months of age, and surgical repair for cleft palate should occur by 12 months of age. Ankyloglossia, caused by an abnormally short or thickened frenulum, is an oral cleft variant common in infants and children.

Key Points in the History

- Ankyloglossia can cause breastfeeding difficulty in infants and speech articulation disorders in older children.

- There may be a family history of oral clefts, especially if associated with syndromes that are genetically inherited such as van der Woude syndrome and velocardiofacial syndrome. Up to 40% of children may have a cleft lip or palate that is not associated with a genetic syndrome.

- Maternal factors such as folic acid deficiency and exposure to cigarette smoke, alcohol, corticosteroids, and/or anticonvulsants (phenytoin, valproic acid) may result in cleft lip or palate.

- An infant with cleft lip and palate may cough, gag, and/or show increased work of breathing during feeds.

- Difficulty feeding with a cleft lip or palate results from a decreased ability to form a tight seal around a standard nipple. The poor seal results in insufficient force to generate a strong suck reflex.

211

- Hearing loss and middle ear disease is highly prevalent in children with cleft palate due to chronic otitis media with effusion (OME) from eustachian tube dysfunction. However, children with isolated cleft lip do not have chronic OME.

- Velopharyngeal dysfunction in children with oral clefts may result in increased nasal resonance, language delay, and speech articulation disorders.

Key Points in the Physical Examination

- Ankyloglossia can lead to a variable degree of limited tongue elevation and mobility.

- Cleft lips are divided into three types: microform, incomplete, and complete.

  - A microform cleft lip consists of a simple notch in the vermilion border of the lip.

  - In an incomplete cleft lip, the defect extends part way through the lip.

  - In a complete cleft lip, the defect extends into the floor of the nose.

- Cleft lip can be unilateral or bilateral, located on the lateral border of the lip (common) or medial surface (rare).

- There is variability in the extent of involvement of the soft and hard palates in cleft palate, but the uvula is always involved.

- Children with cleft lip and palate may have significant dental deformities.

- A submucosal cleft has an intact oral mucosa overlying unfused palatal tissue and is often associated with a bifid uvula.

- The presence of a bifid uvula should prompt investigation for a submucosal cleft, but up to 10% of bifid uvulas occur in isolation.

- A bluish, translucent strip of tissue called the zona pellucida is present in the midline of a submucosal cleft. This diagnosis is not easily visualized but can be palpated as a notch in the posterior region of the soft palate.

PHOTOGRAPHS OF SELECTED DIAGNOSES

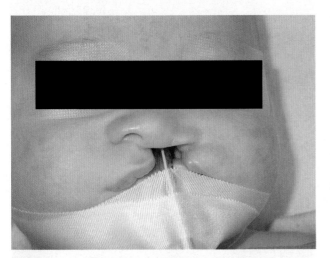

Figure 27-1 **Cleft lip in a child immediately prior to repair.** (Courtesy of Wellington Davis, MD.)

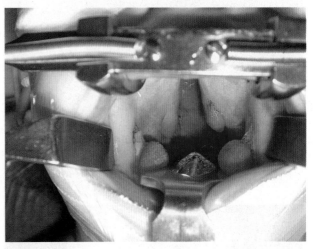

Figure 27-2 **Cleft palate visualized intraoperatively.** (Courtesy of Wellington Davis, MD.)

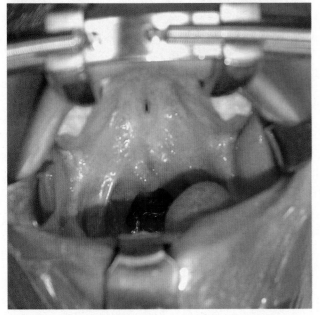

Figure 27-3 **Operative photo of a submucosal cleft palate with a small palatal perforation.** (Courtesy of Wellington Davis, MD.)

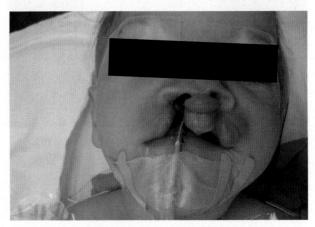

Figure 27-4 **Bilateral cleft lip and palate.** (Courtesy of Scott VanDuzer, MD.)

SECTION 7 • MOUTH

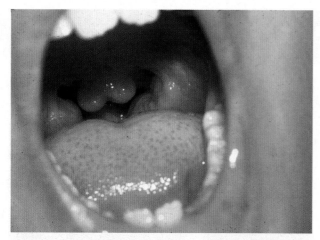

Figure 27-5 **An isolated bifid uvula without other oral clefting.** (Courtesy of the late Peter Sol, MD.)

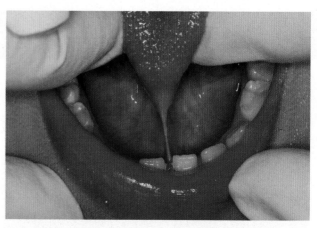

Figure 27-6 **Ankyloglossia.** Note the short lingual frenulum extending to the anterior tip of the tongue. (Courtesy of Theodore P. Croll, DDS.)

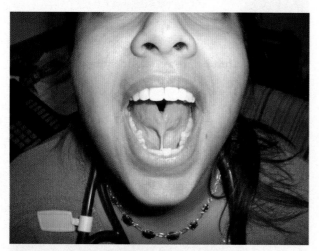

Figure 27-7 **Ankyloglossia.** Note the elevation of the sides but not the middle of the tongue. (Courtesy of Paul S. Matz, MD.)

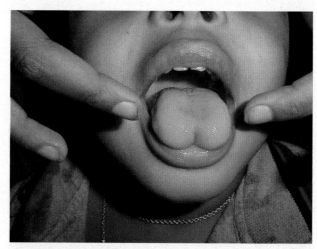

Figure 27-8 **Ankyloglossia.** Note the notched or heart-shaped tongue visible on protrusion of the tongue. (Courtesy of Michael Lemper, DDS.)

DIFFERENTIAL DIAGNOSIS

DIAGNOSIS	ICD-10	DISTINGUISHING CHARACTERISTICS	DISTRIBUTION	ASSOCIATED FINDINGS	COMPLICATIONS	PREDISPOSING FACTORS	TREATMENT GUIDELINES
Ankyloglossia (Tongue Tie)	Q38.1	Short, thickened frenulum Limited tongue elevation and mobility	Frenulum beneath tongue	N/A	Feeding difficulty Speech articulation disorder Poor hygiene	N/A	Frenotomy (also known as frenulectomy, frenectomy) by a trained general pediatrician or pediatric otolaryngologist for feeding difficulty or speech dysfunction
Cleft Lip	Q36.9 with cleft palate: Q37.9	Microform: notch at the vermilion border Incomplete: extension partway through the lip Complete: extension through nasal floor	Lateral lip vs medial lip	Velopharyngeal dysfunction Dental deformity Cleft palate	Feeding difficulty Speech articulation disorder	Maternal drug exposure: anticonvulsants, alcohol, cigarette smoke, corticosteroids Genetic factors	Multidisciplinary team: General pediatrician Cleft surgeon Speech pathologist First-stage repair at 3 months of age
Cleft Palate	Q35.9	Variable involvement of soft and/or hard palate Uvula always involved	Unilateral vs bilateral	Velopharyngeal dysfunction Dental deformity Other characteristics of genetic syndromes associated with cleft palate	Difficulty feeding Hypernasal speech Chronic otitis media with effusion	Maternal drug exposure: anticonvulsants, alcohol, cigarette smoke, corticosteroids Genetic factors	Multidisciplinary team: General pediatrician Cleft surgeon Speech pathologist Dentist Audiologist/ otolaryngologist First-stage repair at 12 months of age
Submucosal Cleft	Q35.9	Intact oral mucosa overlying unfused palatal tissue	Hard and soft palate	Zona pellucida	Speech disturbance	N/A	Speech pathologist

Other Diagnoses to Consider

- Van der Woude syndrome

- Kallman syndrome

- Stickler syndrome

- Velocardiofacial syndrome

- Treacher Collins syndrome

- Crouzon syndrome

When to Consider Further Evaluation or Treatment

- An infant or child may be a candidate for frenotomy if ankyloglossia interferes with feeding or speech.

- Prompt evaluation and follow-up with a multidisciplinary team is recommended for patients with cleft lip and/or palate:

  - General pediatricians ensure coordination of subspecialty services and anticipatory guidance.

  - Consult a surgeon trained in cleft lip and palate reconstruction assessment of surgical repair.

  - Speech therapists will educate parents about proper feeding techniques.

  - Audiology or otolaryngology may be helpful in the management of chronic OME.

- Consultation with pediatric dentistry, genetics, and occupational therapy should be considered, depending on symptoms associated with the cleft lip and/or palate.

SUGGESTED READINGS

Eppley BL, van Aalst JA, Robey A, et al. The spectrum of orofacial clefting. *Plast Reconstruct Surg.* 2005;115(7):101e–114e.
Marazita ML, Mooney MP. Current concepts in the embryology and genetics of cleft lip and palate. *Clin Plastic Surg.* 2004;31:125–140.
Sidman JD, Muntz HR. Cleft lip and palate. In: Wetmore RF, Muntz HR, McGill TJ, eds. *Pediatric Otolaryngology: Principles and Practice Pathways.* 2nd ed. New York: Thieme; 2012:Chap 34.
Tinanoff N. Cleft lip and palate. In: Kliegman RM, Stanton BF, St. Geme JW, Schor NF, Behrman RE, eds. *Nelson Textbook of Pediatrics.* 19th ed. Philadelphia, PA. Saunders Elsevier; 2011:Chap 302.
Viera AR. Unraveling human cleft lip and palate research. *J Dent Res.* 2008;87(2):119–125.
Webb AN, Hao W, Hong P. The effect of tongue-tie division on breastfeeding and speech articulation: A systematic review. *Int J Pediatr Otorhinolaryngol.* 2013;77:635–646.

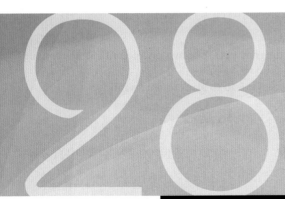

Tongue Discoloration and Surface Changes

Christopher O'Hara

Approach to the Problem

The surface of the tongue may develop changes in color or texture because of intrinsic or extrinsic factors. Discolorations may be related to chewed, ingested, or topical products, or certain infections. It is important to be familiar with some of the more common, benign tongue abnormalities that may present in the pediatric patient so that reassurance and appropriate guidance may be given to families.

Key Points in the History

- Syphilis and lichen planus may be associated with white plaques on the tongue.

- The use of antibiotics, immunosuppressive agents, systemic steroids, or inhaled corticosteroids may predispose patients to oral thrush.

- Immunodeficiency, recent radiation, or cytotoxic therapy predisposes patients to oral thrush and oral hairy leukoplakia. Hairy leukoplakia is caused by Epstein–Barr virus and is seen more commonly in adults affected by human immunodeficiency virus (HIV), but is rare in children affected by HIV.

- White plaques associated with lichen planus are more common in patients with thyroid disease, particularly hypothyroidism.

- Geographic tongue is seen less commonly in smokers.

- Chewing betel leaf, which is common in some Southeast Asian countries, may stain the tongue red. Chewing betel quid, also known as betel paan (a mixture of betel leaf with or without tobacco, spices, areca nut, and slaked lime), is associated with oral leukoplakia.

- Medications, such as antibiotics, antifungal agents, antimalarial drugs (primarily on the hard palate), psychotropic agents (including selective serotonin reuptake inhibitors), phenothiazines, benzodiazepines, and phenytoin, may cause tongue discoloration.

- Argyria is an irreversible blue gray mucocutaneous staining caused by exposure to silver and includes ingestion of a silver-containing supplement known as colloidal silver.

- Use of coffee, tea, tobacco, and cola products may cause brown discoloration of the tongue.

- Ingestion of bismuth-containing products may lead to black tongue staining.

- Minocycline-associated pigmentary changes may persist for years.

- Darkly pigmented adults and children are more likely to have pigmented fungiform papillae of the tongue.

- Dark pigmentation of the fungiform papillae may be seen in iron deficiency.

- Hairy tongue, or elongated filiform papillae in the midline tongue, is associated with the following: tobacco, tea, coffee, antibiotics, griseofulvin, or certain mouthwashes containing an oxidizing agent, such as sodium perborate, sodium peroxide, or hydrogen peroxide.

- Hairy tongue has been linked to herbal tea ingestion in an infant.

- Fixed drug eruptions occur at the same location on the tongue with each exposure.

- Adult females are more prone to fixed drug eruptions on the tongue.

- Glossitis may be precipitated by the use of cytotoxic agents.

Key Points in the Physical Examination

- A white plaque that wipes off easily may be due to milk or food. If it cannot be scraped off easily, bleeds, or leaves a denuded surface after scraping, the white plaque is usually the result of a fungal infection.

- Lichen planus, an immunological disorder, may cause lacy white plaques on the buccal mucosae and may coexist with oral candidiasis.

- White sponge nevus is a rare autosomal dominant condition that starts in childhood and is characterized by bilateral white plaques on the buccal mucosae, and sometimes on the lateral border of the tongue and other mucosal surfaces. The cornified layer may peel away from the underlying mucosa. It may be painful if secondarily infected.

- Linea alba is caused by repeated trauma from biting or chewing and appears as a thin white line on the lateral margins of the tongue (or the buccal mucosae) bilaterally.

- White tongue plaques associated with nail dystrophy and reticular skin pigmentation are hallmarks of Zinsser–Cole–Engman syndrome, also known as dyskeratosis congenita, a rare, X-linked disorder associated with bone marrow failure.

- The white plaques of oral hairy leukoplakia generally cannot be scraped off and are often located on the lateral surface of the tongue.

- A tongue with small smooth areas of denuded papillae surrounded by annular loops of normal papillae is characteristic of a geographic tongue.

- The enlarged papillae of strawberry tongue may briefly persist after the redness has resolved.

- The raised papillae of strawberry tongue may be visualized better with indirect lighting from the side.

- A red tongue that is smooth indicates glossitis, whereas a red tongue with enlarged papillae is more consistent with strawberry tongue.

- Median rhomboid glossitis is a reddened and smooth rhomboid-shaped area of papillary atrophy just anterior to the circumvallate papillae.

- Patches of hyperpigmentation on the tongue may be a normal variant in darkly pigmented individuals.

- Pigmented fungiform papillae of the tongue have three distinct forms. One involves all of the papillae within a well-defined area, usually the anterolateral tongue. Another form involves three to seven hyperpigmented papillae scattered across the dorsal surface. The third involves hyperpigmentation of all the fungiform papillae on the dorsal surface of the tongue.

- Hairy tongue discoloration may be brown, black, green, or yellow depending on the particles, chromogenic bacteria, or fungi that are entrapped; hence, it is no longer known as "black hairy tongue."

PHOTOGRAPHS OF SELECTED DIAGNOSES

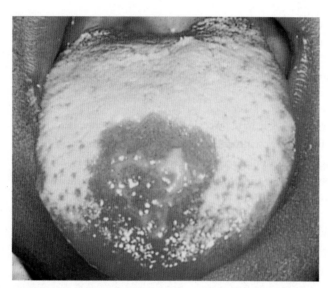

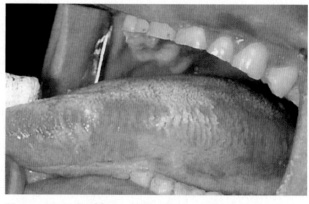

Figure 28-2 Oral hairy leukoplakia. Raised white plaques on the lateral surface of the tongue. (Used with permission from Weber J, Kelley J. *Health Assessment in Nursing.* 2nd ed. Philadelphia, PA: Lippincott Williams & Wilkins; 2003:244.)

Figure 28-1 White plaques from oral thrush. This patient had lingual involvement only, but many children will have plaques located diffusely throughout the oral cavity. (Used with permission from Weber J, Kelley J. *Health Assessment in Nursing.* 2nd ed. Philadelphia, PA: Lippincott Williams & Wilkins; 2003.)

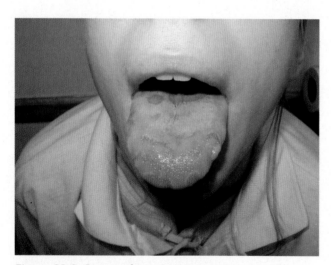

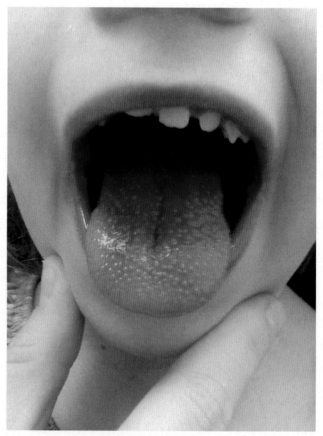

Figure 28-3 Geographic tongue. Irregular areas of denuded papillae are surrounded by normal tongue mucosa. (Courtesy of Paul S. Matz, MD.)

Figure 28-4 Strawberry tongue. Note the prominent fungiform papillae in this child with streptococcal pharyngitis. (Courtesy of Naline Lai, MD.)

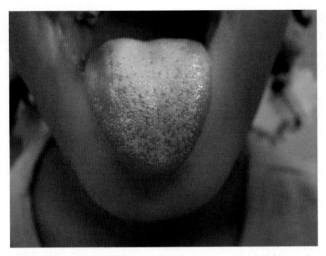

Figure 28-5 **Strawberry tongue.** The prominent white papillae appear like strawberry seeds in a child with streptococcal pharyngitis. (Courtesy of Esther K. Chung, MD, MPH.)

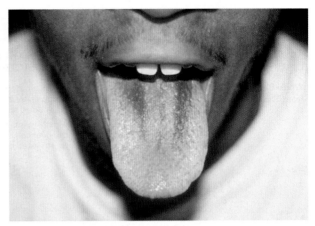

Figure 28-6 **Black tongue.** A teenager with black tongue staining after bismuth ingestion. (Courtesy of Kathleen Cronan, MD.)

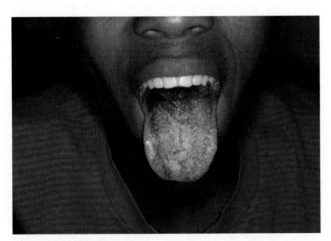

Figure 28-7 **Black tongue.** A teenager experiencing black tongue discoloration after exposure to bismuth. (Courtesy of Jan Edwin Drutz, MD.)

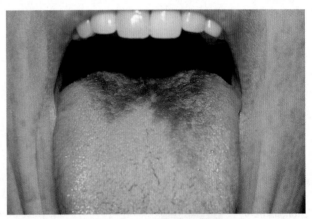

Figure 28-8 **Black hairy tongue.** Note the elongation of the filiform papillae in the posterior tongue. This patient had black discoloration, but the color of the pigmentation is variable. (Used with permission from Goodheart HP. *Goodheart's Photoguide of Common Skin Disorders.* 2nd ed. Philadelphia, PA: Lippincott Williams & Wilkins; 2003:228.)

SECTION 7 • MOUTH

DIFFERENTIAL DIAGNOSIS

DIAGNOSIS		ICD-10	DISTINGUISHING CHARACTERISTICS	DISTRIBUTION	DURATION
White Plaques from Thrush		B37.0	When scraped off, the tongue bleeds or reveals a denuded surface Mostly in infants—peak prevalence is in the fourth week of life	Localized plaques may occur throughout oral cavity Thrush may present as erythematous patches that are painful or cause a burning sensation.	Persistent unless treated
Geographic Tongue		K14.1	White areas of normal papillae surrounding reddened areas of atrophic papillae	Dorsal surface, widespread Appears to migrate across the tongue as it waxes and wanes	Hours to weeks but may wax and wane for months to years
Strawberry Tongue		K14.0	Reddened dorsal surface with enlarged fungiform papillae White or yellow papillae resembling seeds on a strawberry's surface	Usually generalized and found on the anterior two-thirds of the dorsal and lateral tongue surfaces	Erythema associated with Kawasaki disease resolves along with other symptoms of the illness Papillae may remain enlarged after the illness resolves.
Blackening of Tongue from Medication		Y88.0	Typically black discoloration of dorsal surface without changes in size or distribution of papillae	Affects dorsal surface Staining due to amalgam tattoo is seen near dental filling	Typically resolves within days of discontinuation of the offending agent Some cases have prolonged staining.

ASSOCIATED FINDINGS	COMPLICATIONS	PREDISPOSING FACTORS	TREATMENT GUIDELINES
Yeast diaper dermatitis in infants	Oral thrush may be associated with esophageal candidiasis in immunosuppressed states. Oral graft-versus-host disease may present with white plaques. Some evidence for spread to mother during breastfeeding causing candidal mastitis	Antibiotic use Antimalarial agents Erythema multiforme Fifth disease Immune suppressed states Inhaled steroids Lichen planus (rare) Oral hairy leukoplakia Secondary syphilis (rare) Stevens–Johnson syndrome Viral stomatitis	Nystatin suspension or for older children clotrimazole troches until plaques are gone for 48 hours
Fissured tongue Atopic diseases Psoriasis Pain, rarely	Cases that are associated with pain may have a concomitant fungal infection.	Case reports associated with lithium treatment, tenofovir, and bevacizumab	Reassurance May use topical steroid if painful or antifungal if associated with candida Case reports of successful therapy using either tacrolimus or cyclosporine A
Conjunctival erythema in Kawasaki disease and adenoviral infection Palatal petechiae in group A streptococcal pharyngitis White coating seen initially in scarlet fever resolves in 4–5 days	Rheumatic fever in some cases of group A streptococcal pharyngitis Coronary artery ectasia in untreated Kawasaki disease Neurobehavioral manifestations of B12 deficiency in pernicious anemia Fungiform papillary glossitis is associated with atopic disease.	Adenoviral infection Antiepileptic drug hypersensitivity (a reaction to one of the aromatic antiepileptic drugs—phenytoin, carbamazepine, phenobarbital, and primidone) Candy tongue Ehrlichiosis Fungiform papillary glossitis Glossitis Kawasaki disease Pernicious anemia Streptococcal pharyngitis Toxic shock syndrome *Yersinia pseudotuberculosis*	Group A streptococcal pharyngitis requires antibiotic treatment (e.g., penicillin) to prevent rheumatic fever.
Staining of the dentitia and/or the oral and gingival mucosae Nearby dental filling	Lead poisoning or other heavy metal poisoning Drug abuse or addiction when associated with smoking heroin Iron deficiency and hemochromatosis are associated with hyperpigmentation of the papillae.	Adriamycin Arsenic Bismuth Capecitabine Charcoal (Activated) Chlorhexidine Clofazimine Crack cocaine Cyclophosphamide Doxorubicin Fluconazole Gold Hydroxychloroquine Hydroxyurea Inhaled heroin smoke Ketoconazole Lansoprazole with clarithromycin Linezolid Mercury Methyldopa Phenobarbital Risperidone (orally disintegrating form) Ribavirin with pegylated interferon Silver Tegafur Terbinafine Tobacco Zidovudine	Brushing the tongue Discontinuation of the offending agent Chelation therapy if associated with lead poisoning

SECTION 7 • MOUTH

(continued)

DIFFERENTIAL DIAGNOSIS *(continued)*

DIAGNOSIS	ICD-10	DISTINGUISHING CHARACTERISTICS	DISTRIBUTION	DURATION
Hairy Tongue	K14.3	Elongated filiform papillae in the midline dorsally with a plaque of discoloration over this (the color depends on the offending agent) Discoloration is the result of chromogenic bacteria, fungi (*C. albicans*), or trapped particles beneath hyperplastic layers of keratin on the filiform papillae	Medial aspect of dorsal surface just anterior to circumvallate papillae	Persists without discontinuation of offending agent

ASSOCIATED FINDINGS	COMPLICATIONS	PREDISPOSING FACTORS	TREATMENT GUIDELINES
Halitosis Gagging sensation Dysgeusia	Discomfort may be associated with gagging sensation. Higher incidence of oral disease related to poor hygiene Social stigma due to appearance May be a manifestation or precursor of graft-versus-host disease	Alcohol Antidepressants Benzodiazepines Chloramphenicol Coffee Erlotinib Linezolid Olanzapine Penicillins Phenothiazines Poor oral hygiene Smoking Tea Tetracyclines Tricyclic Xerostomia and drugs that induce it	Smoking cessation Brushing the tongue with a soft toothbrush promotes desquamation of the elongated papillae Successful therapy with topical tretinoin or fluconazole in case reports

<table>
<tr><td>

Other Diagnoses to Consider

</td><td>

- Addison disease

- Dermatopathia pigmentosa peticularis

- Dyschromatosis universalis hereditaria

- Dyskeratosis congenita, X-linked (Zinsser–Cole–Engmann syndrome)

- Glossitis

- Hemochromatosis

- Laugier–Hunziker syndrome

- Malignant melanoma

- McCune–Albright syndrome

- Oral melanoacanthoma

- Peutz–Jeghers syndrome

- Von Recklinghausen disease (neurofibromatosis I)

</td></tr>
<tr><td>

When to Consider Further Evaluation or Treatment

</td><td>

- False-negative cultures have been seen in as many as 25% of individuals with oral candidiasis.

- Thrush outside of infancy (barring risk factors such as antibiotic or inhaled steroid use) and recurrent thrush are indications for immunological evaluation, including HIV testing.

- Rare cases of painful geographic tongue may be treated with oral rinses of mucosal anesthetic solutions, such as diphenhydramine, or with topical steroid creams, with the latter being less well tolerated.

- Strawberry tongue is one potential finding in Kawasaki disease. A detailed history and physical examination should be performed to prove or disprove Kawasaki disease so that appropriate therapy may be initiated.

- Black tongue staining and concurrent staining of the gingiva may occur with ingestion of heavy metals such as silver, lead and mercury, arsenic, gold, platinum, and bismuth.

- Brown black discoloration of the lateral edges of the tongue and the gingivae may be seen in Addison disease.

- Smoking heroin has been associated with dark oral plaques. Dentists may be the first clinicians to see this finding.

- Blue-green staining of the gingiva may occur with exposure to copper.

- Orange staining of the gingiva may occur with exposure to cadmium.

</td></tr>
</table>

- Hairy tongue has been associated with trigeminal neuralgia, including disease that lateralizes to the affected side of the face. It is postulated that the pain associated with movement or manipulation of the tongue prevents normal desquamation of the filiform papillae.

- If brushing the tongue does not successfully treat hairy tongue, other therapies such as topical 40% urea, retinoids, salicylic acid, CO_2 laser therapy, or electrodessication may be tried.

- Hairy tongue has been associated with graft-versus-host disease either as a precursor lesion or as a frank manifestation.

SUGGESTED READINGS

Akay BN, Sanli H, Topcuoglu P, Zincircioğlu C, and Heper AO. Black hairy tongue after allogeneic stem cell transplantation: An unrecognized cutaneous presentation of graft-versus-host disease. *Transplant Proc.* 2010;42:4603–4607.

Dubach P, Caversaccio M. Amalgam tattoo. *N Engl J Med.* 2011;364(15):e29.

Ferreira AO, Marinho RT, Velosa J, Costa JB. Geographic tongue and tenofovir. *BMJ Case Rep.* April 17, 2013.

Hubiche T, Valenza B, Chevreau C, et al. Geographic tongue induced by angiogenesis inhibitors. *The Oncologist.* 2013;18:e16–e17.

Khasawneh FA, Moti DF, and Zorek JA. Linezolid-induced black hairy tongue: a case report. *J Med Case Rep.* 2013;7:46.

Körber A, Voshege N. Black hairy tongue in an infant. *CMAJ.* 2012;184(1):68.

Müller S. Melanin-associated pigmented lesions of the oral mucosa: Presentation, differential diagnosis and treatment. *Dermatol Ther.* 2010;23:220–229.

Reamy BV, Derby R, Bunt CW. Common tongue conditions in primary care. *Am Fam Physician.* 2010;81(5):627–634.

Thompson DF, Kessler TL. Drug-induced hairy tongue. *Pharmacotherapy.* 2010;30(6):585–593.

Swellings Within the Mouth

Nancy D. Spector and Darshita P. Bhatia

Approach to the Problem

Children of all ages may present with a variety of swellings within the mouth, ranging from benign lesions to very serious infections. Differentiating mouth swellings may be difficult owing to a lack of available diagnostic and laboratory testing. Common benign lesions can be diagnosed using characteristic locations and distinguishing physical features. Serious swellings of the mouth will typically present with associated systemic signs of illness. Peritonsillar abscess and Ludwig angina have potentially life-threatening complications.

Key Points in the History

- Bohn nodules and Epstein pearls are present in newborns (see Chapter 24: Mouth Sores and Patches and Chapter 25: Focal Gum Lesions).

- Mucoceles and ranulas arise acutely, rupture spontaneously, and are painless and asymptomatic.

- Systemic signs of infection, such as fever and throat pain, help differentiate benign swellings of the mouth from more serious infections.

- Peritonsillar abscess is generally preceded by acute tonsillopharyngitis.

- Patients with Ludwig angina have a history of high fever and an inability to handle secretions.

Key Points in the Physical Examination

- Epstein pearls are smooth, nontender, translucent, pearly white, 1- to 3-mm cysts on the palate near the midline of the roof of the mouth. When such lesions occur on the gums, they are referred to as Bohn nodules.

- Mucoceles and ranulas are fluid-filled, nontender, mobile, and glisten and have a bluish hue.

- Mucoceles are most common on the lower lip.

- Ranulas are found on the floor of the mouth.

- Peritonsillar abscess is characterized by swelling of tissues lateral and superior to the affected tonsil, anterior and medial displacement of the affected tonsil, and displacement of the uvula toward the contralateral side.

- Patients with peritonsillar abscess can have a muffled, or "hot potato," voice.

- Ludwig angina always involves the bilateral submandibular spaces.

- Ludwig angina is characterized by elevation and posterior displacement of the tongue.

- Trismus, or difficulty in opening the mouth, is a frequent finding in patients with peritonsillar abscess and Ludwig angina.

PHOTOGRAPHS OF SELECTED DIAGNOSES

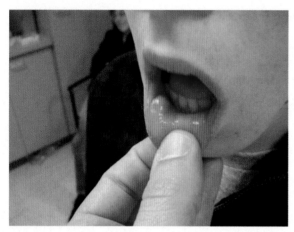

Figure 29-1 **Mucocele.** Fluid-filled pseudocyst protruding from lower lip. (Courtesy of Paul S. Matz, MD.)

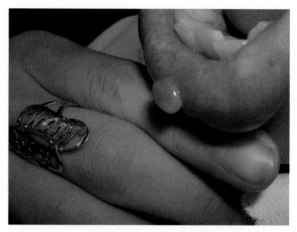

Figure 29-2 **Mucocele.** Fluid-filled pseudocyst protruding from lower lip. (Courtesy of Michael Lemper, DDS.)

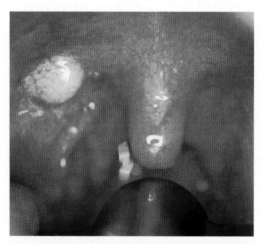

Figure 29-3 **Mucocele of soft palate.** Whitish pseudocyst on the right side of the soft palate. (Used with permission from Handler SD, Myer CM. *Atlas of Ear, Nose and Throat Disorders in Children.* Ontario: BC Decker; 1998:85.)

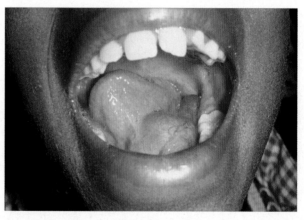

Figure 29-4 **Ranula.** Fluid-filled mass on the floor of the mouth. (Courtesy of Kathleen Cronan, MD.)

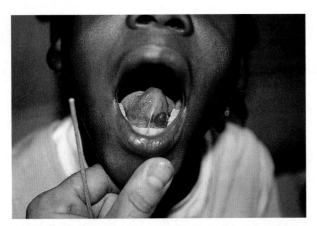

Figure 29-5 Ranula. Fluid-filled cyst on the base of the tongue. (Courtesy of George A. Datto, III, MD.)

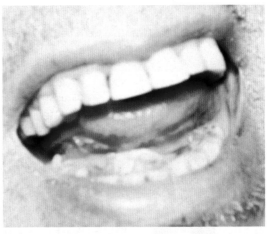

Figure 29-6 Ludwig angina. Note elevation of tongue secondary to swelling of the floor of the mouth. (Used with permission from Greenberg MI. *Greenberg's Atlas of Emergency Medicine.* Philadelphia, PA: Lippincott Williams & Wilkins; 2005:7.)

DIFFERENTIAL DIAGNOSIS

DIAGNOSIS	ICD-10	DISTINGUISHING CHARACTERISTICS	DISTRIBUTION	DURATION/CHRONICITY
Epstein Pearl	K09.8	Newborns Circumscribed, pearly white, 1- to 3-mm cyst	Alveolar ridge or midline hard palate	May be present for weeks before spontaneous rupture
Mucocele	K11.6	Pseudocyst resulting from mucus extravasation into the surrounding tissues Minor salivary gland in origin Acute onset of painless, asymptomatic swelling May fluctuate in size May rupture spontaneously	Common on the lower lip Less common on the upper lip, palate, buccal mucosa, tongue, or the floor of the mouth	Recurrence rate of 14% May be present for weeks to months before rupture
Ranula	K11.6	Pseudocyst resulting from mucus extravasation into the surrounding tissues Major salivary gland in origin Nontender, mobile, glistening, broad-based enlargement Bluish hue May fluctuate in size May rupture spontaneously	Floor of the mouth	Recurrence rate of 14% May be present for weeks to months before rupture
Peritonsillar Abscess (See Chapter 30: Throat Redness)	J36	Throat pain, fever, dysphagia, "hot potato voice," and drooling Occurrence of trismus in 63% of cases Tonsils are erythematous, enlarged, and covered with exudate.	Swelling of the tissues lateral and superior to the tonsil with medial and anterior displacement of the tonsil	Develops over several days after acute tonsillopharyngitis Recurrence rate of 6%–36%
Ludwig Angina	K12.2	Acute life-threatening cellulitis Trismus, high fever, halitosis, inability to handle secretions Feels woody on palpation Unable to depress tongue Caused by gingival bacteria (anaerobic streptococci, *Bacteroides* sp., fusobacteria, and spirochetes)	Bilateral involvement of the submandibular spaces	Develops over several days

ASSOCIATED FINDINGS	COMPLICATIONS	PREDISPOSING FACTORS	TREATMENT GUIDELINES
None	None	None	No intervention required
None	None	Trauma to the salivary gland and excretory duct Obstruction of salivary gland duct flow Trauma to salivary glandular parenchymal cells	No intervention required
None	Large ranulas may interfere with speech, swallowing, or respiration.	Trauma to the salivary gland excretory duct Obstruction of salivary gland duct flow Trauma to salivary glandular parenchymal cells	Generally, no intervention required Consider consultation with otolaryngology for surgical removal for ranulas that interfere with speech, swallowing, or respiration.
Tender cervical adenopathy	Airway compromise Aspiration if spontaneous rupture of abscess Spread of infection resulting in retropharyngeal abscess, parapharyngeal abscess, mediastinitis Septic thrombi leading to osteomyelitis, meningitis, or brain abscess	Acute tonsillopharyngitis	Antibiotics Pain management Consider hospitalization Consider consultation with otolaryngology for possible drainage
Erythema of overlying neck skin, pitting edema, and tenderness	Spread of infection resulting in mediastinitis Laryngeal or subglottic edema Respiratory distress Difficult intubation	Poor oral hygiene Dental extractions Sialadenitis	Immediate hospitalization, evaluation for airway compromise, antibiotics, consultation with otolaryngology

SECTION 7 • MOUTH

Other Diagnoses to Consider

- Hemangioma

- Lymphangioma

- Fibroma

- Parulis (gum abscess)

When to Consider Further Evaluation or Treatment

- Most mucoceles and ranulas rupture spontaneously and will not require further intervention.

- Large ranulas that interfere with speech, swallowing, or respiration should be referred for evaluation by otolaryngology.

- Peritonsillar abscesses require antibiotic administration and pain management in a hospital setting in addition to concurrent consultation with otolaryngology for possible drainage.

- Ludwig angina is a life-threatening condition that requires immediate hospitalization, evaluation for airway compromise, intravenous antibiotics, and consultation by otolaryngology.

SUGGESTED READINGS

Brierly DJ, Chee CKM, Speight PM. A review of paediatric oral and maxillofacial pathology. *Int J of Paediatr Dent.* 2013;23(5):319–329.
Cathcart RA. Inflammatory swellings of the head and neck. *Surgery.* 2012;30(11):597–603.
Delaney J, Keels MA. Pediatric oral pathology. *Pediatr Clin North Am.* 2000;47(5):1125–1147.
Krol DM, Keels MA. Oral conditions. *Pediatr Rev.* 2007;28:15–22.
Patel NJ, Sciubba J. Oral lesions in young children. *Pediatr Clin North Am.* 2003;50:469–486.

Throat Redness

Colette R. Desrochers

Approach to the Problem

Throat redness is a familiar complaint to the general pediatrician or family practitioner. Erythema of the posterior oropharynx suggests an inflammatory or infectious process, but can also be caused by exposure to environmental allergens, airborne irritants, or acid from chronic laryngopharyngeal reflux. The majority of pediatric infections involving the posterior oropharynx are of viral origin. Careful attention to details provided in the patient's history, and to findings observed on the physical examination, will help to identify patients for whom additional testing, such as group A streptococcus rapid antigen detection, should be performed. It is imperative to recognize the acutely ill patient with pharyngeal erythema, and direct the medical evaluation and treatment plan accordingly. For patients with a persistent or recurrent complaint of throat redness, one must broaden the differential diagnosis to include less common etiologies or pathogens.

Key Points in the History

- Pharyngitis may cause neck pain and stiffness.

- Throat redness associated with upper respiratory tract symptoms (rhinorrhea, cough, and conjunctivitis) and/or lower gastrointestinal tract manifestations (vomiting with diarrhea) are characteristic of viral infection and rarely represent a bacterial throat infection.

- Throat pain due to postnasal drip is often worse at night or in the early morning, but improves during the day.

- Infection with adenovirus is associated with conjunctivitis and/or otitis media.

- In group A streptococcal pharyngitis, symptom onset is typically acute. Sore throat, dysphagia, fever, headache, abdominal pain, and vomiting commonly occur.

- Younger children with streptococcal pharyngitis may present with fever, headache, vomiting, abdominal pain, and decreased oral intake. They may not identify sore throat as a primary complaint.

- Incidence of group A beta-hemolytic streptococcal pharyngitis peaks in the late winter and early spring.

- Epidemics of group A beta-hemolytic streptococcal pharyngitis occur in patients who live in close quarters such as military units, dormitories, mental health facilities, schools, homeless shelters, and group homes.

- Otalgia, with referred pain due to sensory innervation of the glossopharyngeal and vagus nerves supplying both the throat and the ear, can be a presenting symptom of streptococcal pharyngitis.

- Retropharyngeal abscesses are most common in children between 2 and 4 years of age.

- Consider infectious mononucleosis, due to Epstein–Barr virus (EBV) infection, in adolescents with fever, throat pain, enlarged posterior lymph nodes, and significant fatigue.

- Adolescents may not disclose sexual risk behaviors; therefore, test teens with persistent pharyngitis for sexually transmitted diseases, such as gonorrhea.

- Candida may be associated with inhaled steroid use for persistent asthma, or seen in patients who are immunosuppressed or immunocompromised.

- Mycoplasma infection is usually associated with cough.

- Increased throat pain after meals or when supine suggests pain related to gastroesophageal reflux.

- Chronic mouth breathing associated with obstructive sleep apnea leads to dry, irritated mucosae and a sore throat, which is worse in the morning and improves throughout the day as the patient drinks fluids. Asking about ambient room temperatures, especially in the winter months, can provide useful history to support this diagnosis.

Key Points in the Physical Examination

- Severe viral pharyngitis and streptococcal pharyngitis may present with fever, pharyngeal erythema with or without exudates, and cervical lymphadenopathy.

- Hoarseness suggests vocal cord inflammation due to a viral process, or laryngopharyngeal reflux.

- Children younger than 3 years of age with throat redness and exudate are more likely to have viral pharyngitis than group A beta-hemolytic streptococcal infection.

- Children with a peritonsillar abscess may have pharyngeal erythema accompanied by unilateral tonsillar hypertrophy, uvular deviation toward the unaffected side, fever, and trismus (the inability to open the mouth fully). In addition, patients typically have a "hot potato" voice, speaking as if they have a mouthful of hot potatoes, due to an inflamed throat.

- Ulcerations are typically seen with viral pharyngitis and stomatitis. Ulcerations on the tonsillar pillars suggest the diagnosis of herpangina caused by coxsackievirus or echovirus. Ulcerations from herpes simplex virus are typically more anterior but may occur posteriorly and in association with gingivitis.

- Infectious mononucleosis may present with pharyngeal and tonsillar erythema, fever, difficulty swallowing, and posterior cervical lymphadenopathy. Fatigue is a prominent symptom, and may persist in up to 22% of cases beyond 2 to 3 weeks of illness.

- Drooling results from the inability to swallow one's secretions. Watch for drooling in patients with severe pharyngitis, pharyngeal ulcerations, or a retropharyngeal abscess.

- Sitting in a tripod position, inspiratory stridor, difficulty breathing, and dehydration are collective findings that require evaluation for epiglottitis.

- Diphtheria is a rare cause of pharyngitis in well-immunized populations. An asymmetric gray pharyngeal membrane, which extends beyond the borders of the anterior tonsillar pillars onto the soft palate and/or the uvula, suggests this diagnosis.

PHOTOGRAPHS OF SELECTED DIAGNOSES

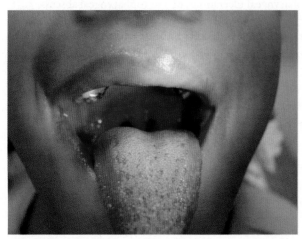

Figure 30-1 Group A streptococcal pharyngitis. Note the marked erythema posteriorly in this patient with scarlet fever. (Courtesy of Esther K. Chung, MD, MPH.)

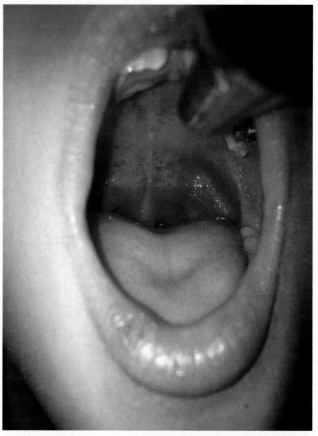

Figure 30-2 Group A streptococcal pharyngitis. Note the marked erythema of the uvula and tonsillar pillars and the palatal petechiae. (Courtesy of Naline Lai, MD.)

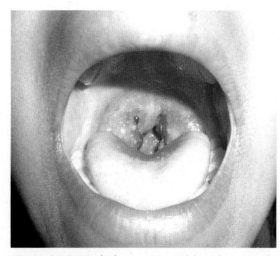

Figure 30-3 Viral pharyngitis. Mild erythema and erythematous papules on both tonsils. (Courtesy of Paul S. Matz, MD.)

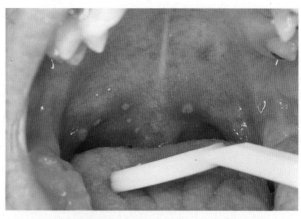

Figure 30-4 Erythematous ulcers on the posterior pharynx. Ulcerations on the tonsillar pillars suggest the diagnosis of herpangina caused by coxsackievirus or echovirus. (Used with permission from Neville BW, Damm DD, White DK. *Color Atlas of Clinical Oral Pathology.* 2nd ed. Baltimore, MD: Williams & Wilkins; 1998.)

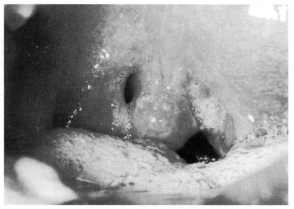

Figure 30-5 Peritonsillar abscess of the left tonsil. (Used with permission from Handler SD, Myer CM. *Atlas of Ear, Nose and Throat Disorders in Children.* Ontario: BC Decker; 1998:90.)

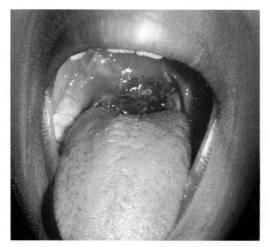

Figure 30-6 Peritonsillar abscess of the right tonsil. Note the swelling and distortion of the area around the right tonsil. (Courtesy of the late Peter Sol, MD.)

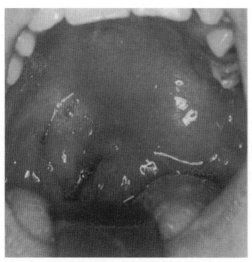

Figure 30-7 Peritonsillar abscess. Note the erythema and swelling on the left and the right deviation of the uvula. (Courtesy of Seth Zwillenberg, MD.)

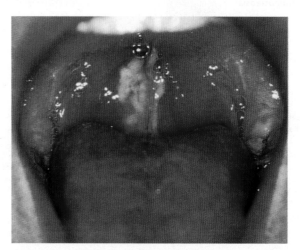

Figure 30-8 Acute tonsillitis secondary to infectious mononucleosis. Note the marked tonsillar enlargement with erythema and the large white-gray patches. (Used with permission from Handler SD, Myer CM. *Atlas of Ear, Nose and Throat Disorders in Children.* Ontario: BC Decker; 1998:91.)

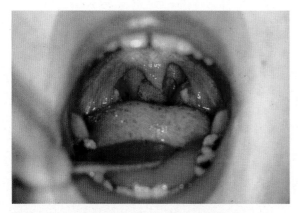

Figure 30-9 Acute tonsillar inflammation due to infectious mononucleosis. Note the tonsillar enlargement with erythema and white exudates. (Courtesy of the late Peter Sol, MD.)

DIFFERENTIAL DIAGNOSIS

DIAGNOSIS		ICD-10	DISTINGUISHING CHARACTERISTICS	DISTRIBUTION	ASSOCIATED FINDINGS
Streptococcal Pharyngitis		J02.0	Posterior pharyngeal erythema Palatal petechiae Tonsillar enlargement Erythema	Posterior oropharynx	Fever Throat pain Cervical and submandibular lymphadenopathy Abdominal pain Headache
Herpangina		B08.5	Discrete erythematous ulcers Painful gray ulcers on an erythematous base	Posterior oropharynx, tonsillar pillars, soft palate	Fever Headache Malaise Hand and foot papulovesicles (coxsackievirus A infections)
Infectious Mononucleosis		B27.0	Pharyngeal and tonsillar erythema with or without exudate	Posterior oropharynx	Fever Fatigue Tonsillar hypertrophy Posterior cervical lymphadenopathy
Peritonsillar Abscess		J36.0	Unilateral tonsillar enlargement Uvular deviation Progressive severity of sore throat despite initial antibiotic treatment of tonsillitis	Tonsils, soft palate, posterior pharynx	Fever Trismus "Hot potato" voice Pain referred to ipsilateral ear

COMPLICATIONS	PREDISPOSING FACTORS	TREATMENT GUIDELINES
Rheumatic fever Glomerulonephritis Cervical adenitis Peritonsillar and retropharyngeal abscess	Exposure to *Streptococcus pyogenes*	Oral penicillin or amoxicillin for 10 days. Once-daily amoxicillin is acceptable. Azithromycin in penicillin-allergic patients
Aseptic meningitis Neonatal sepsis Hepatitis Myocarditis Chronic meningoencephalitis in immunocompromised host Guillain–Barré syndrome	Exposure to precipitating virus—usually coxsackievirus A, also from coxsackievirus B and echoviruses	Supportive care Topical or oral analgesics
Splenomegaly Hepatomegaly Jaundice Splenic rupture Guillain–Barré syndrome Myocarditis Arthritis Meningoencephalitis	Exposure to EBV	Supportive care Oral steroids if respiratory compromise/airway obstruction due to tonsillar hypertrophy
Spread to retropharyngeal space Stridor, suggesting impending airway obstruction Ludwig angina	Previous tonsillitis Recurrent pharyngitis Recent dental procedures	Oral or parenteral antibiotic therapy with clindamycin, penicillin, penicillin and metronidazole, or a cephalosporin Incision and drainage of abscess

SECTION 7 • MOUTH

Other Diagnoses to Consider

- Sexually transmitted diseases (e.g., syphilis [primary or secondary], primary HIV infection, or those caused by *Neisseria gonorrhoeae,* and *Chlamydia trachomatis*)

- Candidal infection

- *Mycoplasma pneumonia*

- Irritation due to chemical exposure or inhalants

- Gastroesophageal or laryngopharyngeal reflux

- Postnasal drip from allergic rhinitis or viral upper respiratory tract infection

- Obstructive sleep apnea

- Diphtheria

When to Consider Further Evaluation or Treatment

- Patients with persistent streptococcal pharyngitis symptoms after 48 hours of appropriate antimicrobial therapy should be seen to rule out suppurative complications. Broad-spectrum antibiotics should be considered.

- A peritonsillar abscess or cellulitis requires emergent otolaryngology evaluation for possible incision and drainage and parenteral antibiotics.

- Viral pharyngitis and herpangina require repeat evaluation if the symptoms persist for more than 10 days.

- Ulcers may be a presenting manifestation of inflammatory bowel disease.

- Urgent evaluation of infectious mononucleosis and treatment with corticosteroids is warranted if signs of airway compromise are evident.

- The development of jaundice, irritability, mental status change, chest pain, or limp may indicate complications of mononucleosis.

SUGGESTED READINGS

Alcaide ML, Bisno AL. Infections of the head and neck: Pharyngitis and epiglottitis. *Infect Dis Clin N Am.* 2007;21(2):449–469.
Chan TV. Otolaryngology for the internist: The patient with sore throat. *Med Clin N Am.* 2010;94(5):923–943.
Choby B. Diagnosis and treatment of streptococcal pharyngitis. *Am Fam Physician.* 2009;79(5):383–390.
Del Mar C. Once-daily amoxicillin eradicates group A beta-hemolytic strep as well as penicillin twice a day. *Pediatrics.* 2008;153:725–725.
Handler SD, Myer CM. *Atlas of Ear, Nose and Throat Disorders in Children.* Ontario: BC Decker; 1998:90–91.
Schwartz B, Marcy SM, Phillips WR, et al. Pharyngitis—principles of judicious use of antimicrobial agents. *Pediatrics.* 1998;101(suppl 1):171–174.
Shaikh N, Swaminathan N, Hooper E. Accuracy and precision of the signs and symptoms of streptococcal pharyngitis in children: A systematic review. *J Pediatr.* 2012;160:487–493.
Shulman ST, Bisno AL, Clegg HW, et al. Clinical practice guideline for the diagnosis and management of group A streptococcal pharyngitis: 2012 update by the Infectious Diseases Society of America. *Clin Infect Dis.* 2012;55(10):e86–e102.

EIGHT

NECK

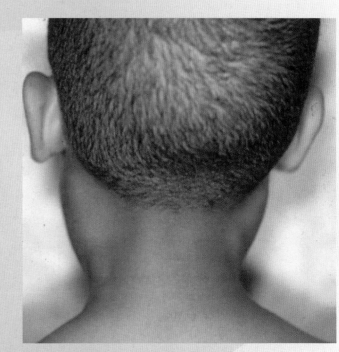

(Courtesy of Ellen S. Deutsch, MD.)

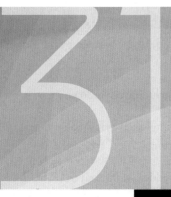

Neck Masses and Swelling

Kristina Toncray

Approach to the Problem

Causes of neck masses and swelling can be broken down into three categories: inflammatory, congenital, and neoplastic; though some may be in more than one category, such as teratoma/dermoid cyst, or infected congenital lesions such as an infected branchial cleft cyst. Clinicians make the majority of diagnoses by taking a careful history and performing a physical examination. Although most neck masses in children are due to inflammatory conditions, followed by congenital conditions, the clinician must be wary of more ominous causes, such as malignancy. Although 80% to 90% of head and neck masses in children are benign, 5% of all malignancies in children are in the head and neck area.

Key Points in the History

- Carefully assess factors such as age; onset, duration, and progression of symptoms; presence or absence of systemic symptoms including fever, fatigue, weight loss, night sweats, joint pain, or swelling; recent upper respiratory tract infection (URI) or sick contacts; animal or food contacts, especially animal bites or scratches or exposure to uncooked meats and unpasteurized milk; immunization status, immunocompromised; recent travel; and medications.

- Acute or subacute enlargement, pain, erythema, fluctuance, and/or recent URI suggest inflammatory conditions.

- Lesions present since birth or shortly thereafter are likely congenital. Think of underlying anatomic anomaly when there is recurrent infection in the same location.

Key Points in the Physical Examination

- Make note of size, location, including sidedness, consistency, mobility, pain, overlying skin changes, and whether the swelling is localized to the neck region or more generalized as in diffuse adenopathy.

- Examine all other nodes and complete a full HEENT (Head, Eyes, Ears, Nose, and Throat) examination, including an oropharyngeal, dental, face, scalp, ear, and eye exam. Perform a general examination, including cardiovascular, pulmonary, abdominal, and extremities examination.

- Consider serial assessments of the neck mass or swelling, ideally performed by the same physician each time.

- Note some diagnosis-specific findings on examination, including the following:

  - Viral adenopathy may be seen in association with findings such as rash, pharyngeal erythema, oral mucosal vesicles, or conjunctival injection.

  - Cervical adenitis is usually rapid in onset, unilateral, tender, warm, and red. The child may have fever, fatigue, and irritability.

  - Patients with bartonella infection usually only have one enlarged node in the area that drains the site of inoculation. A papule or pustule may have been seen at the inoculation site approximately 2 weeks before lymphadenopathy.

  - Branchial cleft cysts are usually deep to the upper third anterior border of the sternocleidomastoid, painless, and with clear drainage from the opening along the sternocleidomastoid. The tract may be palpable.

  - Thyroglossal duct cysts are soft, smooth, nontender, and in the midline, usually below the level of the hyoid. Only 20% are above and 15% are at the level of the hyoid. They typically do not have a primary external opening unless infected. Look for upward movement of the mass with swallowing or tongue protrusion, due to connection with the base of the tongue.

  - Dermoid cysts are usually mobile, though they may adhere to underlying bone, and be nontender. They may be in the midline and confused with thyroglossal duct cysts. Dermoid cysts can be distinguished by depth in that they are generally superficial, by the presence of sebaceous material, and by anatomy as they typically have no connection to the hyoid or tongue.

  - A soft, spongy, compressible swelling with a bluish hue may be a venous malformation.

  - Cystic hygromas can be as small as a few millimeters but are often much larger. They are discrete, soft, nontender, and mobile.

  - Hemangiomas are initially blue or bright red and soft, mobile, and nontender. When regressing, they may have a grayish hue.

  - In congenital torticollis, the face and the chin tilt away from the affected side, while the head tilts toward the ipsilateral shoulder. A mass may be felt.

  - A firm, painless mass is concerning for malignancy. The risk of malignancy increases with increasing node size. Look for associated petechiae, which may indicate malignancy.

PHOTOGRAPHS OF SELECTED DIAGNOSES

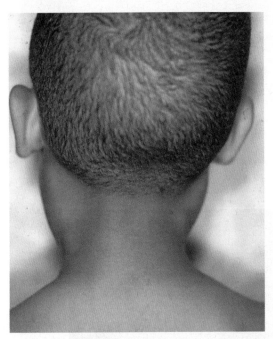

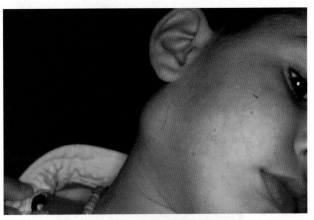

Figure 31-2 Cervical adenitis. This case of acute unilateral adenitis in this 3-year-old child is most likely caused by *Staphylococcus aureus* or group A streptococcus. (Courtesy of Jan Edwin Drutz, MD.)

Figure 31-1 Cervical adenopathy. A posterior view of bilateral adenopathy in a 7-year-old male with a 1- to 2-week history of malaise, sore throat, and low-grade fevers. (Courtesy of Ellen Deutsch, MD.)

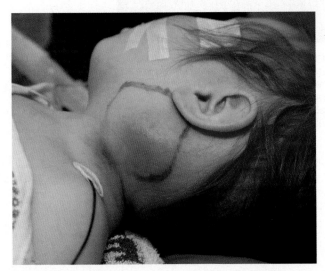

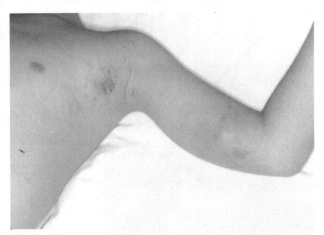

Figure 31-3 Staphylococcal cervical lymphadenitis. (Courtesy of Eden Palmer and Jonathan Perkins, DO.)

Figure 31-4 Cat scratch adenopathy. Epitrochlear and axillary adenopathy that developed proximal to the inoculation site on the finger shown in Figure 31-5. (Courtesy of Mark A. Ward, MD.)

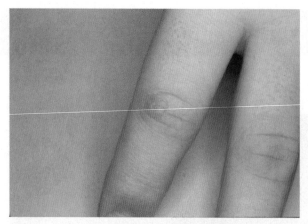

Figure 31-5 Cat scratch inoculation site on the extremity of the 9-year-old child shown in Figure 31-4. (Courtesy of Mark A. Ward, MD.)

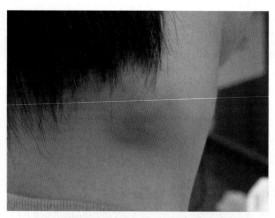

Figure 31-6 Tuberculous adenitis. Note the erythematous swelling in this 13-year-old recent immigrant from southeast Asia who presented with bilateral posterior cervical neck masses. (Courtesy of Esther K. Chung, MD, MPH.)

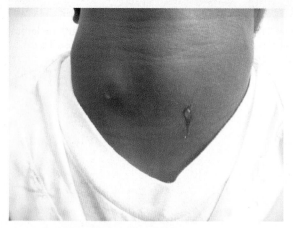

Figure 31-7 Branchial cleft cyst. Draining branchial cleft sinus. (Courtesy of Paul S. Matz, MD.)

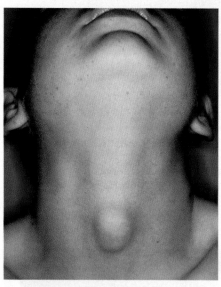

Figure 31-8 Thyroglossal duct cyst. A midline cervical mass presenting in a 6-year-old child. (Used with permission from Snell RS. *Clinical Anatomy.* 7th ed. Baltimore, MD: Lippincott Williams & Wilkins; 2005:CD418.)

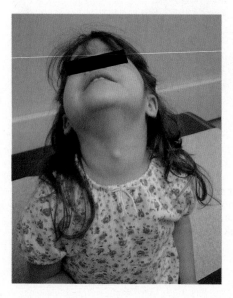

Figure 31-9 Dermoid cyst. A mass found midline overlying the hyoid bone in a 4-year-old child. (Courtesy of Mary L. Brandt, MD.)

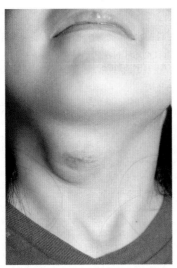

Figure 31-10 Venous malformation. (Courtesy of Eden Palmer and Jonathan Perkins, DO.)

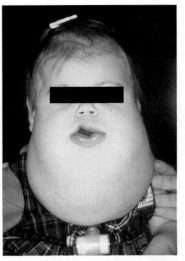

Figure 31-11 Cystic hygroma. A large, soft cervical mass in a 9-month-old infant. Tracheostomy was placed at birth. (Courtesy of Ellen Deutsch, MD.)

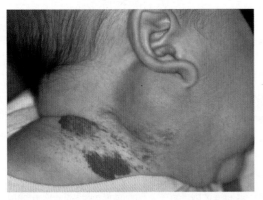

Figure 31-12 Hemangioma. A soft, nontender mass with bluish as well as bright-red aspects of color presents in this 1-month-old infant. (Courtesy of Ellen Deutsch, MD.)

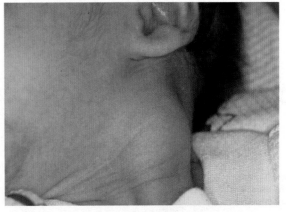

Figure 31-13 Congenital torticollis. A fibrotic mass located in the sternocleidomastoid muscle (SCM) of a 1-month-old infant whose mother was concerned about the infant's head tilt to one side. (Courtesy of Ellen Deutsch, MD.)

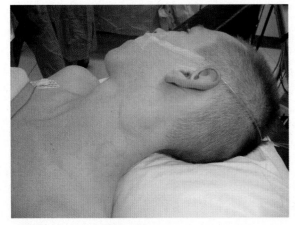

Figure 31-14 Hodgkin lymphoma. Large, fixed cervical masses in a 14-year-old adolescent with weight loss. (Courtesy of Mary L. Brandt, MD.)

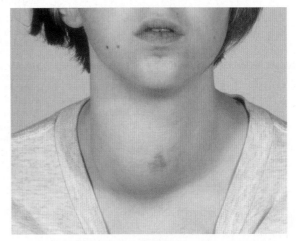

Figure 31-15 Thyroid lymphoma. (Courtesy of Eden Palmer and Jonathan Perkins, DO.)

DIFFERENTIAL DIAGNOSES

DIAGNOSIS	ICD-10	DISTINGUISHING CHARACTERISTICS	ASSOCIATED FINDINGS
INFLAMMATORY			
Cervical Lymphadenopathy	R59.0 Localized enlarged lymph nodes	Palpable lymph nodes common Often a normal finding, especially in those ages 3–5 Location based on location of predisposing infection, if present Not normal in infants Normal cervical lymph nodes up to 1 cm in size	Most commonly associated with predisposing viral/bacterial infection Affects approximately half of children of all ages, majority of those 4–8 years have no associated illness Oculoglandular syndrome: conjunctivitis and enlarged preauricular lymph node Ulceroglandular syndrome: skin lesion and regional lymphadenopathy
Cervical Lymphadenitis	L04.0 Acute lymphadenitis of face, head, and neck	Most common cause of lymph node enlargement in children Most common inflammatory lesion of cervical lymph nodes Usually acute onset of enlarged, painful node in setting of infection; may fluctuate	Usually during or after pharyngitis, tonsillitis, or acute otitis media Caused by *S. aureus* or group A Streptococcus in >80% of cases May be caused by anaerobes in older children, especially in setting of dental disease Usually have leukocytosis and bandemia Note: neonates can have group B Streptococcus "cellulitis–adenitis" syndrome between 3 and 7 weeks of age Patients are usually male and have fever, poor feeding, and adenitis
Chronic Cervical Lymphadenitis	CMI88.1 Chronic lymphadenitis, except mesenteric	Usually large, minimally tender, mildly inflamed, nonfluctuant, no systemic symptoms	Cat scratch/mycobacterial adenitis Enlargement of other lymph nodes Organomegaly
Cat Scratch Disease (*Bartonella henselae*)	A28.1 Cat scratch fever	Fairly common cause of benign lymphadenopathy in children May develop painful regional lymphadenopathy ~2 weeks after a minor scratch Often starts with one or more red papules at site of inoculation Fastidious, slow-growing, gram-negative bacillus seen via indirect immunofluorescent antibody assay, polymerase chain reaction assay, or Warthin–Starry silver stain (nonspecific)	Fever and mild systemic symptoms (fatigue, headache) in ~30% may be seen May present as Parinaud oculoglandular syndrome with conjunctivitis and preauricular or submandibular adenopathy
Mycobacterial Cervical Lymphadenitis	A31.9 Mycobacterial infection, unspecified A18.2 Tuberculous adenitis	Usually not as painful as acute bacterial adenitis and has longer onset than typical bacterial adenitis Firm, mobile Distinguish from typical TB as PPD is negative or only weakly positive, CXR normal	Usually no systemic symptoms

COMPLICATIONS	PREDISPOSING FACTORS	TREATMENT GUIDELINES
Lymphadenitis	Viral illness (i.e., rhinovirus, adenovirus, enterovirus, parainfluenza, influenza, RSV, coxsackievirus, measles, EBV, CMV) Pharyngitis	Observation Early biopsy of nodes that do not resolve Enlarged supraclavicular nodes are pathologic, until proven otherwise Posterior cervical nodes may be due to scalp infection but should be carefully monitored
Sepsis, risk of spread	Bacterial—seeding of lymph nodes from upper respiratory tract or oropharyngeal infection Usually *S. aureus* (MRSA), group A Streptococcus, anaerobes (oral flora) Viral—usually bilateral, shorter duration, self-limited, rarely suppurative	Consider blood culture, complete blood count (CBC), and liver enzymes Oral or parenteral penicillin, cephalosporin, or clindamycin, depending on etiology and degree of illness Tailor treatment based on culture, if available. Warm soaks, drainage if fluctuant; consider ultrasound to help make determination Approximately 10% of children end up needing I&D Send for aspirate or biopsy for Gram stain, culture, acid-fast stain, and mycobacterial culture.
Complications vary depending on underlying etiology	Usually infectious: reactive to viral/bacterial infection, atypical mycobacterial, tuberculous, Bartonella, HIV, Toxoplasma, EBV, CMV infections; hepatitis; sarcoidosis; histoplasmosis; actinomycosis; and malignancy	Labs: CBC with differential tests for mononucleosis, and potentially others (HIV, toxoplasmosis, histoplasmosis, and brucellosis) Chest x-ray, purified protein derivative (PPD) test Full antibiotic course Biopsy (ideally excisional) if does not resolve with antibiotics and if present for 6–8 weeks
Approximately one quarter of affected nodes become suppurative. Skin overlying affected node may be tender, warm, indurated; node may develop central avascular necrosis May cause systemic disease, neurologic or hematologic complications	More likely to be due to a kitten scratch. Often patient does not remember scratch No person-to-person transmission	Usually self-limited Resolves in approximately 8–12 weeks 5-day azithromycin course often recommended to shorten course of illness Needle aspiration may be needed for relief of symptoms; I&D and excision should be avoided as this is associated with persistent drainage and poor wound healing
May be suppurate, then become fluctuant Skin becomes thin and may spontaneously rupture May develop chronic drainage, if not excised while still encapsulated	From environmental contact, rather than person-to-person spread (from contaminated object into mouth)	May resolve on its own Complete excision of node while encapsulated is curative 3–6 months of antibiotic therapy with recurrence, incomplete excision, or chronic drainage

(continued)

DIFFERENTIAL DIAGNOSIS (continued)

DIAGNOSIS		ICD-10	DISTINGUISHING CHARACTERISTICS	ASSOCIATED FINDINGS
CONGENITAL				
Branchial cleft anomalies		Q18.0 Sinus, fistula, and cyst of branchial cleft	90% from second cleft or arch due to occlusion of tract Usually see remnants in anterior border of SCM as painless lateral neck mass or draining opening (but can occur anywhere along line from tonsillar fossa to supraclavicular neck) First: may present as cyst or sinus near external auditory canal, in parotid gland, or adjacent to pinna into anterior neck Third: may see thymic cysts present as neck mass with associated symptoms (dysphagia, hoarseness) in childhood	May be difficult to distinguish from acute lymphadenitis when superinfected May see cysts later in life, but sinus/fistula usually noted in infancy, usually along anterior of sternocleidomastoid
Thyroglossal Duct Cyst		Q89.2 Congenital malformations of other endocrine glands	Most common congenital neck mass (70%) and second most common benign neck mass after lymphadenopathy Ectodermal remnants along the thyroglossal duct, the line of descent of thyroid into neck from base of tongue Rare in newborn period, usually seen in children ages 2–10; up to 1/3 not identified until adulthood 80% at or just below the level of the hyoid	Ectopic thyroid tissue within remnant in ~1/4 of cases May present as painless midline mass or draining sinus One report notes that 35% of patients had previous infection.
Dermoid Cyst		L72.0 Epidermal cyst (among others) D36.0 Benign neoplasm of lymph nodes	Teratoma most common congenital tumor. Dermoid cyst are also known as mature cystic teratoma. Both contain sebaceous material; dermoid can contain sebaceous glands, hair follicles, connective tissue, and papillae Head and neck—second most common location for infants	Often noted prenatally May cause postnatal respiratory distress depending on location
Venous Malformation		Q27.9 Congenital malformation of peripheral vascular system, unspecified	Slow-flow lesion; most common vascular malformation Dysplastic venous channels Blue or purple, soft, compressible, nonpulsatile, usually solitary Often present at birth Grow proportionately; often enlarge at puberty or with trauma	Expand with valsalva maneuver or dependency
Cystic Hygroma		D18.1 Lymphangioma, any site	Benign multiloculated cystic lymphatic malformation (dysplastic proliferation of lymphatic vessels) Soft, compressible, transilluminates, painless Cystic hygroma usually in posterior triangle of neck; twice as likely on left 1 in 12,000 births, with approximately half identified at birth and the majority by the end of the second year of life	Continue to produce lymphatic fluid May be associated with Turner syndrome, Noonan syndrome, and trisomies 13, 18, and 21 Microcystic, macrocystic, or mixed; microcystic usually more infiltrative

COMPLICATIONS	PREDISPOSING FACTORS	TREATMENT GUIDELINES
Treat superinfection with antibiotics and warm soaks Probing and dye studies are usually unnecessary and can cause infection	May be familial in the rare cases of bilateral anomalies 4th–8th week gestation: four pairs of branchial arches and intervening clefts form that eventually become head and neck structures	Treat by complete excision as early as possible; waiting leads to further risk of infection Recurrence rate: <7% after resection Defer resection until infection resolved as resection during infection has increased complication risk of injury to adjacent structures
Commonly becomes infected Papillary adenocarcinoma found in up to 10% of adults undergoing excision (<1% in all patients)	4th–7th week gestation, thyroid diverticulum develops at foramen cecum at base of tongue, descends to final location in anterior midline of neck. Duct involutes after thyroid gland reaches final destination by week 8	Treatment: Sistrunk procedure—complete excision of cyst and sinus tract up to the base of tongue including central portion of the hyoid bone Risk of recurrence after resection is <10% (greater, if previously infected or resection incomplete)
May become infected May occasionally become malignant	Develops along embryonic fusion lines when ectodermal cells become buried below the skin surface	Excise completely to diagnose, for cosmesis, and to ensure no rare malignant transformation Note: Perform CT ± MRI for midline cysts over nasal bridge to determine potential penetration of calvarium
Phleboliths often noted in imaging—may cause pain and swelling May cause distortion of facial features Stasis may cause local or general coagulopathy Bleeding or clotting rare	Consider hereditary syndrome, if multifocal	Sclerotherapy shrinks lesion and helps with symptoms; often require multiple treatments Resection for some
May get infected or suddenly enlarge due to bleeding Enlarge and can compress/stretch nearby anatomic structures including airway May cause speech problems due to dental or jaw complications Usually grow proportionally, though can grow faster with trauma, infection, or hemorrhage	Failure of primordial lymphatic buds to establish route of drainage into venous system Two-thirds of those with cervicofacial malformation require tracheostomy	Controversial whether can regress. Treat those that are painful, cause deformity, or compromise nearby structures Complete excision is treatment of choice: Usually at 2–6 months unless complications arise. May lead to cranial nerve paralysis, infection, seroma. May recur, especially if excision incomplete Sclerotherapy for macrocystic type Other options: radiation, CO_2 laser, embolization for bleeding. Aspiration only for emergency decompression (risk recurrence, hemorrhage, infection) Prophylactic antibiotics if >3 infections per year

(continued)

SECTION 8 • NECK

DIFFERENTIAL DIAGNOSIS *(continued)*

DIAGNOSIS	ICD-10	DISTINGUISHING CHARACTERISTICS	ASSOCIATED FINDINGS
CONGENITAL *(Cont'd)*			
Hemangioma	D18.01 Hemangioma skin and subcutaneous tissue	Benign vascular tumor; true vascular neoplasm (rather than a malformation) Most common head/neck lesion of infancy: 2.5% of newborns. 2/3 in head and neck, though 20% of infants may have multiple sites (brain, liver, GI tract, airway) 30% present in first week of life; most noticeable after first month "Proliferative phase": Usually larger over first year, then up to 80% spontaneously involute by 5 years. Those that do not completely involute by then may continue to over the next 5 years	PHACES: Segmental/trigeminal hemangioma plus one of the following: posterior fossa brain malformation, arterial cerebrovascular anomalies, cardiac defects (often coarctation), eye/endocrine abnormalities Distinguish from RICH (rapidly involuting congenital hemangioma) and NICH (noninvoluting congenital hemangioma) that are fully grown at birth
Congenital Torticollis	Q68.0 Congenital deformity of sternocleidomastoid muscle	Shortening of sternocleidomastoid muscle due to fibrosis: pulls head and neck toward affected side Collagen and fibroblasts form fibrous tumor around atrophied muscle Usually noticed at 2–8 weeks of age	Evaluate older children for cervical rotary subluxation, ocular torticollis, midbrain lesions
NEOPLASTIC			
Lymphoma	R22.1 Localized Swelling, Mass and Lump, Neck C81 Hodgkin Lymphoma C85.91 Non-Hodgkin lymphoma, unspecified, lymph nodes of head, face, and neck	Most common head/neck malignancy in children Hodgkins lymphoma (40%): usually painless rubbery/mobile cervical/supraclavicular adenopathy; may aggregate to form bulky masses, cause pain if hemorrhage into node. Rare before age 5; male predominance 2–3:1. Non-Hodgkins lymphoma (60%): 10% of childhood cancers; 10% in head and neck. Usually age 7–11; male predominance 3:1. Often extranodal, presents aggressively	May have pallor, bruising, petechiae, hepatosplenomegaly

COMPLICATIONS	PREDISPOSING FACTORS	TREATMENT GUIDELINES
May ulcerate, become infected, necrose Periorbital hemangioma can cause vision-related complications 3–5% may produce severe complications: bleeding, platelet-trapping (leading to thrombocytopenia and coagulopathy), airway compromise, heart failure May have residual discoloration or redundant skin	Up to 20% of low birth weight preterm infants Females/males 3:1	Treat usually with watchful waiting, though treatment modalities exist For large/complicated hemangiomas: propranolol (found to reduce color, volume, and elevation; watch for bradycardia, hypotension, hypoglycemia) sclerotherapy, vincristine, interferon-α, steroid injection (best if small and localized), chemotherapy, radiation, laser therapy Consider excision if obstruction, recurrent bleeding, and/or ulceration present Imaging only for questionable, atypical, or large lesion or for surgical planning
	Likely originates prenatally (associated with developmental dysplasia of the hip and tibial torsion) and therefore not due to obstetrical complications	Most treated with PT: Massage, range of motion, and stretching; positional changes that force looking to contralateral side Surgery (transection of middle third of muscle) between ages 1 and 2 if facial hemihypoplasia develops (usually within 6 months without treatment)—gradually resolves after treatment
Neoplastic lymphoma is often diffuse at time of diagnosis	Non-Hodgkin lymphoma more often in the immunocompromised	Chemotherapy Radiation Extensive surgical resection is warranted only in localized low-grade lymphomas.

- Less common causes of infection/lymphadenopathy:

  - Viral: VZV, HSV, HIV, measles, and mumps

  - Bacterial: anaerobes, enteric bacteria (Acinetobacter, *E. coli*, Proteus, Salmonella, Shigella), zoonoses (Brucella, *Francisella tularensis, Yersinia pestis, Yersinia enterocolitica*), spirochetes, Rickettsiae, and leptospirosis

  - Mycobacterial: tuberculosis

  - Fungal: Aspergillus, Histoplasma, Cryptococcus, and coccidiomycosis

  - Protozoa: Toxoplasma, Leishmania, and Trypanosoma

- Immunodeficiencies (Hyper IgE, leukocyte adhesion deficiency, chronic granulomatous disease)

- Pyriform sinus

- Other vascular anomalies (e.g., fast-flow AV malformations)

- Benign tumors: lipoma, fibroma, benign thyroid nodules, and neurofibromas

- Other malignant neoplasms

  - Neuroblastoma, thyroid carcinoma, melanoma, neurogenic tumors, and rhabdomyosarcoma

- Cervical rib

- Kawasaki disease

- Ectopic thyroid

- Connective tissue/autoimmune diseases (lupus, juvenile idiopathic arthritis, and dermatomyositis)

- Serum sickness

- Enlargement of supraclavicular or posterior cervical nodes

- Systemic symptoms concerning for malignancy (e.g., night sweats, weight loss)

- Painless, firm, immobile nodes

- Generally, a node larger than 2 cm

- A single, enlarged node (>1 cm) that does not improve/resolve within 4 to 6 weeks with appropriate antibiotic therapy

SUGGESTED READINGS

Abramowicz S. Padwa BL. Vascular anomalies in children. *Oral Maxillofac Surg Clin N Am.* 2012;24(3):443–455.

American Academy of Pediatrics. *Red Book: 2012 Report of the Committee on Infectious Diseases.* 29th ed. Elk Grove Village, IL: American Academy of Pediatrics; 2012:269–271, 736–767.

Dickson PV, Davidoff AM. Malignant neoplasms of the head and neck. *Sem Pediatr Surg.* 2006;15(2):92–98.

Friedmann AM. Evaluation and management of lymphadenopathy in children. *Pediatr Rev.* 2008;29(2):53–60.

Gross E, Sichel JY. Congenital neck lesions. *Surg Clin North Am.* 2006;86(2):383–392.

Gujar S, Gandhi D, Mukherji SK. Pediatric head and neck masses. *Topics Magn Resonan Imag.* 2004;15(2):95–101.

Kliegman R, Behrman R, Jenson H, et al. Nontuberculous mycobacteria. In: *Nelson Textbook of Pediatrics.* 19th ed. 2011:1011–1016.

Kliegman R, et al. Cat-scratch disease (Bartonella henselae). In: *Nelson Textbook of Pediatrics.* 19th ed. 2011:983–986.

Koch BL. Cystic malformations of the neck in children. *Pediatr Radiol.* 2005;35(5):463–477.

CHEST

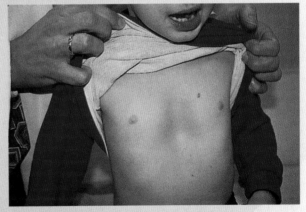

NINE

(Courtesy of George A. Datto, III, MD.)

Abnormal Chest Shape

Amy E. Renwick

Approach to the Problem

Several elements contribute to chest shape, including muscles, bones (ribs, sternum, clavicles, and spine), and underlying organs. Deficiency, hypertrophy, or malformation of any of these structures may produce abnormalities in the appearance of the chest wall. Abnormalities in lung form or function may cause changes in the chest shape; conversely, alterations in the size or shape of the thorax may significantly affect pulmonary function. Rarely, chronic cardiac enlargement may produce a prominence in the precordial chest wall. Pectus excavatum is the most common pediatric chest wall deformity; most of the others are quite rare.

Key Points in the History

- Pectus excavatum and pectus carinatum are more common in males.

- Family history is often positive in patients with pectus excavatum.

- Asymmetry in the immediate neonatal period may be the result of intrauterine compression.

- Children who have symptoms of severe exercise intolerance with abnormal chest shape may have underlying pulmonary or cardiac disease.

- Surgery of the chest wall increases the risk of developing deformities.

Key Points in the Physical Examination

- Tall stature, arachnodactyly, and joint laxity suggest Marfan syndrome in patients with pectus excavatum or pectus carinatum.

- Syndactyly and brachydactyly are associated with Poland syndrome. Poland syndrome is more common in males. Patients have absence of the pectoralis muscle, more often on the right.

- Short stature and webbed neck with shield chest (broad, with widely spaced nipples) may be seen in Turner or Noonan syndrome. Patients with Noonan syndrome also may have pectus excavatum or pectus carinatum.

- Narrow shoulders with various anomalies of the clavicles and upper extremities occur in Holt–Oram syndrome (which is also associated with cardiac and sternal defects) and cleidocranial dysplasia (in which underdeveloped or absent clavicles, delays in fontanel closure, and tooth eruption also may be seen).

- A narrow or bell-shaped thorax is associated with many osteochondrodysplasias, such as achondroplasia, cleidocranial dysplasia, and Jeune thoracic dystrophy (small chest, short ribs and shortened bones in extremities). It may also be seen in patients with neuromuscular disorders.

- Skin overlying a sternal cleft may be thin, scarlike, and hyperpigmented.

PHOTOGRAPHS OF SELECTED DIAGNOSES

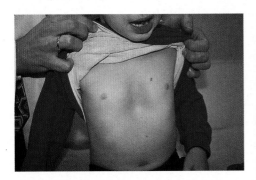

Figure 32-1 **Pectus excavatum.** Anterior view of child with pectus excavatum. (Courtesy of George A. Datto, III, MD.)

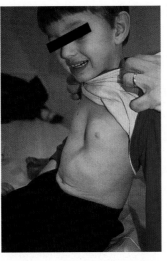

Figure 32-2 **Pectus excavatum.** Lateral view of child with pectus excavatum. (Courtesy of George A. Datto, III, MD.)

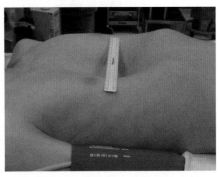

Figure 32-3 **Pectus excavatum.** Severe pectus in an adolescent with significant exercise intolerance. (Courtesy of Christopher D. Derby, MD.)

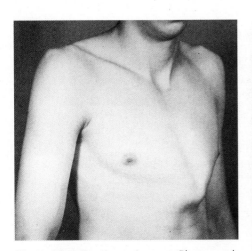

Figure 32-4 **Pectus carinatum.** Photograph of (a)symmetric chondrogladiolar pectus carinatum in a 19-year-old man. (Adapted with permission from Shamberger RC. Chest wall deformities. In: Shields TW, ed. *General Thoracic Surgery*. 4th ed. Baltimore, MD: Williams & Wilkins, 1994:529–557.)

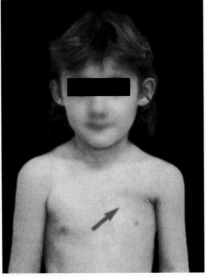

Figure 32-5 **Poland syndrome.** Absence of pectoralis major muscle. (Used with permission from Staheli LT. *Practice of Pediatric Orthopedics*. Philadelphia, PA: Lippincott Williams & Wilkins; 2001:192.)

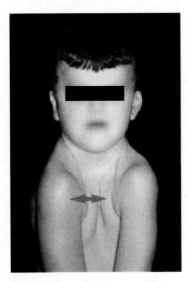

Figure 32-6 **Cleidocranial dysplasia.** Narrow chest with drooping shoulders. (Used with permission from Staheli LT. *Practice of Pediatric Orthopedics*. Philadelphia, PA: Lippincott Williams & Wilkins; 2001:192.)

SECTION 9 • CHEST

DIFFERENTIAL DIAGNOSIS

DIAGNOSIS	ICD-10	DISTINGUISHING CHARACTERISTICS	DISTRIBUTION	DURATION/ CHRONICITY
Pectus Excavatum	Congenital Q67.6 Acquired M95.4 Rachitic E64.3	Sternal depression Sternum may rotate to right, making right-sided structures smaller Deformity worsens during puberty	Midline in sternum	Chronic, may worsen over time
Pectus Carinatum	Congenital Q67.7 Acquired M95.4 Rachitic E64.3	Sternal protrusion Generally noted later in childhood than pectus excavatum	Midline sternum	Chronic, worsens over time
Barrel Chest	M95.4	Anteroposterior diameter of chest increased relative to transverse diameter. (Normal ratio is 1:1 in infancy, with transverse diameter increasing with age.)	Entire chest	Chronic
Shield Chest	M95.4	Wide chest with broadly spaced nipples	Entire chest	Chronic
Poland Sequence	Q79.8	Unilateral deficiency of pectoralis muscles and breast structures Usually right-sided	Most often right-sided	Chronic
Sternal Cleft	Q76.7	Complete or partial separation of sternum May manifest as U-shaped or V-shaped depression, or with bulge from underlying structures May change with respiration Pulsations of heart may be visible. If there is overlying skin, it is often thin and hyperpigmented.	Midline over sternum	Chronic
Cleidocranial Dysplasia	Q74.0	Absent or hypoplastic clavicles, resulting in abnormal shoulder movement Narrow thorax	Generally bilateral clavicles and entire thorax	Chronic

ASSOCIATED FINDINGS	COMPLICATIONS	PREDISPOSING FACTORS	TREATMENT GUIDELINES
Increased incidence of scoliosis, congenital heart disease May be associated with Marfan syndrome, homocystinuria, Noonan syndrome, and other genetic disorders	Rarely interferes with cardiac or respiratory function, though some children have exercise limitations May be a significant cosmetic problem Can give false appearance of cardiomegaly on chest x-ray	Excessive growth of costal cartilage Male:female prevalence ratio 3:1	Treatment is often not necessary. Surgical correction may have psychological benefits. Significant physiological benefits of surgery are uncertain.
As for pectus excavatum	Rarely interferes with cardiac or respiratory function, though some children have exercise limitations May be a significant cosmetic problem	Excessive growth of costal cartilage More common in males	Treatment is often not necessary. Surgical correction may have psychological benefits. Physiological benefits of surgery are controversial.
Digital clubbing	According to underlying cause	Severe asthma or other obstructive lung disease (e.g., meconium aspiration syndrome) Genetic disorders such as spondyloepiphyseal dysplasia, Smith–McCort dysplasia, Costello syndrome	Address underlying cause if possible.
Turner syndrome Noonan syndrome	According to underlying cause	N/A	N/A
May also have rib defects. Ipsilateral syndactyly of hand	Respiratory problems when significant rib defects are present Breast tissue also is typically absent on affected side.	Male:female prevalence ratio 3:1 Abnormal blood flow through subclavian artery	Breast reconstruction may be considered, particularly for females
Usually an isolated anomaly Ectopia cordis Pentalogy of Cantrell Facial hemangiomas Cleft lip or palate	None (unless associated defects)	None	Surgical repair in infancy
Variety of other skeletal anomalies Delayed closure of sutures and anterior fontanel Abnormal teeth Delayed tooth eruption Hearing impairment Osteoporosis	Respiratory problems in infancy	Autosomal dominant inheritance	Extensive dental work often necessary Monitor for hearing loss Measure bone mineral density starting in early adolescence

SECTION 9 • CHEST

Other Diagnoses to Consider

- Vertebral deformities

- Acute or healed injuries

- Isolated rib anomalies

- Isolated clavicular anomalies

- Other genetic syndromes or congenital malformations

- Chest wall masses

When to Consider Further Evaluation or Treatment

- Perceived limitations of exercise tolerance in patients with pectus excavatum or pectus carinatum can be evaluated with pulmonary function testing or exercise tolerance testing.

- Surgical intervention may be considered for patients with significant psychosocial concerns relating to pectus excavatum or pectus carinatum.

- Surgery to correct severe pectus excavatum may improve subjective exercise tolerance and some measures of cardiac and pulmonary function.

- Patients with sternal cleft should be evaluated for other midline abnormalities.

- Sternal clefts are usually repaired in infancy.

- Breast reconstruction may be performed for patients, especially females, with Poland syndrome.

- Patients with cleidocranial dysplasia should have a hearing evaluation, and often require extensive dental work.

SUGGESTED READINGS

Grissom LE, Harcke HT. Thoracic deformities and the growing lung. *Semin Roentgenol.* 1998;33:199–208.
Jayaramakrishnan K, Wotton R, Bradley A, Naidu B. Does repair of pectus excavatum improve cardiopulmonary function? *Interact Cardiovasc Thorac Surg.* 2013;16:865–870.
Jones KL, Jones MC, Casanelles MD. Recognizable patterns of malformation. In: *Smith's Recognizable Patterns of Human Malformation.* 7th ed. Philadelphia, PA: Elsevier Saunders; 2013:78–82, 164–167, 400–401, 420–421, 526–528.
McGuigan RM, Azarow KS. Congenital chest wall defects. *Surg Clin North Am.* 2006;86:353–370.
Myers NA. An approach to the management of chest wall deformities. *Prog Pediatr Surg.* 1991;27:170–190.
Nuss D, Kelly Jr RE. Congenital chest wall deformities. In: Holcomb III GM, Murphy JP, eds. *Ashcraft's Pediatric Surgery.* 5th ed. Philadelphia, PA: WB Saunders; 2010:249–265.
Ravitch M. *Congenital Deformities of the Chest Wall and Their Operative Correction.* Philadelphia, PA: WB Saunders; 1977.
Staheli LT. *Fundamentals of Pediatric Orthopedics.* 4th ed. Philadelphia, PA: Lippincott Williams & Wilkins; 2007:112.

Breast Swelling and Enlargement

D'Juanna White-Satcher

Approach to the Problem

It is important to consider the age of the patient and his or her stage of pubertal development when assessing the potential cause of breast enlargement, as it is common for an individual's breasts to develop at different rates. Disorders involving breast swelling most often present during the pubertal years, although they may occur in infancy and early childhood. Many patients may be uncomfortable disclosing breast concerns during an initial patient history; therefore, related abnormalities may be only coincidentally identified during routine physical examination. A breast examination should be performed as part of every well child care visit.

Some of the most common breast concerns, such as breast asymmetry and gynecomastia, may not be true diseases but rather normal physiological variants. Breast enlargement and swelling may also be congenital, infectious, or hormonal in etiology. In male patients, the most common cause of breast tissue development is benign physiologic gynecomastia.

Key Points in the History

- Breast tissue development occurring in females less than 8 years of age is generally considered to be abnormal, although there may be racial or ethnic variations noted.

- Benign gynecomastia often begins as unilateral breast enlargement and involves the right side twice as often as the left.

- Breast tissue in gynecomastia tends to be tender and/or painful soon after the onset of breast enlargement.

- Development of gynecomastia either before puberty begins or after puberty is completed would not be consistent with benign physiologic gynecomastia.

- In a teenager with gynecomastia, the history should include a list of any medications or recreational drugs that the patient might be using, as drugs may be the cause of gynecomastia. Some drugs associated with gynecomastia include anabolic steroids, marijuana, heroin, isoniazid (INH), metronidazole, dilantin, ketoconazole, ranitidine, and omeprazole.

- Rapid, painful growth of breast tissue in females in early adolescence is seen with a diagnosis of juvenile breast hypertrophy.

- A history of significant chest wall trauma in the prepubertal female may predispose to underdevelopment of the breast on the side of the trauma and thus contribute to breast asymmetry.

- A history of breastfeeding, nipple piercing, or breast trauma often precedes the development of a breast infection.

Key Points in the Physical Examination

- There is considerable variability in the size, shape, and consistency of breasts among individuals.

- An individual's breasts may develop at different rates, which can result in a different Tanner stage for each breast.

- Although breast asymmetry may be a normal physiological variant, a physical exam ination that includes inspection and palpation should be done to rule out a mass lesion in the larger breast.

- Erythema, warmth, and tenderness of the breast would support the diagnosis of an infectious process, such as mastitis or breast abscess.

- In the evaluation of premature thelarche, the patient must be examined for other signs of pubertal development, such as the presence of pubic hair, axillary hair, or a growth spurt.

- In an overweight patient, fatty tissue may be confused with breast development. A physical examination that includes palpation is necessary to determine whether breast tissue is present.

- Physiologic gynecomastia in males, if it occurs, usually presents when a male is in Tanner stages II–III for pubic hair and genitalia.

PHOTOGRAPHS OF SELECTED DIAGNOSES

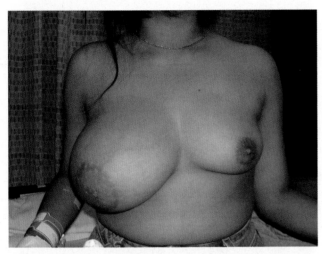

Figure 33-1 Breast asymmetry. Adolescent female with Tanner stage III breast development and significantly asymmetric breasts. (Courtesy of Mary L. Brandt, MD.)

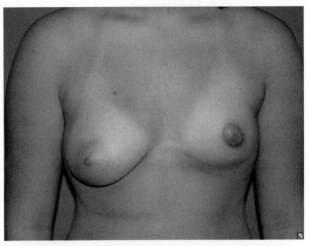

Figure 33-2 Breast asymmetry. Note the left breast is smaller, although with a normal appearance. (Courtesy of Jeff Friedman, MD.)

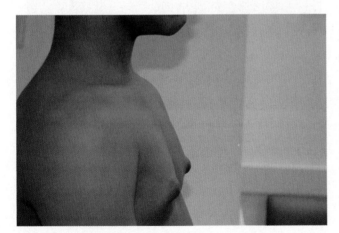

Figure 33-3 Gynecomastia. Thirteen-year-old boy with gynecomastia Tanner stage II breasts. (Courtesy of D'Juanna White-Satcher, MD, MPH.)

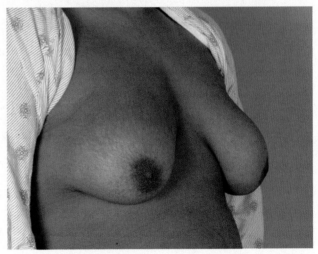

Figure 33-4 Gynecomastia. Fourteen-year-old boy with cosmetically significant benign gynecomastia—both breasts in Tanner stage III. (Courtesy of Lior Heller, MD.)

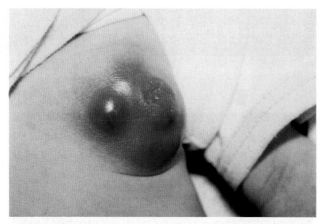

Figure 33-5 **Mastitis.** Ten-day-old female infant with swelling and erythema of the left breast. (Used with permission from Fleisher GR, Ludwig S, Baskin MN, et al. *Pictorial Review of Pediatrics.* Baltimore, MD: Lippincott Williams & Wilkins; 1998:185.)

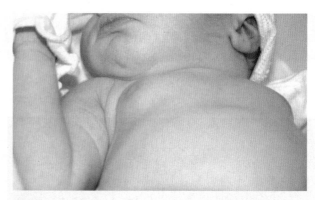

Figure 33-6 **Neonatal breast hypertrophy.** Two-week-old female infant with right breast hypertrophy. (Courtesy of D'Juanna White-Satcher, MD, MPH.)

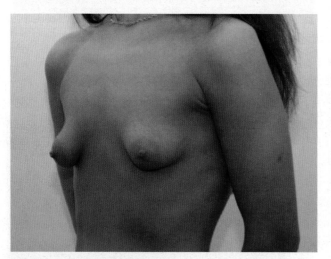

Figure 33-7 **Tuberous breast.** Note hypoplasia and sagging of breast tissue at chest wall on right breast. (Courtesy of David A. Horvath, MD.)

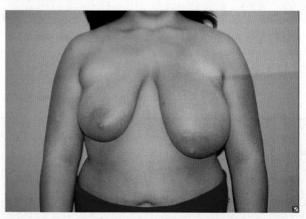

Figure 33-8 **Juvenile breast hypertrophy.** Note pendulous left breast in this 13-year-old girl. Also, the patient presents with asymmetric breasts. (Courtesy of Jeff Friedman, MD.)

DIFFERENTIAL DIAGNOSIS

DIAGNOSIS	ICD-10	DISTINGUISING CHARACTERISTICS	DURATION	ASSOCIATED FINDINGS	PREDISPOSING FACTORS	TREATMENT GUIDELINES
Breast Asymmetry	Q83.8	Size difference between breasts No palpable mass in larger breast	May resolve after puberty 25% persists into adulthood	Left breast is more often larger	May have history of prepubertal trauma or surgery involving the smaller breast	Breast pads Cosmetic surgery, if severe, after breast development is complete
Gynecomastia	N62	Rubbery or firm breast tissue Size may vary from a small nodule beneath areola to a size resembling female Tanner stage II–III breast	Physiological: 1–2 years Nonphysiological: may resolve if causal agent removed	More prevalent in obese patients	Physiological: puberty, family history Nonphysiological: variety of therapeutic and recreational drugs, liver disease, Klinefelter syndrome, and hormone-secreting tumor	Surgery, if not resolved after puberty or after discontinuation of involved medicine or resolution of medical condition
Mastitis/Neonatal Mastitis	N61/ P39.0	Erythema, warmth, induration, pain Unilateral Fever may be present	Resolves with appropriate therapy	N/A	Breast or nipple trauma Breastfeeding	Antibiotics Warm compresses
Premature Thelarche	E30.8	Breast development in a non-African-American girl <8 years (<6 years in African American) No other signs of pubertal development present	Evolves into normal pubertal development	No other signs of pubertal development should be present	Family history Exogenous estrogen exposure	N/A
Pseudogynecomastia (Lipomastia)	N62	No breast tissue present Fatty tissue or excessive muscular development in breast region	Lifelong unless weight loss occurs	Obesity	Obesity	Weight loss, although may not completely resolve
Neonatal Breast Hypertrophy	P83.4	Unilateral or bilateral Present at birth or shortly thereafter	Weeks to 2–3 months of age	May be associated with white milky discharge	Present in 70% of newborns	Self resolves
Tuberous Breast	Q83.9	Breast base is limited in size but nipple-areola is overdeveloped	Lifelong	None	Although congenital, it becomes notable with puberty	Surgical after full breast development for cosmesis
Juvenile Breast Hypertrophy	N62	Rapid growth Painful May be associated with thinning of skin and overlying venous distension Can be unilateral	N/A	Can result in psychological problems/self-esteem issues	Puberty Family history	Hormonal manipulation and/or surgery may be considered after complete breast development
Polymastia/Polythe-lia (Supernumerary Nipple; Accessory Breast)	Q83.3/ Q83.1	Unilateral or bilateral	Since birth May not become notable until puberty or lactation	Occasionally associated with genitourinary or cardiovascular anomalies	Family history	Surgical excision if desired for cosmetic reasons

Other Diagnoses to Consider

- Fibroadenoma

- Trauma

- Foreign body

- Breast cyst

- McCune–Albright syndrome

- Klinefelter syndrome

- Neoplastic disorders

When to Consider Further Evaluation or Treatment

- If surgical intervention is being considered, it should be delayed until breast development is complete, usually after 18 years of age.

- Patients with breast tissue enlargement greater than 4 cm before the onset of puberty should be evaluated for potential underlying pathology.

- In a patient with isolated premature thelarche, one should consider obtaining a bone age, especially if a growth spurt has been noted.

- In a patient with premature thelarche who has other secondary signs of sexual maturation, further evaluation for precocious puberty is recommended.

SUGGESTED READINGS

Diamantopoulos S, Bao Y. Gynecomastia and premature thelarche: a guide for practitioners. *Pediatr Rev.* 2007;28(9):e57–e66.
DiVastas A, Weldon C, Labow B. The breast: examination and lesions. In: Emana SJ, Laufer MR, Goldstein DP, eds. *Pediatric and Adolescent Gynecology.* 6th ed. Philadelphia, PA: Lippincott Williams & Wilkins; 2011:405–419.
Greydanus D, Matytsina L, Gains M. Breast disorders in children and adolescents. *Prim Care Clin Office Pract.* 2006;33(2):455–502.
Macdonald HR. Breast disorders. In: Neinstein LS, ed. *Adolescent Health Care: A Practical Guide.* 5th ed. Philadelphia, PA: Lippincott Williams & Wilkins; 2007:754–763.

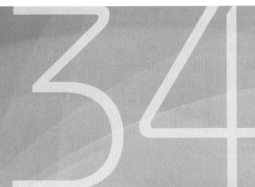

Chest Lumps

Barbara W. Bayldon and Tomitra Latimer

Approach to the Problem

Chest wall lumps should be divided into those of skeletal origin, by far the most common, and those of nonskeletal origin. Skeletal causes of lumps include trauma, accidental or nonaccidental, rickets, and, less commonly, malignancy, infection or congenital anomalies. Nonskeletal lumps represent abnormalities of other chest wall elements resulting in accessory nipples, precocious puberty, male gynecomastia, hemangiomas, or infection. Skeletal lumps, other than a prominent xyphoid process, should all be evaluated by medical imaging, and child physical abuse should be considered in the differential diagnosis of traumatic or unexplained injuries.

Key Points in the History

- In neonates, skeletal anomalies likely represent a clavicle callus from a missed clavicle fracture, or a congenital skeletal anomaly.

- Although dark-skinned infants and toddlers are most at risk, rickets should be considered in any infant, especially breast-fed infants, who have not had vitamin D supplementation, and older children with intake less than the equivalent quantity of vitamin D (400 IU) found in 1,000 ml of vitamin D fortified milk.

- The most common infant nonskeletal lump is an accessory nipple.

- Rib fractures in an infant or child, usually posterior, strongly suggest child physical abuse. Significant force is needed to fracture children's ribs since the thoracic cage is compliant and elastic when young. Children with acquired skeletal lumps should be evaluated for nonaccidental trauma. In preadolescents, trauma represents the most likely cause of a skeletal anomaly, usually resulting from a motor vehicle accident or fall from a height.

- Preadolescents may have either precocious thelarche or, especially when obese, pseudoprecocious puberty. Precocious puberty is much less frequent.

- Adolescent males may complain of lumps that reflect gynecomastia.

- Bone malignancies rarely present in the first decade.

273

- Congenital and asymptomatic lumps are usually benign. Pectus carinatum is rare and is often not diagnosed at birth but can be associated with an underlying ventriculoseptal defect.

- Growth over time raises concern for infection, malignancy, or trauma.

- A hemangioma will grow over time and then involute.

- Pain, redness, or other associated symptoms raise the concern of infection, malignancy, or trauma.

Key Points in the Physical Examination

- Tenderness or erythema at the location is concerning for trauma, infection, and malignancy.

- Concurrent additional areas of skeletal tenderness, bruising, or other unexplained marks on the skin are suggestive of child physical abuse. A complete musculoskeletal and skin examination should be performed.

- Rickets is characterized by a bilateral "rachitic rosary" (enlarged costochondral junctions) and can be accompanied by thickened wrists and ankles, and genu varus or valgus as well as frontal bossing, delayed fontanelle closure, and teeth eruption.

- Newborn clavicle fractures are associated with brachial plexus injury 10% of the time, so a careful ipsilateral upper extremity neurologic examination should be done.

- Supernumerary nipples are located along the milk (or mammary) line and are usually smaller than normal nipples and ill-formed.

- Pseudoprecocious puberty, a condition in which fat deposition mimics breast development (the areola is small, and the nipple is flat), needs to be differentiated from true precocious puberty.

PHOTOGRAPHS OF SELECTED DIAGNOSES

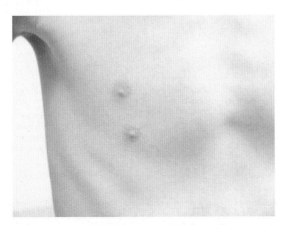

Figure 34-1 Supernumerary nipple. Fully developed nipple in embryonic milk line. (Courtesy of Philip Siu, MD.)

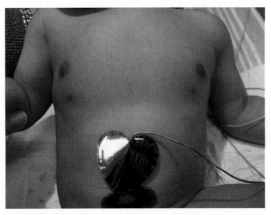

Figure 34-2 Supernumerary nipples. Bilateral supernumerary nipples in a newborn. (Courtesy of Esther K. Chung, MD, MPH.)

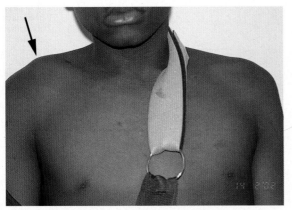

Figure 34-3 Clavicular fracture. Distal clavicular fracture with swelling over child's acromioclavicular joint. (Used with permission from Fleisher GR, Ludwig S, Baskin MN, eds. *Atlas of Pediatric Emergency Medicine*. Philadelphia, PA: Lippincott Williams & Wilkins; 2004:362.)

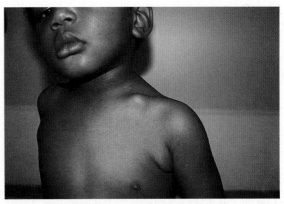

Figure 34-4 Pseudoarthrosis of clavicle (nonunion of fracture with healing) of clavicle. Painless swelling of mid-clavicle. (Courtesy of George A. Datto, III, MD.)

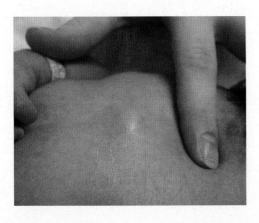

Figure 34-5 Prominent xyphoid process. Firm, painless palpable xyphoid process in an infant. (Courtesy of Esther K. Chung, MD, MPH.)

DIFFERENTIAL DIAGNOSIS

DIAGNOSIS	ICD 10	DISTINGUISHING CHARACTERISTICS	DISTRIBUTION	DURATION/ CHRONICITY	ASSOCIATED FINDINGS	COMPLICATIONS	PREDISPOSING FACTORS	TREATMENT GUIDELINES
Super-numerary Nipple	Q83.3	Small ill-shaped nipple	Milk (or mammary) line	Congenital	None	None, except cosmetic	Congenital	None, except if opting for surgical removal
Clavicle Fracture	Clavicle fracture S42.0 Clavicle fracture due to birth injury P13.4	Crepitus or swelling over clavicle	Clavicle	Short	Brachial plexus injury	Malalignment, long-term brachial plexus deficits	Trauma	No intervention in neonates In older children, consider figure 8 splint
Rickets	E55.0	Rachitic rosary	Costochondral junctions	Months	Bowing of legs, splayed wrists	Hypotonia and delayed motor milestone, hypocalcemic seizures	Inadequate intake of vitamin D, or lack of necessary enzyme or renal wasting, depending on etiology	Initiation of adequate intake of vitamin D with maintenance of calcium intake to avoid hungry bone syndrome, or in cases of genetic abnormality, calcitriol
Rib Fractures	S22.3	Pain, tenderness, shallow breathing	Anywhere over ribs but more likely lower ribs, with child physical abuse more likely to be posterior	Short	With child physical abuse, look for other fractures and marks such as bruises, retinal hemorrhages in young children	Ineffective breathing, pulmonary contusion, or abdominal organ injury	Trauma If have underlying defect, such as cancer or osteogenesis imperfecta, trauma may be minimal	Ensure adequate breathing, pain control
Prominent Xyphoid Process	Q76.9	Prominent bony protrusion at the lower part of sternum	Lower sternum	Congenital	None	None	None	No treatment needed
Precocious Thelarche	E30.8	Breast bud	Nipple area	Months	Other signs of puberty	If associated with precocious puberty, short stature	If central precocious puberty, activation of the hypothalamus–pituitary–gonadal axis	Usually none. Serial examinations are recommended to see if this becomes associated with precocious puberty.

Other Diagnoses to Consider

- The most important diagnoses to rule out are a child physical abuse or, less often, malignancy or infection.

- Malignancies include the following:

  - Osteosarcoma is the most common bone malignancy

  - Ewing sarcoma

  - Rhabdomyosarcoma

  - Metastatic disease

- Bifid rib

- Osteochondroma

- Osteomyelitis (very rare in the chest)

- An underlying heart condition may cause a precordial bulge.

- Osteogenesis imperfecta may be a cause of pathologic fracture. Look for blue sclera, and also explore family history and the patient's past history of any fractures.

- Poland syndrome: absence of the pectoralis muscle, the ipsilateral ribs, and/or syndactyly

When to Consider Further Evaluation or Treatment

- Most noncongenital lumps deserve further evaluation.

- A lump associated with pain, erythema, and soft tissue swelling or any constitutional symptoms should raise concern for trauma, infection, or malignancy. A prompt evaluation should be done.

- Precocious puberty, breast development before 7 years of age in Caucasian girls and before 6 years of age in African American girls deserves further evaluation and/or referral. Older definitions of precocious puberty use age 8 years as the cutoff for evaluation.

- Gynecomastia in prepubertal males, other than in infancy, should be considered pathologic.

- Medical imaging is important for evaluation of possible fractures, malignancies, and rickets. When evaluation of the bones is desired, it is important to specify this to the radiologist.

- Whenever child physical abuse is suspected, a skeletal survey is indicated. In young children, an ophthalmologic examination is also warranted.

SUGGESTED READINGS

Casey CF, Slawson DC, Neal LR. Vitamin D supplementation in infants, children, and adolescents. *Am Fam Physician.* 2010;81(6):745–748.
Jewell JA, McElwain LL, Blake AS. Picture of the month. Nutritional rickets. *Arch Pediatr Adolesc Med.* 2006;160(9):983–985.
Kocher MS, Kasser JR. Orthopedic aspects of child abuse. *J Am Acad Orthop Surg.* 2000;8(1):10–20.
Nield LS, Kamat D. Refracture of the clavicle in an infant: case report and review of clavicle fractures. *Clin Pediatr.* 2005;44(1):77–83.
Nimkin K, Kleinman PK. Imaging of child abuse. *Pediatr Clin North Am.* 1997;44:615–635.
Schweich P, Fleisher G. Rib fractures in children. *Pediatr Emerg Care.* 1985;1(4):187–189.
Yaw KM. Pediatric bone tumors. *Semin Surg Oncol.* 1999;16(2):173–183.

ABDOMEN

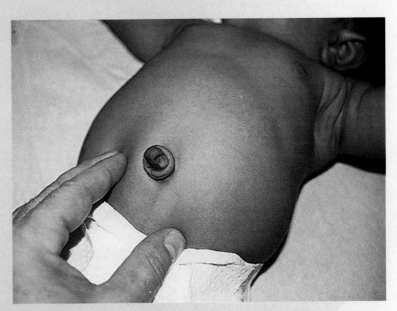

(Courtesy of George A. Datto, III, MD.)

Abdominal Midline Bulges

Alison Nair and Lee R. Atkinson-McEvoy

Approach to the Problem

An abdominal mass in an infant or child has a long differential diagnosis and includes a spectrum of conditions. These conditions range from those that are benign and self-resolving to those that are life threatening and require urgent intervention. These illnesses involve the many organ systems contained in the abdominal cavity, and the pathophysiology of each disease is diverse.

The etiology of some bulges is related to normal processes that occur during fetal development that fail to complete. For example, omphaloceles and gastroschisis can result from the normal process of gastrointestinal development that begins outside the fetus and then reenters the abdomen. Urachal cysts are remnants of the allantois that forms the umbilicus in fetal development. Diastasis recti and umbilical hernias are due to failure of abdominal wall musculature to fully close. In the majority of cases, these midline bulges resolve spontaneously.

Key Points in the History

- Diastasis recti is common in newborns.

- Umbilical hernias are more prevalent in preterm (up to 75% of <1,500 g birth weight) and African American infants (20% vs 3% of Caucasian neonates).

- Omphaloceles are often associated with chromosomal disorders, including trisomy 13, 18, and 21, and with Beckwith–Wiedemann syndrome, whereas gastroschisis often occurs in isolation.

- Hypertrophic pyloric stenosis presents at about 2 to 6 weeks of life with projectile nonbilious vomiting.

- Persistent urachus and other urachal anomalies can present with a persistently draining umbilical cord.

- About 1% to 2% of patients have a positive family history in patients with Wilms tumor.

**Key Points
in the Physical
Examination**

- Diastasis recti presents as a midline, vertical ridge that can extend between the xiphoid process and the umbilicus, when an infant cries.

- An epigastric hernia is often located in the middle abdomen above the umbilicus and may occur in multiples.

- Umbilical granulomas can have a seropurulent discharge on yellow- or pink-colored tissue and are distinguished from umbilical polyps in that they usually resolve following treatment with silver nitrate.

- The classic finding for hypertrophic pyloric stenosis is a firm, movable, olive-shaped mass in the midepigastrium about 2 cm in length.

- Persistent urachus may have urine or stool in the drainage, if present.

PHOTOGRAPHS OF SELECTED DIAGNOSES

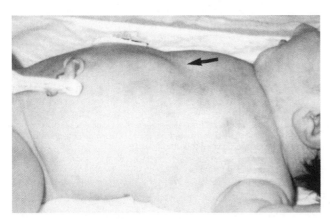

Figure 35-1 Diastasis recti. (Used with permission from Fletcher MA. *Physical Diagnosis in Neonatology.* Philadelphia, PA: Lippincott–Raven Publishers; 1998:357.)

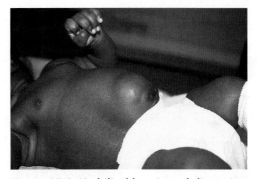

Figure 35-2 Umbilical hernia and diastasis recti. (Courtesy of George A. Datto, III, MD.)

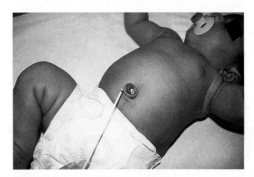

Figure 35-4 Umbilical granuloma following treatment with silver nitrate. (Courtesy of George A. Datto, III, MD.)

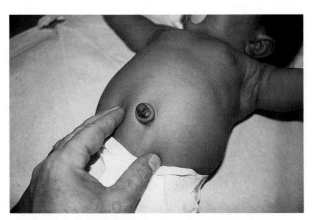

Figure 35-3 Umbilical granuloma. Pink granulation tissue at the base of the umbilicus. (Courtesy of George A. Datto, III, MD.)

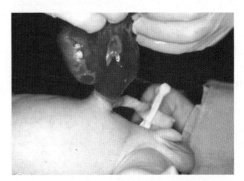

Figure 35-6 Gastroschisis. (Courtesy of Douglas Katz, MD.)

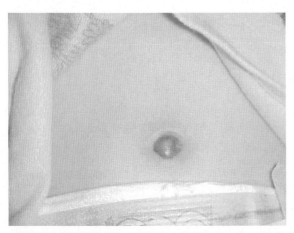

Figure 35-5 Infected urachal cyst. Infected urachal cyst in a 3-month old infant. (Courtesy of Ben Alouf, MD.)

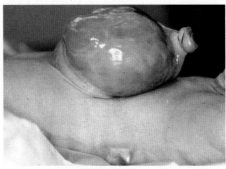

Figure 35-7 Omphalocele. (Courtesy of Douglas Katz, MD.)

DIFFERENTIAL DIAGNOSIS

DIAGNOSIS	ICD-10	DISTINGUISHING CHARACTERISTICS	DISTRIBUTION	DURATION/ CHRONICITY
Diastasis Recti	Q79.5	Enlarged fascial ridge between the rectus abdominis muscles	Midline, vertical ridge between the xiphoid process and the umbilicus that becomes pronounced with increased intra-abdominal pressure	Congenital lesions usually resolve as the rectus muscles develop
Umbilical Hernia	K42.9	Herniation of peritoneal contents due to imperfect closure or weakness of the umbilical ring	Soft, skin-covered protuberance at the umbilicus	Observation; tends to resolve by 12–18 months
Epigastric Hernia	K43.9	Small ventral hernia usually containing preperitoneal fat caused by a defect in the decussating fibers of the linea alba	Less than 1 cm, firm, skin-covered mass located in the middle abdomen above the umbilicus	Does not resolve without surgical intervention
Umbilical Granuloma	P83.6	Yellow- or pink-colored, raised tissue with seropurulent discharge May be confused with an umbilical polyp which is firm, red tissue with mucoid secretion	Located in umbilicus	N/A
Urachal Cyst	Q64.4	Group of anomalies including patent urachus, urachal cyst, urachal sinus, and urachal diverticulum	Midline mass below the umbilicus that persistently drains as an erythematous tender mass	N/A
Gastroschisis	Q79.3	Extrusion of abdominal structures through a small defect to the right side of an intact umbilical cord	Collection of abdominal contents without an overlying sac May include portions of the gastrointestinal tract, genital organs, and other solid organs	N/A
Omphalocele	Q79.2	Collection of abdominal contents covered by a sac, including the umbilicus May include portions of the gastrointestinal tract, genital organs, and other solid organs	Midline	N/A
Hypertrophic Pyloric Stenosis	Q40.0	Hypertrophy and stenosis of the pyloric opening resulting in firm, movable, olive-shaped mass	Located in the midepigastrium and approximately 2 cm in length	Onset of symptoms generally at 2–3 weeks of age
Wilms Tumor	C64	Smooth, firm, flank or abdominal mass	Found in the flank or abdomen	N/A

ASSOCIATED FINDINGS	COMPLICATIONS	PREDISPOSING FACTORS	TREATMENT GUIDELINES
Umbilical hernia	No fascial defect, so not a true hernia and no risk for incarceration	N/A	Observation
Associated with diastasis recti	Risk of incarceration	Increased prevalence in infants with low-birth weight and among African Americans	Surgical intervention if incarcerated, if persists past age 4–5, or if associated with a large sac of skin apparent when the hernia is reduced
20% of patients present with multiple epigastric hernias	Risk of incarceration, 25% over lifetime	N/A	Refer for surgical evaluation and resection at time of presentation.
		N/A	Silver nitrate cauterization followed by excision, if persists
Associated with bladder outlet obstruction	Failed closure of the allantoic duct	N/A	Refer to specialist for surgical evaluation and excision.
Usually occurs as isolated defect	Short gut syndrome complicates many cases following surgical intervention.	Associated with younger aged mothers	Urgent surgical evaluation and repair is necessary after birth.
Associated with chromosomal disorders, including Trisomy 13, 18, 21, and Beckwith–Wiedemann syndrome May be associated with malrotation May have associated cardiac, renal, skeletal, or pulmonary anomalies	Preoperative concern for rupture of membrane covering intestinal contents Preoperative and postoperative gastrointestinal infection and sepsis are concerns.	N/A	Urgent surgical evaluation and repair is necessary after birth.
N/A	Associated with nonbilious vomiting, poor weight gain, and hyperchloremic metabolic alkalosis	More common in males; those who are first-born	Refer for urgent surgical evaluation and repair. Requires careful fluid, electrolyte, and acid–base management preoperatively
Associated with abdominal pain, vomiting, hematuria, or hypertension	N/A	Associated with WAGR syndrome, Denys–Drash syndrome and Beckwith–Wiedemann syndrome 1%–2% of patients have a family history of Wilms tumor.	Refer to specialist for surgical resection, chemotherapy, and possible radiotherapy.

Other Diagnoses to Consider

- Intestinal duplication

- Polycystic kidney disease

- Neuroblastoma

- Omphalomesenteric cyst or fistula

- Hepatic masses (hepatic hemangioma, hepatic mesenchymal hamartoma, hepatoblastoma, and choledochal cyst)

- Hydrocolpos/hydrometrocolpos, fused hymen resulting in the formation of a mass after menarche

- Ovarian mass, when large, may be palpable in the midline

When to Consider Further Evaluation or Treatment

- Epigastric hernias are at high risk of incarceration. Patients with these should be referred to pediatric surgery for further evaluation.

- Umbilical hernias have a 5% risk of strangulation, incarceration, or evisceration. Hernias smaller than 1.5 cm in diameter are twice as likely to become incarcerated.

- Umbilical hernias that present with symptoms, are very large, or persist beyond 4 to 5 years of age and are generally repaired.

- Silver nitrate can be used to cauterize an umbilical granuloma. If it persists, surgical resection can be considered.

- Ultrasound can be used to confirm the diagnosis of pyloric stenosis. In pyloric stenosis, the loss of electrolytes requires fluid and electrolyte resuscitation and acid–base management preoperatively.

- Hepatic, flank, and pelvic masses often require multidisciplinary approaches to diagnosis and management.

SUGGESTED READINGS

Brodeur AE, Brodeur GM. Abdominal masses in children: Neuroblastoma, Wilms' tumor, and other considerations. *Pediatr Rev.* 1991;12:196–206.
Geller E, Kochan PS. Renal neoplasms of childhood. *Radiol Clin North Am.* 2011;49(4):689–709.
Ipp LS, Taubel D, Walters H, et al. Adolescent with an abdominal mass. *Adolesc Med State Art Rev.* 2012;23(2):285–289.
Kelly KB, Ponsky TA. Pediatric abdominal wall defects. *Surg Clin North Am.* 2013;93(5):1255–1267.
Ladino-Torres MF, Strouse PJ. Gastrointestinal tumors in children. *Radiol Clin North Am.* 2011;49(4):665–677.
Pomeranz A. Anomalies, abnormalities, and care of the umbilicus. *Pediatr Clin North Am.* 2004;51(3):819–827.
Salameh JR. Primary and unusual abdominal wall hernias. *Surg Clin North Am.* 2008;88(1):45–60.
Schwartz MZ, Shaul DB. Abdominal masses in the newborn. *Pediatr Rev.* 1989;11:172–179.

Enlarged/Distended Abdomen

Brent D. Rogers and Colette C. Mull

Approach to the Problem

An increase in the girth of a child's abdomen, abdominal distension, may be physiologic (e.g., swallowed air, lumbar lordosis in toddlers) or pathologic (e.g., intestinal obstruction, functional or mechanical). It occurs at all ages and in healthy, acutely ill, and chronically ill children. Abdominal distension can be the result of accidental and nonaccidental trauma. For example, a pneumomediastinum may occur in a child on a ventilator, or a pneumoperitoneum may be the result of blunt trauma. The mechanisms that result in abdominal distension are intraluminal or extraluminal accumulation of air or fluid, intra-abdominal mass, organomegaly, ascites, and abdominal wall hypotonia. Rapid recognition of pathologic abdominal distension is essential to reducing morbidity and mortality. Imaging studies and laboratory tests often have a role in determining the etiology of a child's enlarged abdomen.

Key Points in the History

- A child typically complains of minimal pain with an ileus, but significant pain with an intestinal obstruction.

- Assume bilious vomiting is secondary to intestinal obstruction until proven otherwise.

- Delayed passage of meconium (after 48 hours of life) in the newborn period is highly concerning for Hirschsprung disease, gastrointestinal structural abnormality, cystic fibrosis, and hypothyroidism.

- Hematemesis, melena, and jaundice are clinical features of portal hypertension.

- Failure to thrive, rapid weight loss or gain, fever, fatigue, irritability, and bone pain suggests malignancy.

- Absence of historical details in an ill child with abdominal distension is a red flag for nonaccidental trauma.

- Gastrointestinal infections, pneumonia, and peritonitis with recent history of surgery may be associated with paralytic ileus.

- Ovulation may precede onset of menses, and therefore pregnancy should be considered in all pubertal females with lower abdominal distension. Cyclical distension, with or without abdominal pain, may represent hemato(metro)colpos.

- Pica-induced bezoars should be considered in neurologically or psychologically impaired children.

- Children with hemolytic disease are at risk for distension from splenomegaly.

- A prenatal history of oligohydramnios may result in distal urinary obstruction in the newborn, whereas polyhydramnios is associated with upper intestinal obstruction.

- History of abdominal surgery puts a child at risk for adhesions and small-bowel obstruction.

- Family history should include asking about metabolic diseases, early infant death among relatives, polycystic kidney disease, and cystic fibrosis.

- Constipation and ileus can be caused by misuse of medications (e.g., tricyclic antidepressants, antihistamines, antidiarrheal agents), ingestion of herbal products contaminated with belladonna alkaloids (e.g., teas, meat seasonings, stews), and exposure to anticholinergic substances through recreational drug use (e.g., smoking jimsonweed, use of jimsonweed-laced heroin).

- A history of greasy, foul-smelling stools in the setting of abdominal distension suggests malabsorption.

Key Points in the Physical Examination

- Ascites, flatus, and ileus present with symmetrical abdominal distension.

- Malignancy, constipation, pregnancy, and organomegaly may present with more localized abdominal distension.

- Visible peristaltic waves may be seen with intestinal obstruction.

- To detect abdominal organomegaly, it is important to begin palpation in the lowest part of the abdomen and then proceed upward toward the chest.

- Bowel sounds are decreased or absent in ileus and hyperactive in intestinal obstruction.

- Consider a rectal examination in the evaluation of abdominal distension as the presence of hard stool is suggestive of functional constipation or a pelvic mass. An empty rectal vault in the setting of constipation is suggestive of Hirschsprung disease.

- Pallor and nail clubbing are physical findings that suggest chronic malabsorption.

- Spider nevi, palmar erythema, and jaundice suggest chronic liver disease.

- Prominent abdominal superficial veins may represent portal hypertension or an obstruction in systemic venous return.

PHOTOGRAPHS OF SELECTED DIAGNOSES

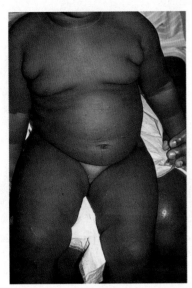

Figure 36-1 Obesity. Enlarged abdomen from increased adiposity. (Courtesy of George A. Datto, III, MD.)

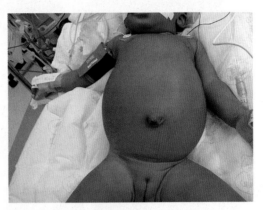

Figure 36-2 Ascites. Large distended abdomen in an infant. (Courtesy of Vani V. Gopalareddy, MD.)

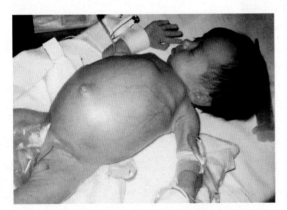

Figure 36-3 Abdominal distension resulting from hepatomegaly in a child with untreated galactosemia. Note that the distension is more prominent in the upper abdomen. (Used with permission from Fletcher MA. *Physical Diagnosis in Neonatology.* Philadelphia, PA: Lippincott–Raven Publishers; 1998:353.)

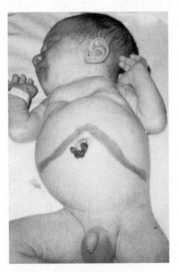

Figure 36-4 Abdominal distension resulting from massive hepatosplenomegaly in an infant with congenital cytomegalovirus infection. Note that the distension is more prominent in the upper abdomen. (Used with permission from Fletcher MA. *Physical Diagnosis in Neonatology.* Philadelphia, PA: Lippincott–Raven Publishers; 1998:354.)

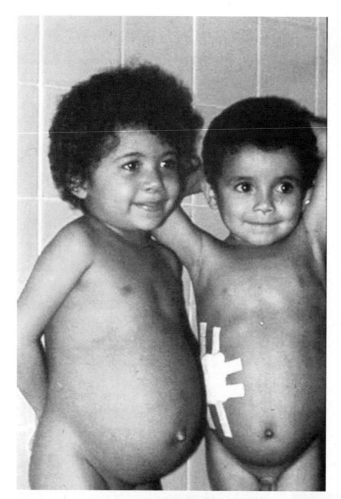

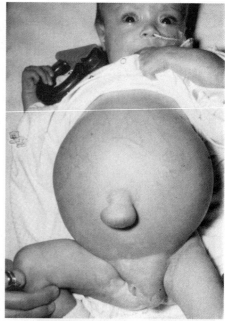

Figure 36-6 Female infant with cirrhosis due to biliary atresia. Note abdominal distension, umbilical hernia, and labial swelling due to massive ascites. McMillan JA, Feigin RD, DeAngelis C, et al. *Oski's Solution*. Philadelphia, PA: Lippincott, Williams & Wilkins; 2006.

Figure 36-5 Two young boys suffering from visceral leishmaniasis (*Leishmania chagasi*) from Brazil. Both have abdominal distension due to hepatosplenomegaly. (Courtesy of WHO. Photograph by Dr. P. Marsden. WHO/TDR/Marsden.)

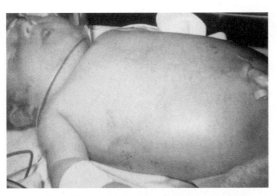

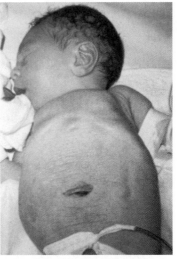

Figure 36-7 Abdominal distension in an infant with anasarca. Note that the distension is more prominent in the flanks. (Used with permission from Fletcher MA. *Physical Diagnosis in Neonatology.* Philadelphia, PA: Lippincott-Raven Publishers; 1998:355.)

Figure 36-8 Abdominal distension at the flanks in an infant with prune belly syndrome. (Used with permission from Fletcher MA. *Physical Diagnosis in Neonatology.* Philadelphia, PA: Lippincott-Raven Publishers; 1998:355.)

DIFFERENTIAL DIAGNOSIS

DIAGNOSIS	ICD-10	DISTINGUISHING CHARACTERISTICS	DISTRIBUTION
Constipation	K59.0	Indentable abdominal mass Hard stool in rectum	Left lower quadrant (LLQ) and suprapubic pain and enlargement May feel stool-filled bowel in LLQ May be generalized if more severe
Paralytic Ileus	K56.0	Resonant percussion note	Generalized
Small-Bowel Obstruction	K56.6	Acute abdominal distension	Generalized
Ascites	R18	Dull percussion note Fluid wave Bulging of flanks in newborns	Generalized
Necrotizing Enterocolitis	P77	Premature infants Septic appearing	Generalized
Hepatomegaly	R16.0	Enlarged liver span determined by palpation or percussion	Right upper quadrant, but if severe may appear to be generalized enlargement of the abdomen
Splenomegaly	R16.1	Palpable edge in left upper quadrant	Left upper quadrant
Wilms Tumor	C64	Asymptomatic flank mass Median age of presentation: 3 years	Flank
Neuroblastoma	C74.9	Large abdominal mass Lymphadenopathy Median age: 2 years	Flank or abdomen

DURATION/ CHRONICITY	ASSOCIATED FINDINGS	PREDISPOSING FACTORS	TREATMENT GUIDELINES
Chronic—often begins in toddler age	External or internal hemorrhoid Anal fissures Rectal bleeding Encopresis	Diet low in fiber Psychological factors	Bowel catharsis—oral, nasogastric, or rectal Medications, such as polyethylene glycol 3350 (has stool softening and laxative effects) and lactulose should be started in those that have failed dietary changes. Long-term maintenance program with a high-fiber diet and/or medication
Acute	Periumbilical pain Decreased bowel sounds	Abdominal surgery Gastroenteritis Peritonitis Trauma Medication or anesthesia reaction Sepsis	Bowel rest Nasogastric suction
Acute	Bilious vomiting Obstipation	Prior abdominal surgery Malrotation	Urgent surgical intervention
Acute or nonacute	Ankle swelling	Liver disease Cardiac disease Infections Lymphoma Ovarian pathology	Treat underlying condition Spironolactone Salt restriction Albumin and lasix
Acute	Apnea Lethargy Vomiting	Prematurity, although up to 10% of cases occur in full-term infants	Bowel rest Parenteral nutrition Antibiotic therapy Surgery for bowel injury
Acute or nonacute	Jaundice Pruritus Skin findings Ascites	Infection Storage disease Malignancy Autoimmune Vascular disease Tumor	Treat underlying conditions, if possible. Fat-soluble vitamin supplements Screen for varices.
Acute or nonacute	Superficial abdominal venous distension when associated with portal hypertension Pallor	Infection Hematologic disorder Neoplasm Storage diseases Portal hypertension Autoimmune disorder	Treat underlying condition. Portosystemic shunts Splenectomy Avoidance of contact sports
Acute	Hypertension Hematuria Abdominal pain Vomiting	Beckwith–Wiedemann syndrome WAGR syndrome—Wilms tumor, aniridia, genitourinary abnormalities, and mental retardation	Refer to oncologist to treat underlying condition.
Acute	Bone pain Proptosis and ecchymosis Opsoclonus myoclonus Horner syndrome	1%–2% may have an inherited form, but the large majority are considered sporadic	Refer to oncologist to treat underlying condition.

Other Diagnoses to Consider

- Ruptured appendicitis

- Intussusception

- Hirschsprung disease, toxic megacolon

- Malrotation with volvulus

- Incarcerated hernia

- Surgical adhesions

- Obstructed bladder

- Polycystic kidney disease

- Hydronephrosis

- Ovarian mass, cyst

- Pregnancy

- Hematocolpos

- Neoplasms, lymphoma

- Trauma

- Pulmonary hyperinflation

  - Bronchiolitis

  - Asthma exacerbation

- Anasarca

- Abdominal distension in a newborn accompanied by bilious vomiting is a surgical emergency. An upper gastrointestinal series must be emergently performed to rule out malrotation with or without volvulus.

- If intussusception is suspected, an obstruction series should be performed to rule out perforation, and then an ultrasound and/or air enema should be obtained to make the diagnosis.

- The presence of ascites warrants consultation with pediatric gastroenterology and an ultrasound to identify the cause. A diagnostic paracentesis may be necessary.

- CT scan may be required when history, physical exam, laboratory studies, and other imaging have failed to identify the etiology of abdominal distension.

SUGGESTED READINGS

Avner JR. Abdominal distention. In: Fleischer GR, Ludwig S, et al., eds. *Textbook of Pediatric Emergency Medicine*. 6th ed. Philadelphia, PA: Lippincott Williams & Wilkins; 2010:153–159.
Belamarich PF. Abdominal distention. In: McInerny TK, Adam HM, Campbell DE, et al., eds. *American Academy of Pediatrics Textbook of Pediatric Care*. Elk Grove Village, IL: American Academy of Pediatrics; 2008:1369–1376.
Juang D, Snyder CL. Neonatal bowel obstruction. *Surg Clin North Am.* 2012;92:658–711.
Lambert SM. Pediatric urological emergencies. *Pediatr Clin North Am.* 2012;59:965–976.
Pepper VK, Stanfill AB, Pearl RH. Diagnosis and management of pediatric appendicitis, intussusception, and Meckel diverticulum. *Surg Clin North Am.* 2012;92:505–526.
Schonfeld D, Lee LK. Blunt abdominal trauma in children. *Curr Opin Pediatr.* 2012;24:314–318.

BACK

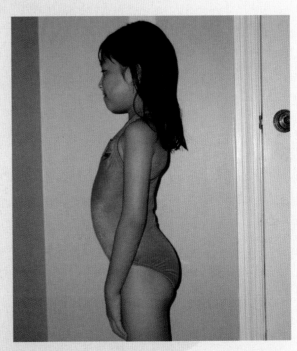

(Courtesy of Esther K. Chung, MD, MPH.)

37

Curvature of the Back

Shareen F. Kelly

Approach to the Problem

Physicians use the plane and the position of a curve relative to the spine to describe curvatures of the back. The term scoliosis implies lateral spinal curvature in the coronal plane and necessarily involves a rotational component as well. The rotational component is visualized most often as a rib hump viewed posteriorly when the spine is flexed. Scoliosis is described by the severity and position of the rib hump and can be measured in various ways. Kyphosis is an exaggerated curve of the thoracic spine in the sagittal plane with the apex of the curve directed posteriorly. Lordosis refers to a marked curvature that occurs in the sagittal plane of the lumbar spine with the apex of the curve directed anteriorly. Curvature of the spine can present with varying severity and may progress with age and growth. Beyond skeletal maturity, scoliosis generally does not progress; however, kyphosis and lordosis may progress into adulthood.

Key Points in the History

- Family history of scoliosis is present in approximately 30% of new cases of scoliosis.

- Sports participation and day-to-day functioning usually are not affected by the curvature of scoliosis.

- Complaints of back pain are not characteristic of idiopathic scoliosis and should prompt the physician to rule out other diseases.

- Progressive scoliosis is more likely in nonambulatory patients than ambulatory patients.

- The curvature of idiopathic scoliosis is more likely to progress during times of rapid growth.

- Rapidly progressing curves are more likely to require treatment.

- Kyphosis can be postural or structural in nature.

- Postural kyphosis is generally flexible and corrected with adjustment of posture.

- Fixed kyphosis may cause pain with neck motion.

- Radicular pain, changes in bowel or bladder function, sensory abnormalities, and problems with balance and/or coordination all point to an underlying neurologic problem.

- Constitutional symptoms—including prolonged fever, weight loss, night sweats, and malaise—may provide clues regarding malignancies or inflammatory diseases.

Key Points in the Physical Examination

- Bony deformities detected upon palpation along the spine suggest vertebral anomalies or spinal dysraphism.

- Skin overlying the spine marked with hemangiomas, hair tufts, clefts, and/or other macular discolorations may be the only clinical clue to occult spinal dysraphism.

- The most common presentation of idiopathic scoliosis is that of a thoracic curve with a right thoracic rib hump when viewed from behind on the Adams forward bend test.

- Scoliosis may be evaluated with the help of a handheld scoliometer; curves greater than 7 degrees or those likely to progress should be evaluated by radiographs.

- Radiographic evaluation includes calculation of the Cobbs angle; the decision to brace or proceed with surgery is based on degree of curvature and likelihood of progression.

- Lower extremity muscular weakness, tightness of hamstrings, and decreased deep tendon reflexes are suggestive of a neurological abnormality.

- Patients with more advanced sexual maturity ratings are less likely to have progression of their scoliosis.

- Range of motion assessment is critical in children with kyphosis or lordosis.

PHOTOGRAPHS OF SELECTED DIAGNOSES

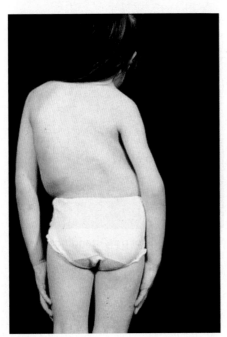

Figure 37-1 Scoliosis. (Used with permission from SIU/Biomedical Communications/Custom Medical Stock Photography.)

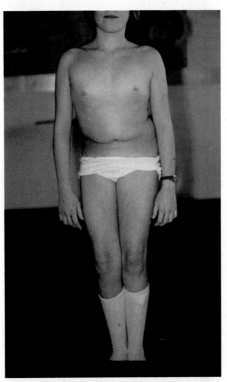

Figure 37-2 Scoliosis, anterior view. Note the pelvic tilt and abnormal skin folds. (Courtesy of the late Peter Sol, MD.)

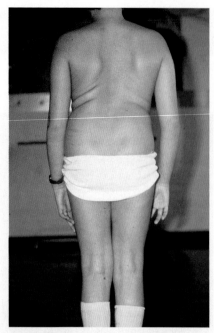

Figure 37-3 Scoliosis, posterior view. Note the abnormal skin folds and scapular position. (Courtesy of the late Peter Sol, MD.)

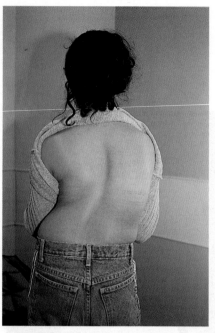

Figure 37-4 Scoliosis, standing. Dramatic spinal curvature in an adolescent. (Courtesy of George A. Datto, III, MD.)

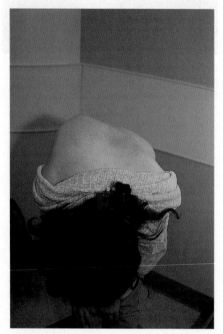

Figure 37-5 Scoliosis, bending forward. Note the marked asymmetry of the back. (Courtesy of George A. Datto, III, MD.)

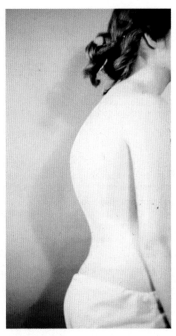

Figure 37-6 Kyphosis. (Courtesy of Martin I. Herman, MD.)

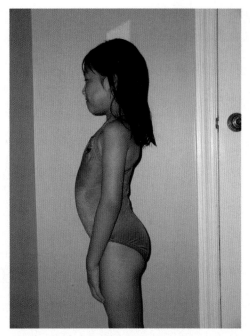

Figure 37-7 Lordosis. Note the thoracolumbar curvature on side view of this child in her normal stance. (Courtesy of Esther K. Chung, MD, MPH.)

DIFFERENTIAL DIAGNOSIS

DIAGNOSIS	ICD-10	DISTINGUISHING CHARACTERISTICS	DISTRIBUTION	DURATION/CHRONOCITY
Scoliosis	M41.1 (Juvenile idiopathic scoliosis)	Lateral curvature of the spine Right (most often) thoracic rib hump on Adams forward bend test	Female:male ratio is 4:1. Idiopathic scoliosis presents most often in adolescence.	Curve progresses through puberty Usually no decrease in function
Kyphosis	M40	Convex curvature of the upper thoracic spine Best viewed from the side with the child standing	Postural kyphosis more common in prepubertal children Structural kyphosis may affect any age.	Postural kyphosis corrects with physical therapy. Structural kyphosis may progress into old age.
Lordosis	M40.5	Concave curvature of the lumbar spine Best viewed from the side while child is standing or when child is lying supine on a firm, flat surface	All age groups Physiologic lordosis most often occurs in prepubertal children.	Depends on underlying cause—physiologic lordosis will resolve with growth

ASSOCIATED FINDINGS	COMPLICATIONS	PREDISPOSING FACTORS	TREATMENT GUIDELINES
Asymmetry of clavicles and/or scapulae Asymmetry of back skin folds Leg length discrepancy Asymmetric iliac crests when standing upright	Severe cases (mostly nonambulatory) may result in restrictive lung disease and/or cor pulmonale.	Most often idiopathic Congenital scoliosis may result from vertebral anomalies.	Observation for mild curves Bracing for moderate and progressive curves Surgical spinal fusion for extreme curves
Postural kyphosis often seen with compensatory lordosis Fixed kyphosis is often painful.	When associated with osteoporosis, may be painful and may cause symptoms of compression	Postural kyphosis: poor posture Scheuermann disease	Depending on etiology—bracing or surgical correction or no treatment
Buttocks appear more prominent. Curve may correct with forward bending. May be associated with hip flexor muscle contractures May be compensatory curve for hyperkyphosis	Pain Decreased flexibility and movement	Poor posture, obesity, hip flexor contracture Congenital lordosis: vertebral or neuromuscular problems Acquired lordosis: diskitis or spondylolisthesis	Physical therapy Treatment of associated deformities, such as kyphosis

Other Diagnoses to Consider

- Marfan syndrome

- Ehlers–Danlos syndrome

- Leg length discrepancy

- Spasm of the spinous or paraspinous muscles with compensatory splinting

- Bone dysplasias

- Metabolic diseases, including rickets, osteoporosis, homocystinuria, and osteogenesis imperfecta, may be associated with scoliosis.

- Spinal tumors

- Neuromuscular disorders

- Spondylolisthesis

When to Consider Further Evaluation or Treatment

- Left-sided thoracic scoliosis in an otherwise normal teenager should prompt further evaluation to rule out an underlying lesion.

- A tall, thin child with scoliosis and Marfanoid features should have genetic, cardiac, and ophthalmologic evaluations.

- Congenital scoliosis mandates orthopedic evaluation.

- Scoliosis associated with constitutional symptoms warrants evaluation to uncover possible rheumatologic disorders or malignancies.

- Scoliosis associated with significant back pain should be investigated by an orthopedic specialist.

- Kyphosis that progresses quickly should be referred to an orthopedic specialist.

SUGGESTED READINGS

Rosenberg JJ. *Pediatrics in Review.* 2011;32:397–398.

Staheli L. *Fundamentals of Pediatric Orthopedics.* Philadelphia, PA: Lippincott-Raven Publishers; 2008:242–255.

Stewart DG, Skaggs DL. Consultation with the specialist: adolescent idiopathic scoliosis. *Pediatrics in Review.* 2006;27:299–305.

Vernacchio L, Trudell EK, Hresko MT, Karlin LI, Risko W. A quality improvement program to reduce unnecessary referrals for adolescent scoliosis. *Pediatrics.* 2013;131(3):e912–20.

Ward T, Davis HW, Hanley EN. Orthopedics. In: *Atlas of Pediatric Physical Diagnosis.* 5th ed. New York, NY: Gower Medical Publishing; 2007:719–802.

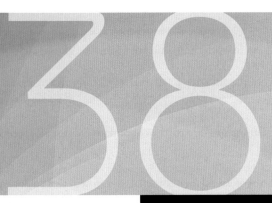

Midline Back Pits, Skin Tags, Hair Tufts, and Other Lesions

Darshita P. Bhatia and Nancy D. Spector

Approach to the Problem

Congenital midline back lesions such as sacral dimples, skin tags, hairy patches, hemangiomas, dermal sinuses, and lipomas are present in approximately 5% to 7% of infants. It is important to recognize and diagnose midline back lesions as they may correlate with a spinal dysraphism. Spinal dysraphisms are characterized as open or closed. Open lesions involve protrusion of the spinal cord or nerves through defects in the meninges or vertebral column. Examples of open lesions are spina bifida with meningocele or spina bifida with myelomeningocele. Closed lesions (occult dysraphisms) are improperly formed nervous system structures covered by skin. Examples of closed lesions are spina bifida occulta or isolated tethered cord. Closed lesions may have overlying cutaneous stigmata that signal an underlying defect. Spinal dysraphisms, such as tethered cord or dermal sinus, are important to identify early in order to prevent serious neurologic and infectious complications. Acquired midline back lesions, such as pilonidal cysts, occur in adolescence and may only be identified after infection.

Key Points in the History

- Midline back lesions are typically present at birth.

- Back lesions combined with the presence of neurologic symptoms such as bowel or bladder incontinence, extremity weakness, parasthesias, or gait abnormalities strongly suggest spinal dysraphism.

- Back lesions without the presence of neurologic symptoms do not rule out an underlying spinal defect.

- Long-standing tethered cord may result in asymmetric lower extremity growth and neurologic sequelae.

- Erythema, warmth, and tenderness surrounding a midline back lesion in an adolescent may suggest an infected pilonidal cyst.

- An infected congenital dermal sinus tract may be the cause of recurrent meningitis.

- Simple sacral dimples are located <2.5 cm from the anus and are within the gluteal cleft.

- Atypical sacral dimples are >2.5 cm from the anus, have a diameter >5 mm, and may be associated with other cutaneous markers.

- Vascular nevi—salmon patches, nevus flammeus—are patches of pink to red discolorations of the skin.

- Hemangiomas on the back are soft masses of vascular endothelial overgrowth that may have a blue or reddish discoloration.

- Lumbosacral hypertrichosis or "hairy patch" is often V-shaped and poorly circumscribed. Hair can be dark or light with a silky texture. This must be distinguished from the normal sacral hair seen in newborns.

- Subcutaneous lipomas on the back are palpated as homogeneous, soft masses that are flesh colored.

- Skin tags are small outgrowths of skin that may be located on the back.

- Dermoid sinuses present as small skin openings that lead to a narrow duct. Protruding hair, hairy patches, or vascular nevi may be present nearby.

- Deviation of the gluteal cleft suggests an underlying mass, such as a lipoma or myelomeningocele.

PHOTOGRAPHS OF SELECTED DIAGNOSES

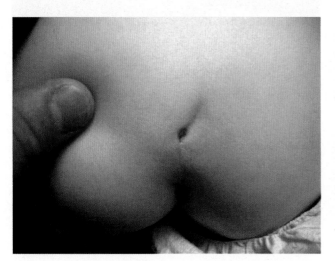

Figure 38-1 Sacral dimple. Shallow dimple visible within the gluteal fold. (Courtesy of Paul S. Matz, MD.)

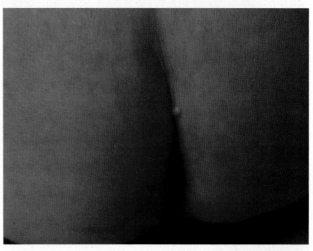

Figure 38-2 Sacral skin tag with no underlying spinal pathology. Note the isolated nodule within the gluteal fold. (Courtesy of Esther K. Chung, MD, MPH.)

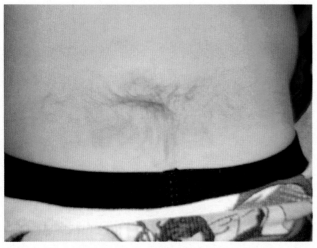

Figure 38-3 Hair tuft. (Courtesy of Joseph Piatt, MD.)

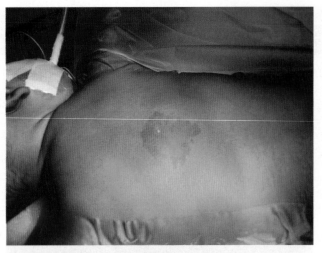

Figure 38-4 Infected dermal sinus connected to intramedullary dermoid cyst. Thoracic sinus associated with purulent discharge. (Courtesy of Joseph Piatt, MD.)

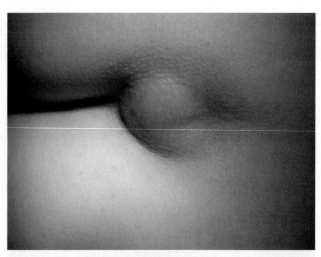

Figure 38-5 Infected pilonidal cyst. A large erythematous fluctuant mass visible at the superior portion of the gluteal fold. (Courtesy of Scott VanDuzer, MD.)

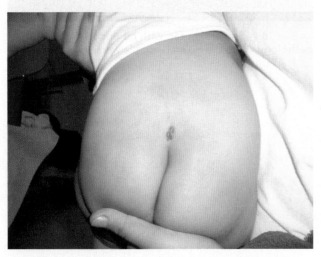

Figure 38-6 Sacral hemangioma. Vascular malformation visible overlying sacral spine. (Courtesy of Paul S. Matz, MD.)

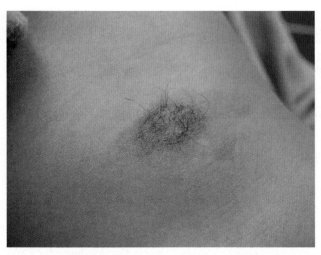

Figure 38-7 Lumbar hemangioma. This midline lesion was associated with a dermal sinus and an underlying tethered cord. (Courtesy of Esther K. Chung, MD, MPH.)

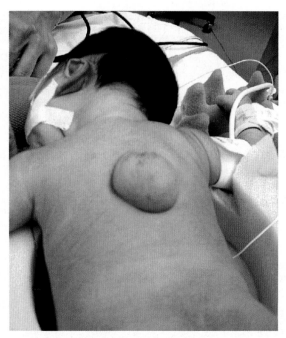

Figure 38-8 Thoracic meningocele. Large skin-covered thoracic mass in an infant. (Courtesy of Joseph Piatt, MD.)

DIFFERENTIAL DIAGNOSIS

DIAGNOSIS		ICD-10	DISTINGUISHING CHARACTERISTICS	DISTRIBUTION
Sacral Dimple or Pit		L05.91	Small indentation of the skin, often circular May be shallow or deep ("bottomless")	Simple: <2.5 cm from anus, <5 mm diameter Atypical: >2.5 cm from anus, >5 mm diameter, "bottomless"
Vascular Nevi		Q82.5	Patches of pink to red skin discoloration	May occur anywhere on the back and other parts of the body
Hemangioma		D18.00	Lesion caused by proliferating vascular endothelium Rapid growth in infancy followed by involution	May occur anywhere on the back and other parts of the body
Hair Tufts/Patches		Q84.2	Cluster of hair, silky texture, dark or light	Mid or lower back, V-shaped
Lipoma		D17.9	Flesh-colored mass of adipose cells	May occur anywhere on the back and other parts of the body
Skin Tag		Q82.8	Small growth of skin	Found anywhere on body
Dermal Sinus		Q06.8	Small skin opening (often indistinguishable from sacral dimple) that leads to a narrow duct that can track through the dura	Along entire midline neuroaxis, above the gluteal cleft
Pilonidal Sinus/Cyst		L05.91	Small sinus tract in the skin containing hair and debris May be erythematous and tender if infected	Intergluteal cleft, usually lateral
Spina Bifida		Q05.9	Occult: defect of vertebral bodies without protrusion of meninges or spinal cord Meningocele: sacral mass with protruding meninges Myelomeningocele: sacral mass with protruding meninges and nervous tissue	Along entire midline neuroaxis

ASSOCIATED FINDINGS	PREDISPOSING FACTORS	TREATMENT GUIDELINES
Potential for occult spinal dysraphism with atypical dimples	Unknown	Lumbosacral ultrasound for atypical dimples or dimples associated with other cutaneous stigmata Lumbosacral MRI is also an option.
Potential for occult spinal dysraphism if located above gluteal cleft in midline back or associated with a second midline back lesion	Unknown	Ultrasound/MRI for midline back lesion above the gluteal cleft or associated with second midline lesion
Potential for occult spinal dysraphism	Unknown	Ultrasound/MRI for high or midline back lesions
Potential for occult spinal dysraphism	Unknown	Ultrasound/MRI for distinct patches of hair
Highly associated with occult spinal dysraphism if located midline above gluteal cleft	Unknown	Ultrasound/MRI for high or midline back lesions
Potential for occult spinal dysraphism if located on midline back	Unknown	Ultrasound/MRI for high or midline back lesions
Highly associated with spinal dysraphism if midline and above gluteal cleft	Unknown	Ultrasound/MRI for high or midline lesions IV antibiotics and hospitalization if concern for meningitis
Rarely occult spinal pathology Infection	Pubertal hormones, obesity, local trauma, and poor hygiene increase the risk of hair and debris causing obstruction that may lead to cyst formation and infection	Incision and drainage, intravenous or oral antibiotics for infection
Occult: other cutaneous stigmata Meningocele: tethered cord, hydrocephalus Myelomeningocele: neurologic symptoms such as incontinence, paralysis, absence of reflexes, lack of sensation, and lower extremity deformities	Inadequate folic acid supplementation during pregnancy	Occult: Imaging with ultrasound/MRI, if imaging indicates abnormalities of the spinal cord, refer to pediatric neurosurgeon for further evaluation Meningocele/Myelomeningocele: Immediate transfer to an ICU Cover with a sterile, moist dressing until operative repair is performed Long-term follow-up with general pediatrics, neurosurgery, orthopedic surgery, urology, physical therapy, and occupational therapy

SECTION 11 • BACK

- Two or more congenital midline back lesions are strong indicators of spinal dysraphism.

- Atypical sacral dimples warrant further imaging.

- Simple sacral dimples with a visible base do not warrant further imaging.

- Midline back hairy patches, lipomas, skin tags, and hemangiomas may be indicative of occult spinal dysraphism and should be further evaluated with imaging.

- Vascular nevi that are located above the gluteal cleft in the midline back or associated with a second midline back lesion should be imaged.

- Tracts of a dermoid sinus may pass through the dura, increasing the risk for cerebrospinal infection.

- Any child with the presence of neurologic signs and symptoms in combination with a back lesion should be referred immediately for further imaging.

- Infants with spina bifida with meningocele or myelomeningocele should have coordinated care involving general pediatrics, neurosurgery, orthopedic surgery, urology, and physical and occupational therapy.

SUGGESTED READINGS

Ackerman LL, Menezes AH. Spinal congenital dermal sinuses: a 30-year experience. *Pediatrics*. 2003;112:641–647.
Drolet BA. Cutaneous signs of neural tube dysraphism. *Pediatr Clin North Am*. 2000;47(4):813–823.
Guggisberg D, Hadj-Rabia S, Viney C, et al. Skin markers of occult spinal dysraphism in children. *Arch Dermatol*. 2004;140:1109–1115.
Kinsman SL, Johnston MV. Spina bifida occulta. In: Kliegman RM, Stanton BF, St. Geme JW, et al., eds. *Nelson Textbook of Pediatrics*. 19th ed. Philadelphia, PA: Saunders Elsevier; 2011.
Medina LS, Kerry Crone K, Kuntz KM. Newborns with suspected occult spinal dysraphism: a cost-effectiveness analysis of diagnostic strategies. *Pediatrics*. 2001;108:e101.
Sardana K, Gupta R, Garg V, et al. A prospective study of cutaneous manifestations of spinal dysraphism from India. *Pediatr Dermatol*. 2009;26(6):688–695.
Schropp C, Sorensen N, Collman H, et al. Cutaneous lesions in occult spinal dysraphism—correlation with intraspinal findings. *Childs Nerv Syst*. 2006;22:125–131.
Zywicke HA, Rozelle CJ. Sacral dimples. *Pediatr Rev*. 2011;22(3):109–113.

EXTREMITIES

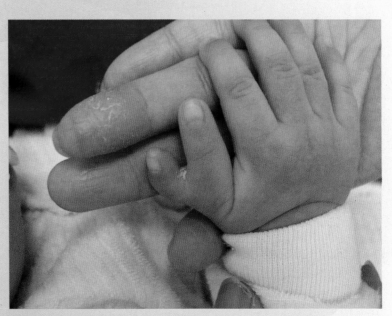

(Courtesy of Esther K. Chung, MD, MPH.)

EXTREMITIES

Nail Abnormalities

Kenya Maria Parks

Pediatricians encounter a vast array of nail disorders in clinical practice. Basic knowledge of the common nail disorders is pivotal for assessment, diagnosis, and referral when necessary. Nail pathology can result from focal or systemic abnormalities. The nail can be directly affected by localized infection, inflammation, mechanical forces, or trauma. Alternatively, nail pathology can result from nutritional deficits, genetic abnormalities, systemic disease, and medication or toxin exposures.

Nails are functional, structural, and cosmetic components of human anatomy. The nail plate is a translucent arrangement of compressed, keratinized dead cells. Nail folds are specialized epithelium that provide structure and protect the nail plate and matrix. The lateral nail fold is the paronychium, and the proximal nail fold is called the eponychium or cuticle. Underlying the eponychium is the nail matrix that contains the germinal cells. It takes 20 days for the fingernail and 80 days for the toenail to emerge from the matrix. Matrix to free edge growth for the fingernail is close to 6 months and 12 to 18 months for the toenail. This growth interval is important to consider for the timing of a potential insult and deciding the treatment course.

Key Points in the History

- Cyanotic congenital heart defects, chronic lung disease, and gastrointestinal disorders are associated with digital clubbing.

- Dermatological disorders such as psoriasis, eczema, alopecia areata, and lichen planus are associated with nail pitting and dystrophy.

- Disease states and certain medications, such as Kawasaki disease, hand–foot–mouth disease, pneumonia, prolonged high fevers, and chemotherapy, can cause a temporary growth arrest in the nail that is later manifested as Beau lines.

- There are benign familial forms of digital clubbing and koilonychias.

- Given the time it takes for nails to emerge from the matrix and grow, a history of medication or toxin exposure should be retrospective and encompassing.

- Nails are porous, and cosmetic products and frequent washing can strip and weaken the nail.

- Nail salons can be the source of fungal and bacterial nail infections.

- Koilonychia is associated with iron deficiency anemia in the adult population.

- Repeated local trauma can impact the growth and integrity of the nail.

Key Points in the Physical Examination

- In digital clubbing, assess for cardiopulmonary pathology such as murmurs or wheezing.

- Lovibond angle, the angle of eponychium to the nail plate, is normally 160 degrees. Clubbing induces angles of greater than 180 degrees.

- Schamroth window is the normal space that is seen when the dorsal aspects of opposing fingers are aligned. This diamond-shaped space is absent in clubbing.

- Dermatologic disorders such as psoriasis, eczema, and lichen planus are associated with nail pitting and dystrophy.

- Inspect the shape, color, texture, and thickness of the nail. Thickened, yellowed nails should raise the suspicion for onychomycosis.

- The nail fold capillaries are dilated in rheumatoid disorders.

- Splinter hemorrhages can be the sign of repeated nail trauma, such as in sports, or more ominously in bacterial endocarditis.

- Local growths, lesions, or cysts can impact the growth and appearance of the nail.

PHOTOGRAPHS OF SELECTED DIAGNOSES

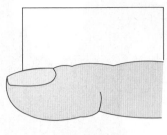 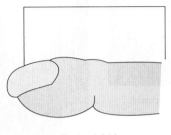 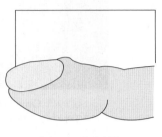

Normal   Early clubbing   Advanced clubbing

Figure 39-1 Nail clubbing. (Left) The angle between the nail and the digit is normally about 20 degrees in a child. (*Center*) Flattened angle represents early stage of clubbing. (*Right*) In advanced clubbing, the nail is rounded over the end of the finger. Note also that the distal phalanx is bulbous and of greater depth than the proximal portion of the finger (interphalangeal depth). (Used with permission from Pillitteri A., *Maternal and Child Nursing.* 4th ed. Philadelphia, PA: Lippincott, Williams & Wilkins; 2003.)

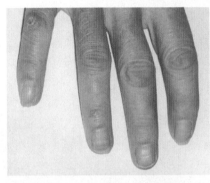

Figure 39-2 Beau lines. Beau lines of a severe illness in past. Illness was 5 weeks ago, 5 mm distal to the lunula (plate grows 1 mm/week). (Used with permission from Berg D, Worzala K. *Atlas of Adult Physical Diagnosis.* Philadelphia, PA: Lippincott Williams & Wilkins; 2006.)

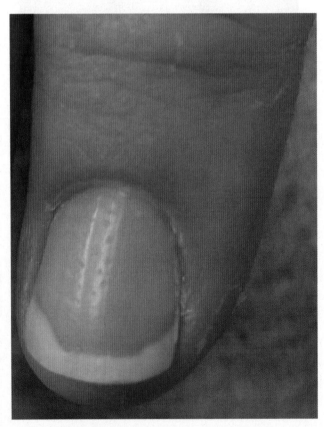

Figure 39-4 Nail pitting. (Courtesy of Dr. Barankin Dermatology Collection.)

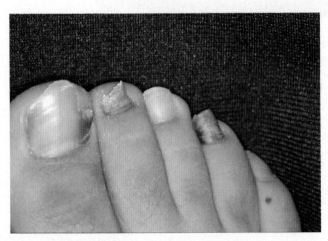

Figure 39-3 Onychomycosis. Note the yellow discoloration and thickening of the nail bed. (Courtesy of Denise W. Metry, MD.)

SECTION 12 • EXTREMITIES

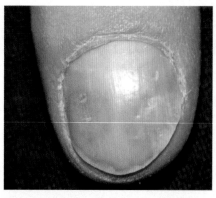

Figure 39-5 Onycholysis. Psoriasis. Pitting and onycholysis are evident in this nail. (Used with permission from Goodheart HP. *Goodheart's Photoguide of Common Skin Disorders.* 2nd ed. Philadelphia, PA: Lippincott Williams & Wilkins; 2003.)

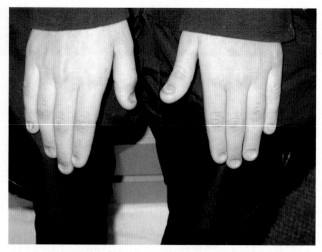

Figure 39-6 Koilonychia/nail spooning. Note the concave shape of the nail bed. (Courtesy of Moise L. Levy, MD.)

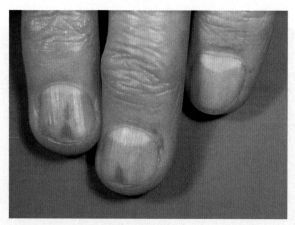

Figure 39-7 Subungual splinter hemorrhages. (Used with permission from Gold DH, Weingeist TA. *Color Atlas of the Eye in Systemic Disease.* Baltimore, MD: Lippincott Williams & Wilkins; 2001.)

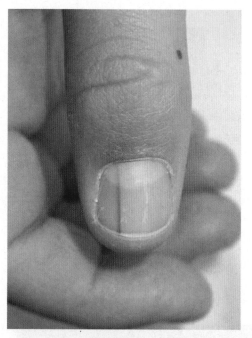

Figure 39-8 Longitudinal melanonychia. Note the longitudinal band of hyperpigmentation with no extension onto surrounding skin. (Courtesy of Moise L. Levy, MD.)

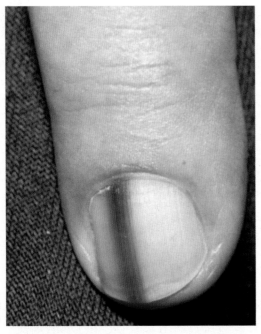

Figure 39-9 Junctional nevus. (Used with permission from Goodheart HP. *Goodheart's Photoguide to Common Skin Disorders.* 2nd ed. Philadelphia, PA: Lippincott Williams & Wilkins; 2003:356.)

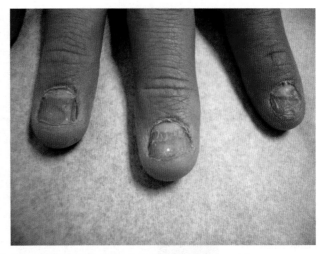

Figure 39-10 Nail dystrophy. A teenager with scaling of the nail suggestive of nail dystrophy. (Courtesy of Paul S. Matz, MD.)

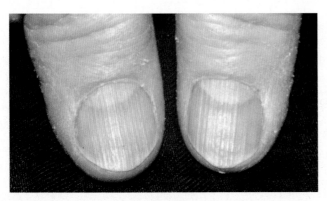

Figure 39-11 Longitudinal ridging. This normal variant is characterized by ridging in all of the nails. (Used with permission from Goodheart HP. *Goodheart's Photoguide to Common Skin Disorders.* 2nd ed. Philadelphia, PA: Lippincott Williams & Wilkins; 2003:233.)

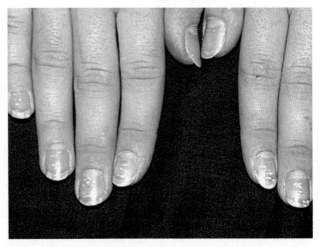

Figure 39-12 Leukonychia striata. (Used with permission from Goodheart HP. *Goodheart's Photoguide to Common Skin Disorders.* 2nd ed. Philadelphia, PA: Lippincott Williams & Wilkins; 2003:240.)

SECTION 12 • EXTREMITIES

DIFFERENTIAL DIAGNOSIS

DIAGNOSIS		ICD-10	DISTINGUISHING CHARACTERISTICS	DISTRIBUTION	DURATION/ CHRONICITY
Clubbing		R68.3	Clubbing refers to the curvature of the nails and widening of the distal phalanx. It represents a usually permanent expansion of the fibrovascular matrix	Most of the time, it will involve all the nails. It can be unilateral.	This is a chronic and irreversible process.
Beau Lines		L60.4	Transverse line or depression that represents an interruption of growth	Will usually affect all the nails. A single nail could be affected when it results from local trauma.	The depression will grow out with the nail.
Onychomycosis		B35.1	Yellowed, discolored, and thickened nails	Toe nails are more commonly affected. It can involve one to all nails.	Continued treatment until the affected nail grows out
Nail Pitting		L60.8	Pitting of the nails is grooves or depressions in the nail.	Commonly involves all the fingernails	Systemic issues usually cause and determine the duration.
Onycholysis		L60.1	The separation of the nail from the distal nail bed	Can involve one or more nails	It can be acute or chronic
Koilonychia		L60.3	Concavity or spooning of the nails	Typically involves all the nails	Usually chronic
Longitudinal Melanonychia/ Pigmented Bands		L60.9 (Nail disorder, unspecified)	Brown to black, longitudinal pigmentation	May be solitary or multiple (most commonly a result of normal ethnic pigmentation in darker-skinned persons)	May be chronic

ASSOCIATED FINDINGS	COMPLICATIONS	PREDISPOSING FACTORS	TREATMENT GUIDELINES
It is associated with chronic pulmonary, cardiac, or gastrointestinal pathology	Complications arise from the underlying systemic issue.	Congenital cyanotic heart disease, chronic lung disease, and gastrointestinal disorders	Address the underlying issue.
None, the insult usually predates the finding.	No direct complications	Trauma, prolonged fever, systemic illness, and chemotherapy	None
Tinea pedis Family members with fungal nail or skin infections Immunodeficiency	Onycholysis	Tight or ill-fitted shoes, trauma, and sport activities	Oral terbinafine, itraconazole, fluconazole
It is often associated with inflammatory skin conditions such as eczema, alopecia areata, and psoriasis.	None	The associated skin disorder	Address the associated or underlying issue.
Onychomycosis	None	Medications, trauma, onychomycosis, infections	Address the local or systemic issue if one exists.
In children it is often idiopathic.	None	Trauma and frequent water immersion. Associated with anemia and hypothyroidism in adults	Address the local or systemic issue if one exists.
Malignant melanoma (very rare) should be suspected whenever a solitary streak suddenly becomes darker and/or wider, edges become blurred, and/or a family history of melanoma exists	Those associated with underlying disease	May be caused by infection (fungal or bacterial) or melanin (nevi, normal ethnic pigmentation) Multiple pigmented bands may also be a feature of Addison disease or Cushing disease, Peutz–Jeghers syndrome, or pernicious anemia.	Depending on etiology, treatment with anti-infectives or treatment of systemic illness

SECTION 12 • EXTREMITIES

Other Diagnoses to Consider

- Nail psoriasis

- Pachyonychia congenital (rare genetic disorder characterized by hypertrophic nail dystrophy)

- Onychomadesis (nail dystrophy)

- Leukonychia

- Muehrcke lines

When to Consider Further Evaluation or Treatment

- Children presenting with nail clubbing should be assessed for potential cardiac, pulmonary, or gastrointestinal issues.

- Immunodeficiency should be considered in cases of severe onychomycosis that are unresponsive to antifungal agents.

- Endocarditis should be considered in cases of painful splinter hemorrhages seen in conjunction with Osler nodes.

- Subungual masses should be carefully evaluated. Consider diagnostic imaging, biopsy, and referral to a dermatologist.

- Fungal cultures should be done in cases of suspected onychomycosis.

SUGGESTED READINGS

Piraccini BM, Iorizzo M. Drug reactions affecting the nail unit: diagnosis and management. *Dermatol Clinic*. 2007;25:215–221.
Piraccini BM, Starace M, Bruni F. Onychomycosis in children. *Expert Rev Dermatol*. 2012;7:569–578.
Shah KN, Rubin AI. Nail disorders as signs of pediatric systemic disease. *Curr Probl Pediatr Adolesc Health Care*. 2012;42:204–211.
Tosti A, Daniel R, Piraccini BM, et al. *Color Atlas of Nails*. Heidelberg: Springer-Verlag; 2010:31–38, 87–88, 103–111.
Zaidi Z, Lanigan SW. Nail disorders. *Dermatology in Clinical Practice*. London: Springer-Verlag, 2010:381–393.

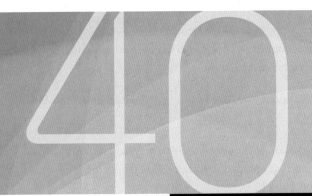

Arm Displacement

LaTanya J. Love

Approach to the Problem

Arm displacement in children frequently occurs as a result of trauma. Dislocation of the upper extremity can also be the result of an underlying congenital musculoskeletal abnormality that causes joint laxity. Consideration should be given to the mechanism of injury when dealing with traumatic dislocations. It is important to identify fractures that could cause a problem with future arm growth and function.

Key Points in the History

- Brachial plexus injuries may lead to shoulder dislocation as early as 3 months of age.

- Risk factors for neonatal brachial plexus injuries include shoulder dystocia, fetal macrosomia, large for gestational age infants, and history of traumatic birth.

- In infants and younger children, pain from a dislocation usually presents as a pseudoparesis, where the child refuses to move the affected extremity.

- Congenital dislocations are frequently seen without a history of trauma and often associated with other defects. When evaluating a patient, it is important to determine whether there is a prior history of dislocation.

- An anterior shoulder dislocation is usually caused by trauma to the abducted, externally rotated and extended arm, and is usually associated with sports-related injuries.

- A posterior shoulder dislocation is less common. This injury is usually from trauma to the anterior shoulder.

- A traction injury of the upper extremity frequently leads to acute radial head subluxation, also known as "nursemaid elbow." Radial head subluxation develops from displacement of the annular ligament, which is unlikely to be displaced after 5 years of age. The peak incidence of nursemaid elbow is between 2 and 3 years of age.

- An elbow dislocation is commonly seen in contact sports, such as wrestling or football, and in noncontact activities, such as gymnastics. This dislocation is most commonly posterior and secondary to falling on an outstretched arm, or a twisting injury to the elbow.

- Fractures of the distal radius are more common in adolescents than in younger children, and the usual history includes a fall on a hyperextended wrist.

- Habitual dislocations can be seen in children who have ligamentous laxity who are also able to voluntarily dislocate their joints.

- Sprengel deformity is a congenital elevation of the scapula, which may have multidirectional joint instability. Patients with a diagnosis of Sprengel deformity should undergo evaluation for other abnormalities of the vertebrae and ribs.

<table>
<tr><td>

Key Points in the Physical Examination

</td><td>

- Physical examination should always include inspection, palpation, range of motion evaluation, neurologic evaluation, and vascular evaluation.

- With an anterior dislocation of the shoulder, there is a loss of shoulder contour, and the arm is held slightly abducted and externally rotated. Axillary nerve damage can be seen following this injury and should be evaluated.

- With a posterior dislocation of the shoulder, there is a loss of shoulder contour, and the arm is held slightly adducted and internally rotated, and the shoulder is unable to be rotated externally.

- With radial head subluxation, a child usually refuses to use arm and holds it in a flexed and pronated position.

- Fractures of the elbow usually present with tenderness over the radial head or proximal ulna along with pain and swelling.

- Sprengel deformity is usually associated with muscle hypoplasia and can result in disfigurement and functional limitation of the shoulder.

</td></tr>
</table>

PHOTOGRAPHS OF SELECTED DIAGNOSES

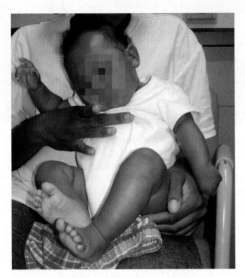

Figure 40-1 Brachial plexus injury. An infant with left arm held in adduction with internal rotation of the arm and pronation of the forearm. (Courtesy of Joseph Piatt, MD.)

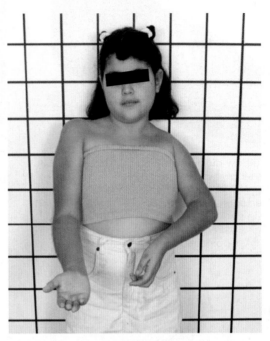

Figure 40-2 Brachial plexus injury. Patient attempting to extend and supinate arms. Compare with the normal movement of right arm. (Courtesy of Shiners Hospitals for Children, Houston, Texas.)

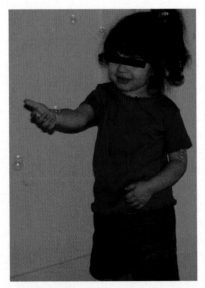

Figure 40-3 Nursemaid elbow. Child holding left arm slightly flexed and pronated toward body. Note child reaching for bubbles freely with right arm, but not with affected arm. (Courtesy of Jeoffrey K. Wolens, MD.)

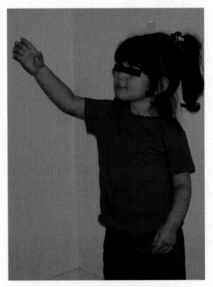

Figure 40-4 Nursemaid elbow. Child holding left arm slightly flexed and pronated toward body. Note child reaching for bubbles freely with right arm overhead, but not with affected arm. (Courtesy of Jeoffrey K. Wolens, MD.)

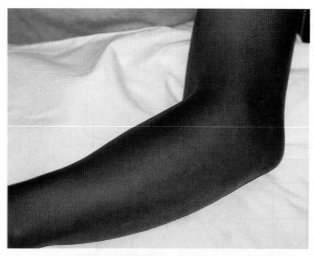

Figure 40-5 Elbow dislocation. This adolescent football player had his elbow hyperextended when tackling another player. Note the sharp contour due to the prominent olecranon displaced posteriorly on the injured side. (Used with permission from Fleisher GR, Ludwig S, Baskin MN. *Atlas of Pediatric Emergency Medicine.* Philadelphia, PA: Lippincott Williams & Wilkins; 2004.)

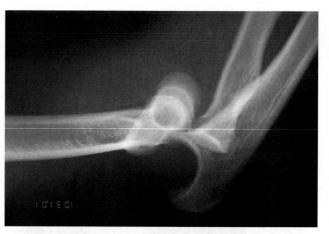

Figure 40-6 Elbow dislocation. This radiograph shows the dislocation shown in Figure 40-5 without an associated fracture. (Used with permission from Fleisher GR, Ludwig S, Baskin MN. *Atlas of Pediatric Emergency Medicine.* Philadelphia, PA: Lippincott Williams & Wilkins; 2004.)

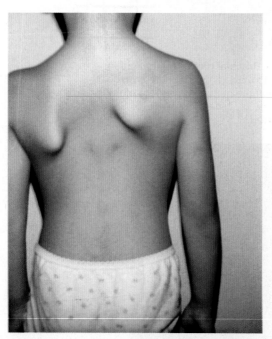

Figure 40-7 Sprengel deformity. Note right-sided deformity with elevation of scapula and asymmetry of shoulders and neck when compared with normal left side. (Courtesy of Shriners Hospitals for Children, Houston, Texas.)

DIFFERENTIAL DIAGNOSIS

DIAGNOSIS	ICD-10	DISTINGUISHING CHARACTERISTICS	COMPLICATIONS	PREDISPOSING FACTORS	TREATMENT GUIDELINES
Brachial Plexus Injury	S14.3XXA Newborn CM P14.0 CM P14.1 CM P14.3	Painless Can be associated with fracture of the distal humerus	N/A	Traction injury during delivery that leads to imbalance of musculature that pulls the shoulder posteriorly Risk factors include fetal macrosomia, shoulder dystocia, and traumatic delivery	Physical therapy Surgical repair if symptoms not resolving within 3 to 9 months
Shoulder Dislocation	Anterior S43.016A Posterior S43.026A	Anterior dislocation—arm held abducted and externally rotated Posterior dislocation—arm adducted and internally rotated	Nerve and vascular injuries are rare but can be complications Rotator cuff tears are uncommon in younger patients. Recurrent dislocations are common	Usually caused by direct trauma to humerus and shoulder	Procedural sedation is generally used. Anterior dislocation: usually starts with scapular manipulation Posterior dislocation: orthopedic surgeon should be consulted. Shoulder immobilizer for 3 weeks
Radial Head Subluxation (Nursemaid Elbow)	S53.006A	Child not using affected arm, and elbow is usually flexed and forearm pronated Occurs in children up to 5 years of age, but most commonly in children 2 to 3 years of age	None	Traction on pronated arm with elbow in extension	Hyperpronate and extend the affected arm. If unsuccessful, then supinate and flex the arm. The physician should feel a "click" over the radial head once it is reduced and the patient should be able to resume using the arm within 10 minutes The arm does not need additional treatment or immobilization after successful reduction.
Radial Head Dislocation	S43.016A	Pain and tenderness to palpation over radial head Swelling	Ulnar fracture Ulnar nerve injury	Hyperextension of elbow Fall onto an outstretched arm	An orthopedic surgeon should be consulted for reduction
Elbow Dislocation	S53.006A S53.106A	Posterior dislocation most common Usually adolescent males	Neurovascular injury	Usually after fall from outstretched hand with forearm supinated and elbow extended	Procedural sedation is highly recommended Posterior dislocations—counter-traction and stabilization of distal humerus while traction to distal arm and flexion of the elbow
Sprengel Deformity	CM Q68.8	Elevation and medial rotation of scapula	None	Congenital and usually arises from interruption of normal caudal migration of the scapula.	Physical therapy to strengthen muscles Surgical treatment is best between 3 and 8 years of age when significant deformity is present.

SECTION 12 • EXTREMITIES

Other Diagnoses to Consider

- Cerebral palsy

- Osteogenesis imperfecta

- Ehlers–Danlos syndrome

- Larsen syndrome

- Familial joint instability syndrome

- Radioulnar synostosis

- Nonaccidental trauma

When to Consider Further Evaluation or Treatment

- Recurrent dislocation is a common complication of shoulder dislocation. All patients with a diagnosis of shoulder dislocation should be evaluated by an orthopedic surgeon after reduction, because of the high incidence of shoulder instability post-reduction.

- In suspected radial head subluxation: a child without history of a traction injury, or a child with a history consistent with radial head subluxation, with focal swelling or tenderness should have radiographs done to evaluate for a potential fracture.

- Radiographs of the arm should be obtained for any patient with a suspected radial head subluxation that is not reducible, in order to rule out fracture of the radius or ulna.

- A visible posterior fat pad on a lateral radiographic image of the elbow in the setting of trauma is usually indicative of a fracture.

- If a patient has generally worsening pain in the forearm with or without paresthesia or decreased sensation, and/or increased pain in the forearm with the passive extension of the muscles, the possibility of a compartment syndrome should be considered.

- If there is suspected nerve injury in association with a fracture, and normal function has not returned after 8 to 12 weeks of symptoms, consider electromyography and further evaluation by a neurologist.

SUGGESTED READINGS

Chasm RM, Swencki SA. Pediatric orthopedic emergencies. *Emerg Med Clin North Am.* 2010;28(4):907–926.

Cramer KE, Scherl SA, eds. *Pediatrics: Orthopedic Surgery Essentials.* Philadelphia, PA: Lippincott Williams & Wilkins; 2004:104–135.

Mariscalco MW, Saluan P. Upper extremity injuries in the adolescent athlete. *Sports Med Arthrosc Rev.* 2011;19:17–26.

Moukoko D, Ezaki M, Wilkes D, et al. Posterior shoulder dislocations in infants with neonatal brachial plexus palsy. *J Bone Joint Surg Am.* 2004;86-A(4):787–793.

Pizzutillo PD, ed. *Pediatric Orthopedics in Primary Practice.* New York: McGraw-Hill; 1997:9–12, 29–32, 37–44, 51–54, 61–64, 325–328.

Staheli L. *Fundamentals of Pediatric Orthopedics.* 4th ed. Philadelphia, PA: Lippincott Williams & Wilkins; 2008:65–73, 268–275.

Staheli L. *Practice of Pediatric Orthopedics.* 2nd ed. Philadelphia, PA: Lippincott Williams & Wilkins; 2006:228–240.

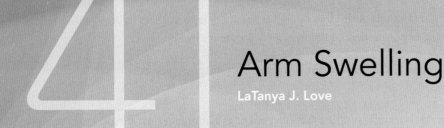

Arm Swelling

LaTanya J. Love

Approach to the Problem

Arm swelling can be a common manifestation of musculoskeletal, infectious, or rheumatologic diseases. The first consideration in a patient presenting with arm swelling is inquiry regarding a previous history of trauma. Traumatic events can result in injuries such as hematomas, sprains, and fractures. A clinician must also consider nonaccidental trauma in immobile children and in children presenting without a history to support a traumatic injury. Other potential diagnoses in patients presenting with arm swelling are infection and tumors. If more than one joint presents with swelling, consideration can be given to associated systemic diseases such as systemic lupus erythematosus, juvenile idiopathic arthritis, or inflammatory bowel disease. It is also very important to differentiate between conditions that might require urgent medical intervention.

Key Points in the History

- Presence of precipitating factors such as trauma or recent illness.

- For infants or patients presenting with an inconsistent history, nonaccidental trauma should be considered.

- Younger children who are not able to express pain may have a history of decreased use of the affected arm.

- Osteomyelitis, septic arthritis, and soft-tissue infections should be considered in patients who also present with subacute arm swelling, erythema, decreased arm movement, and fever. The most common bacteria in bone infections are *Staphylococcus aureus* and Group A streptococcus.

- Predisposing factors for soft-tissue infections include breaks in the skin from bites, abrasions, or preexisting skin conditions.

- It is common for distal radial, ulnar (Colles), greenstick, and buckle (torus) fractures to occur following trauma, such as falling on an outstretched hand, when a child is trying to protect himself/herself from a fall.

- Supracondylar fractures in children can be secondary to high-velocity injuries such as falling from a bicycle or playground equipment, such as monkey bars.

- Younger children usually sustain supracondylar fractures after shorter falls, such as fall from a bed or sofa.

- A ganglion cyst is a cystic swelling that can present as a nontender wrist mass. However, if it occurs near a joint, it can be painful.

- In the arm, osteochondromas are common benign, slow-growing, nonpainful, bone tumors that usually occur at the proximal humerus. Osteochondromas usually stop growing once the child reaches skeletal maturity.

- Children with a history of a bleeding disorder, such as hemophilia, may develop hemarthrosis or hematoma with minimal trauma.

- In a child with a history of a central venous line who presents with acute arm swelling, venous thromboembolism should be considered.

Key Points in the Physical Examination

- If a history of known trauma or nonaccidental trauma is suspected, the practitioner should perform a complete examination looking for other areas of trauma.

- In evaluating a child presenting with arm swelling, it is important to perform a complete neurovascular examination.

- Supracondylar fractures are at risk for nerve damage, so it is important to assess the median, radial, and ulnar nerves. The median nerve can be assessed by asking the patient to make the "OK" sign. The radial nerve can be assessed by asking the patient to make the "thumbs-up" sign. The ulnar nerve can be assessed by asking the patient to abduct all fingers against resistance.

- In distal forearm fractures, clinicians should also evaluate the elbow and wrist for associated fractures.

- Increased pain on passive extension of the fingers, cold hands, and excessive swelling can be suggestive of compartment syndrome in patients with supracondylar fractures.

- Ganglion cysts transilluminate and are typically firm, nontender, mobile nodules over the wrist.

- Osteochondromas and other bone tumors usually present as a discrete, painless, nonmobile mass.

PHOTOGRAPHS OF SELECTED DIAGNOSES

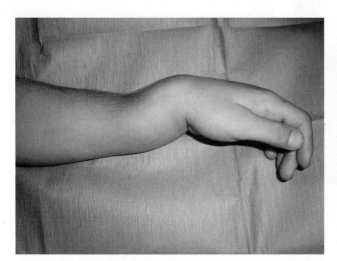

Figure 41-1 Colles fracture. Wrist swelling with obvious deformity. (Courtesy of William Phillips, MD.)

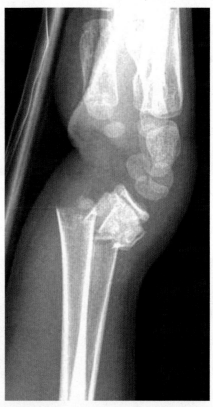

Figure 41-2 Colles fracture. Distal radial fracture with dorsal angulation. (Courtesy of William Phillips, MD.)

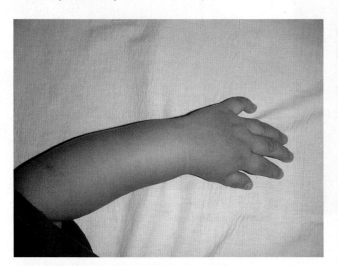

Figure 41-3 Torus fracture. (Courtesy of Michael C. Distefano, MD.)

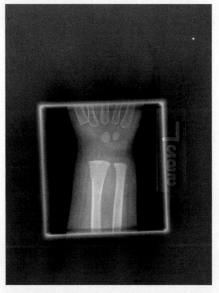

Figure 41-4 Torus fracture. (Courtesy of Michael C. Distefano, MD.)

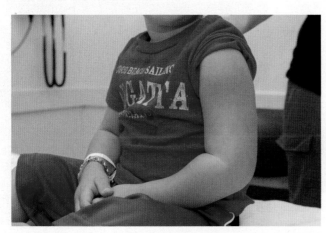

Figure 41-5 Supracondylar fracture. Note the swelling of the left elbow. (Courtesy of Michael C. Distefano, MD.)

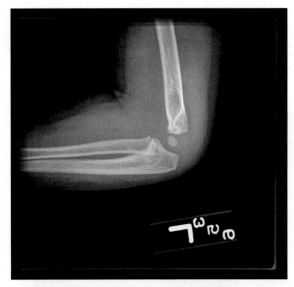

Figure 41-6 **Supracondylar fracture.** Left grade 1 supracondylar fracture (nondisplaced) with associated posterior fat pad. No other radiographic evidence of fracture. (Courtesy of Michael C. Distefano, MD.)

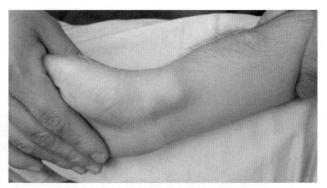

Figure 41-7 **Ganglion cyst.** Localized swelling over the volar surface of the wrist of a school-aged child. (Courtesy of Mary L. Brandt, MD.)

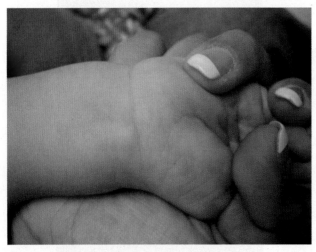

Figure 41-8 **Ganglion cyst.** Localized swelling over the volar surface of the wrist of an infant. (Courtesy of Mary L. Brandt, MD.)

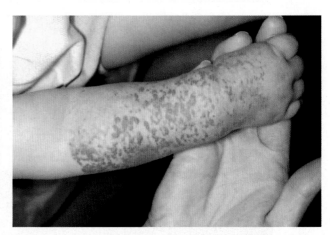

Figure 41-9 **Large hemangioma of right forearm of an infant.** Swelling with raised areas of vascular prominence is present. (Courtesy of Moise L. Levy, MD.)

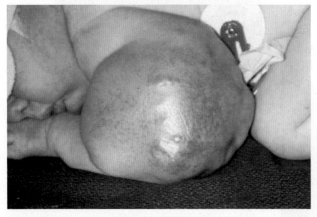

Figure 41-10 **Cavernous hemangioma.** (Courtesy of Jan Edwin Drutz, MD.)

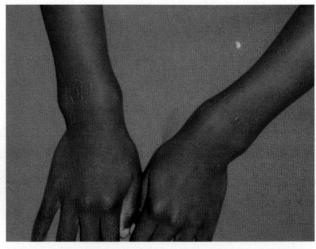

Figure 41-11 **Rickets.** Bilateral wrist swelling secondary to vitamin D deficiency rickets. (Courtesy of Tom Thacher, MD.)

DIFFERENTIAL DIAGNOSIS

DIAGNOSIS	ICD-10	DISTINGUISHING CHARACTERISTICS	DISTRIBUTION	COMPLICATIONS	TREATMENT GUIDELINES
Colles Fracture	S52.539A (closed) S52.539B S52.539C (open)	Distal radial fracture that is typically angulated	Distal forearm	Nerve damage	Nondisplaced and minimally angulated fractures can be splinted in a sugar-tong splint.
Buckle Fracture (Torus Fracture)	S52.119A S52.299A	Distal radial fracture with only minor irregularity in the contour of the cortex	Distal forearm	Reinjury	Splint for 2–4 weeks
Supracondylar Fracture	S42.413A (closed) S42.413B S42.416B (open)	Usually occurs after fall onto an outstretched hand with elbow in hyperextension	Swelling of the entire elbow Fracture of the distal humerus	Neurovascular damage If vascular damage, usually brachial artery involved Compartment syndrome	Nondisplaced or minimally displaced fractures may be immobilized in a posterior splint and sling All displaced fractures require orthopedic evaluation.
Ganglion Cyst	M67.40	May present as firm mass over the wrist or as joint pain Transilluminates	Wrist and tissue adjacent to finger joints	None	May spontaneously regress Aspiration or surgical removal is recommended only for functional impairment or cosmetic concern
Osteochondroma	D16.00 (upper extremity long bone) D16.10 (upper extremity short bone)	Painless mass or a painful mass associated with trauma	Usually proximal humerus	Malignant transformation to a chondrosarcoma	Most are monitored clinically. Surgical excision for painful or rapidly growing lesion
Aneurysmal Bone Cyst	M85.50	Rapidly growing benign lesion Generally occur in adolescents	More common in long bones	Because of rapid growth may destroy bone Lesions that cross growth plate may cause growth arrest	Excision, curettage, and bone grafting

Other Diagnoses to Consider

- Septic arthritis

- Osteomyelitis

- Systemic lupus erythematosus

- Juvenile idiopathic arthritis

- Postinfectious arthritis

- Rickets

- Sickle cell vasooclusive crisis

- Rickets

- Venous thromboembolism

- Klippel–Trenaunay syndrome

- Hemangioma

- Bone tumor

When to Consider Further Evaluation or Treatment

- Recent fever with monoarticular disease can be suggestive of a joint or bone infection and should be evaluated rapidly.

- Fractures in stages of healing that are not consistent with the clinical history, or multiple fractures with different stages of healing, should raise suspicion for child abuse.

- In fractures that are open, or show evidence of neurovascular compromise or compartment syndrome, a prompt evaluation by an orthopedic surgeon is indicated.

- Most ganglion cysts resolve spontaneously. A ganglion cyst that causes significant pain or decreased function may be referred to an interventional radiologist for aspiration or a surgeon for excision.

- Wrist sprains that have not improved with rest, ice, and range of motion exercises should be referred to an orthopedic surgeon.

SUGGESTED READINGS

Chasm RM, Swencki SA. Pediatric orthopedic emergencies. *Emerg Med Clin North Am.* 2010;28(4):907–926.
Cramer CE, Sheri SA, eds. *Pediatrics: Orthopedic Surgery Essentials.* Philadelphia, PA: Lippincott Williams & Wilkins; 2003:104–135.
Gereige R, Kumar M. Bone lesions: Benign and malignant. *Pediatr Rev.* 2010;31:355–363.
Plint AC, Perry JJ, Correll R, et al. A randomized, controlled trial of removable splinting versus casting for wrist buckle fractures in children. *Pediatrics.* 2006;117(3):691–697.

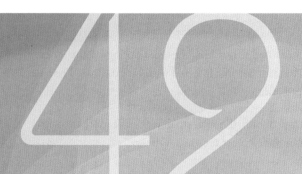

Hand Swelling

Lauren Wilson and Rebecca G. Taxier

Approach to the Problem

Hand swelling can be a result of pathology in the bones, joints, tendons, blood vessels, or soft tissues. Many systemic diseases, such as Kawasaki disease, sickle cell disease (SCD), juvenile idiopathic arthritis (JIA), viral arthritides, and serum sickness, can produce hand swelling. In these cases, hand involvement tends to be symmetric, and other constitutional symptoms lend important clues to the etiology. More localized causes of hand swelling include osteomyelitis, septic arthritis, tenosynovitis, cellulitis, trauma, and soft-tissue tumors. Careful examination of the hand, paying close attention to joint motion, range of motion, and areas of tenderness, swelling, or erythema, can narrow the differential diagnosis based on the anatomic structures involved.

Key Points in the History

- Osteomyelitis in the hands can result from hematogenous spread of infection, direct inoculation as seen with a puncture wound, or contiguous spread from adjacent structures as may be seen with septic arthritis. In infants, osteomyelitis commonly causes swelling of adjacent soft tissues.

- Septic arthritis, most commonly caused by *Staphylococcus aureus*, is usually monoarticular and associated with swelling, erythema, and pain on movement.

- Cellulitis may occur at the site of minor trauma. Patients may also report a "spider bite" that becomes larger and more erythematous, as the initial papular lesion often resembles an insect bite.

- JIA has a variety of manifestations. Of the seven subtypes of JIA, polyarticular rheumatoid factor positive (2%–7% of JIA), systemic (4%–17%), and psoriatic (2%–11%) are most likely to have hand involvement.

- Dactylitis associated with SCD presents with tender, erythematous, and edematous hands or feet in patients. It is frequently the presenting sign, occurring in 25% of affected individuals by 1 year of age and in 40% by 2 years of age. The pathophysiology is thought to be similar to other vasoocclusive crises.

- Clenched fist injuries are caused by the closed fist striking the teeth during a fight. These are not often recognized as bite injuries, but can become infected with mouth flora. They also have a high rate of extensor tendon and joint capsule injuries.

- A boxer's fracture is a fracture of the fourth or fifth metacarpal neck. The mechanism is usually a closed fist striking a hard, immobile object such as a wall.

Key Points in the Physical Examination

- The extremity changes associated with Kawasaki disease (one of the five principal features, in addition to fever) typically manifest initially in the hands as swelling and palmar erythema. The palms may progress to painful induration within the acute phase. Desquamation of the fingertips appears in the convalescent phase, usually as the fever resolves (commonly at 10–14 days, if untreated).

- A sensitive screening examination showing arthritis in the metacarpophalangeal (MCP), proximal interphalangeal, and/or distal interphalangeal joints is the inability to make a completely clenched fist; that is, the fingertips do not meet the palm.

- Psoriatic arthritis is often accompanied by a psoriatic rash; if the rash is absent, arthritis must be accompanied by two of the following criteria: family history of psoriasis in a first-degree relative, dactylitis, and nail pitting. The typical scaly rash of psoriasis is most often found on the elbows, knees, and extensor surfaces.

- In a displaced boxer's fracture, the fourth or fifth knuckle (MCP joint) will appear depressed when examining the partially closed fist. Even when nondisplaced, edema, discoloration, and point tenderness are usually present.

PHOTOGRAPHS OF SELECTED DIAGNOSES

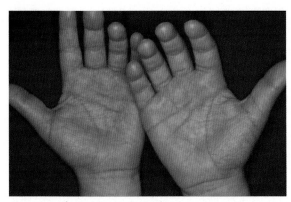

Figure 42-1 Kawasaki disease. The hands of this 4-year-old with 5 days of high fever show diffuse erythema and swelling. (Courtesy of Mark A. Ward, MD.)

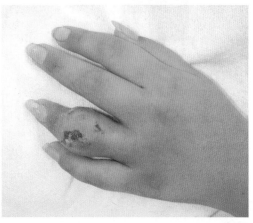

Figure 42-2 Osteomyelitis. Soft-tissue swelling, joint involvement, and fistulous tracts complicate the finger osteomyelitis seen in this 12-year-old female. (Courtesy of Mary L. Brandt, MD.)

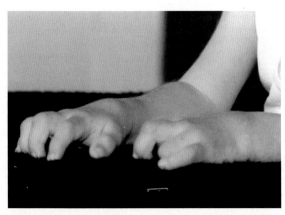

Figure 42-3 Juvenile rheumatoid arthritis. Flexion contractures complicate the polyarticular JIA seen in this 5-year-old. Also, note the swelling of the wrists and the fingers. (Courtesy of Shriners Hospitals for Children, Houston, Texas.)

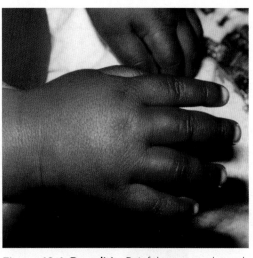

Figure 42-4 Dactylitis. Painful sausage-shaped fingers and symmetrical swelling of the hands characterize the onset of dactylitis in this infant with SCD. (Courtesy of Tom Thatcher, MD.)

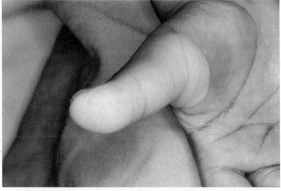

Figure 42-5 Blistering distal dactylitis. A superficial blister with an erythematous base covers the entire distal volar fat pad of this 5-year-old, also extending to the base of the digit. (Courtesy of Mark A. Ward, MD.)

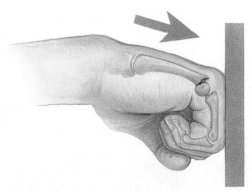

Figure 42-6 Boxer's fracture. The neck of the fourth or fifth metacarpal snaps when a closed fist strikes a hard immobile object. (Used with permission from the Anatomical Chart Company. ACC Systems and Structures Chart Images, p. 2.)

DIFFERENTIAL DIAGNOSIS

DIAGNOSIS		ICD-10	DISTINGUISHING CHARACTERISTICS	DISTRIBUTION
Kawasaki Disease		M30.3	Principal features are fever for at least 5 days, plus four of five of the following: Edema and erythema of hands and feet; nonexudative conjunctivitis; lip and oral mucosal changes; rash; cervical lymphadenopathy (>1.5 cm)	Hand involvement: typically diffuse swelling, sometimes with palmar erythema or induration
Osteomyelitis (OM)		M86.9	Most frequently caused by *S. aureus* Also consider *Kingella kingae*, Group A streptococcus in preschoolers, and *Escherichia coli* or Group B streptococcus in neonates Young infants are more likely to have multifocal disease. Soft-tissue swelling around bone lesions is more frequent in infants.	Most commonly found in metaphysis of tubular bones—femur, tibia, humerus, and phalanges—as well as pelvis
Disseminated Gonococcal Infection (DGI)		A54.49 A54.42	DGI occurs in 1%–3% of all *Neisseria gonorrhoeae* infections. DGI presents in two main forms: tenosynovitis–dermatitis–polyarthralgia triad and purulent arthritis	Tenosynovitis–dermatitis–polyarthralgia: Tenosynovitis often affects wrist, fingers, ankle, and toes Purulent arthritis: Mono- or oligoarticular septic arthritis, usually of knee, wrist, or ankle
Septic Arthritis		M00.9	*S. aureus* is the most common cause of bacterial arthritis in children; streptococci and *K. kingae* also occur; Salmonella frequent in children with SCD Presents with swollen joint(s), pain on passive movement, and fever (not always present)	Usually unifocal and affecting lower extremities Wrist and metacarpal joints rarely affected
Juvenile Idiopathic Arthritis		M08.90	Arthritis lasting at least 6 weeks, with onset before 16 years of age; often a diagnosis of exclusion Seven subtypes: oligoarticular, polyarticular (RF+ and RF−), systemic, psoriatic, and enthesitis-related Typically associated with morning stiffness	Polyarticular RF+, systemic, and psoriatic most likely subtypes to involve hands
Dactylitis (Hand–Foot Syndrome)		D57.00 D57.219 D57.819	Painful, symmetric swelling A type of vaso-occlusive crisis that affects children under 2 years of age with sickle cell disease	Diffuse involvement of metacarpals and proximal phalanges; also involves the feet in a similar fashion
Viral Arthritis		M03.2	**Hepatitis B virus infection:** 10%–25% of patients develop arthritis during febrile prodrome, followed by icterus 1–14 days later	Interphalangeal and metacarpal joints, usually symmetric
		B06.82	**Rubella infection:** Exanthem, palate petechiae, lymphadenopathy (retroauricular, posterior cervical, and occipital)	Interphalangeal and metacarpal joints Also can involve knees and wrists
		M01.5	**Parvovirus:** Nonspecific prodrome, followed by slapped cheek rash (young children) or generalized exanthem 5–7 days later	Postinfectious transient small joint pain with or without frank arthritis Knees may be affected in younger children
Blistering Distal Dactylitis		L08.9	Superficial tender blisters on an erythematous base Usually caused by Group A streptococcus, also reports of *S. aureus* and Group B streptococcus	Usually affects the distal volar fat pad of a finger or thumb

ASSOCIATED FINDINGS	PREDISPOSING FACTORS	TREATMENT GUIDELINES
Acutely: irritability, gastrointestinal symptoms, carditis, arthritis/arthralgias, gallbladder hydrops After 10 days of illness: coronary artery aneurysm, finger and toe desquamation	Age typically 1–5; median age is 2 years All racial groups are affected, but those of Asian and Pacific Island descent are particularly at risk. Seasonal clusters in winter and early spring Risk increases for twins and siblings of index cases	Laboratory evaluation for incomplete Kawasaki disease if three or fewer criteria are met Treatment with intravenous immunoglobulin (IVIG) and aspirin Baseline and follow-up echocardiogram given risk of coronary artery aneurysms
Pseudoparalysis in young infants Deep venous thrombophlebitis in up to 30% Periosteal abscess Avascular necrosis Limb shortening, if growth plate affected	2:1 male-to-female ratio Half under age 5 Risk factors include minor trauma, puncture wounds, adjacent infection (septic arthritis), immunodeficiency, indwelling catheters, sickle cell disease, and sepsis.	Prompt surgical drainage if abscess, sequestrum, or contiguous infection is present Initial empiric IV antibiotic therapy is based on age, comorbidities, and local antibiotic resistance patterns
Dermatitis (usually painless pustular lesions) Acute endocarditis Meningitis (rare)	Unprotected sexual intercourse 3:1 female-to-male ratio Risk factors for dissemination of gonococcal infection: complement deficiency, recent menstruation, pregnancy, or immediate postpartum state	Consult orthopedist for joint washout, if purulent arthritis. Ceftriaxone IV typically first line; however, concerns for increasing resistance Screen for other sexually transmitted infections.
N/A	Immunodeficiency, joint surgery, underlying arthritis, hemoglobinopathy	An orthopedic surgeon should be consulted to assist with joint aspiration. Initial empiric antibiotic therapy is based on clinical status, age, and local antibiotic resistance patterns.
Polyarticular RF+: joint destruction, deformity, uveitis Systemic onset: fevers, rash, leukocytosis, hepatosplenomegaly, macrophage activation syndrome Psoriatic: Dactylitis, psoriatic rash, nail pitting	Heterogenous group of diseases; HLA alleles and environmental causes thought to play a role	NSAIDs Glucocorticoids Disease-modifying antirheumatic drugs (DMARDs) to modulate immune response Physical and occupational therapy
Dactylitis before age 1 is a predictor for other markers of severe sickle cell disease: stroke, pain episodes, recurrent acute chest syndrome, and death	African American background (incidence 1:500) Hispanic American background (1:36,000) Dactylitis more frequent in HbSS	Manage with analgesia, adequate hydration, and warm packs Hydroxyurea is effective in preventing dactylitis.
Pruritic rash 5% develop persistent infection with immune complex-mediated sequelae	Vertical and horizontal transmission IV drug use Contaminated blood products Sexual intercourse	Supportive care
Low-grade fevers, conjunctival injection Postinfectious encephalitis (1 in 6,000)	Developing countries Eliminated from the United States in 2004	Supportive care
Hydrops fetalis in pregnant women Rare: transient aplastic crisis, papular purpuric "gloves and socks syndrome"	Common worldwide Adult females most likely to develop postinfectious arthritis	Supportive care
No systemic symptoms	No known risks Usually no history of trauma	Incision and drainage Systemic antibiotic tailored to causative organism

<table>
<tr><td>

Other
Diagnoses
to Consider

</td><td>

- Henoch–Schönlein purpura

- Lysosomal storage disease (Farber disease, also known as ceramidase deficiency)

- Pachydermodactyly (superficial dermal fibromatosis)

- Soft-tissue tumors

- Serum sickness

- Tuberculous dactylitis

</td></tr>
<tr><td>

When to
Consider
Further
Evaluation
or Treatment

</td><td>

- Orthopedic or plastic surgery consultation should be obtained for significant soft-tissue infections of the hand, particularly with abscess, as tenosynovitis and other deeper involvement can cause permanent functional deficits.

- A hand fracture with any adjacent break in the skin should be treated emergently as an open fracture, requiring orthopedic surgery consultation.

- If septic arthritis is suspected, joint aspiration and irrigation should be performed. Most infections should be treated by arthrotomy (or sometimes arthroscopy) and a surgical washout, in order to minimize the potential for cartilage destruction and subsequent arthritis.

- Dactylitis associated with SCD should be treated like other vaso-occlusive crises with hydration and analgesics.

- Patients with four of five principal features of Kawasaki disease may be treated with IVIG and aspirin after 4 days of fever. Patients with 5 days of fever and suspected Kawasaki disease, but fewer than four features, should have an echocardiogram and additional laboratory testing, and may be treated for incomplete or atypical Kawasaki disease if results support the diagnosis.

</td></tr>
</table>

SUGGESTED READINGS

Faust SN, Clark J, Pallett A, et al. Managing bone and joint infection in children. *Arch Dis Child.* 2012;97:545–553.

McCavit TL. Sickle cell disease. *Pediatr Rev.* 2012;33(5):195–206. Erratum in. *Pediatr Rev.* 2012;33:375.

Newburger JW, Takahashi M, Gerber MA, et al. Diagnosis, treatment, and long-term management of Kawasaki disease: a statement of the Council on Cardiovascular Disease in the Young, American Heart Association. *Pediatrics.* 2004;114(6):1708–1733. Erratum in. *Pediatrics.* 2005;115(4):1118.

Ravelli A, Martini A. Juvenile idiopathic arthritis. *Lancet.* 2007;369:767–778.

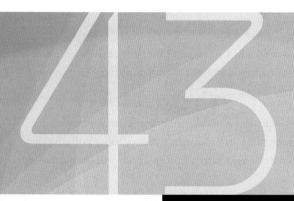

Finger Abnormalities

David Y. Khechoyan and
Larry H. Hollier, Jr

Approach to the Problem

Congenital finger anomalies are common with an incidence of 1 per 500 to 1,000 live births. The most common anomaly is polydactyly (duplication) followed by syndactyly (failure of differentiation). Presence of a congenital hand anomaly should alert the provider to perform a careful history and physical examination to evaluate for other associated malformations or syndromes. Congenital hand malformations are classified by embryologic origin and clinical manifestations. The major categories and representative examples include (1) failure of formation of parts (e.g., phocomelia, radial club hand), (2) failure of differentiation or separation of parts (e.g., syndactyly, clinodactyly, camptodactyly), (3) duplication (e.g., polydactyly), (4) overgrowth (e.g., macrodactyly), (5) undergrowth (e.g., thumb hypoplasia), and (6) congenital constriction band syndrome. A referral to a Pediatric Hand Specialist for further evaluation and surgical treatment is recommended for most congenital hand and digit anomalies.

Key Points in the History

- Approximately 80% of cases of syndactyly are sporadic. Males are affected twice as frequently as females. Complex syndactyly can be found as part of a syndrome, such as Poland or Apert syndrome.

- Clinodactyly is defined as abnormal curvature of the digit in the radioulnar plane. It rarely causes functional limitations. It may be seen as part of a syndromic condition, for example, Down syndrome (Trisomy 21).

- Camptodactyly refers to a congenital finger flexion deformity at the proximal interphalangeal (PIP) joint. There are two variants, one that appears in infancy with equal gender predilection and the other that presents in adolescent girls. Functional impairment is rare. The small finger is most commonly affected.

- Polydactyly is defined as preaxial (radial), central, or postaxial (ulnar). It may occur as an isolated malformation or as part of a syndrome, such as Trisomy 13 syndrome.

- Radial polydactyly (thumb duplication) occurs in 1 in every 12,000 live births with equal incidence in blacks and whites. The most common form of thumb duplication is complete duplication of the proximal and distal phalanges.

- Ulnar polydactyly is more common in blacks and is usually inherited in an autosomal dominant fashion without associated anomalies. In Caucasian patients, ulnar polydactyly may indicate serious chromosomal anomaly or associated malformations and should prompt further investigations.

- Ulnar polydactyly is subdivided into Type A (complete duplication up to the level of metacarpal head) and Type B (small rudimentary digit).

- Macrodactyly, or digital gigantism, reflects enlargement of all tissue elements of an involved digit. The index finger is most commonly affected. Two forms have been described: (1) static, with digit enlargement at birth with subsequent growth proportionate to the child; and (2) progressive, with disproportionate enlargement with age.

- Hypoplastic thumb malformation may be isolated or as part of a broader radial deficiency. When radial deficiency is present, detailed evaluation to exclude associated abnormalities, such as VACTERL (**V**ertebral anomalies, **A**nal atresia, **C**ardiac defects, **T**racheoesophageal fistula and/or **E**sophageal atresia, **R**enal and radial anomalies, and **L**imb defects) syndrome, thrombocytopenia with absent radius (TAR) syndrome, Fanconi anemia, or Holt–Oram syndrome, is critical.

- Congenital constriction band anomalies are typically sporadic, but may be associated with club feet or cleft lip and palate. The malformation may vary from simple constriction to complete congenital digital amputations.

Key Points in the Physical Examination

- Syndactyly may be present as webbing between two adjacent digits that can involve the entire length of the digits (complete syndactyly) or partial length of the digits (incomplete syndactyly). Simple syndactyly refers to a soft tissue connection only, whereas complex syndactyly indicates a soft and skeletal tissue union. Syndactyly most commonly involves the third webspace and is more frequently seen on the ulnar (postaxial) aspect of the hand.

- The most common form of clinodactyly is radial deviation of the small finger at the distal interphalangeal (DIP) joint. This occurs because the middle phalanx is shaped like a trapezoid, delta phalanx, as a result of an abnormal epiphysis.

- Camptodactyly most commonly involves the small finger. The anomaly may reflect longitudinal deficiency of skin, hand intrinsic muscles, extensor mechanism, and bony defects.

- Ulnar polydactyly is subdivided into two variants:

  - Type A ulnar polydactyly refers to complete duplication up to the level of the metacarpal head. This requires more extensive surgical treatment with excision of the well-formed, polydactylous digit and reinsertion of supporting ligaments and hypothenar muscles to the remaining digit.

- Type B ulnar polydactyly refers to a rudimentary polydactylous digit attached to the hand via a soft tissue stalk that contains a neurovascular pedicle. Simple excision of the anomalous, extra digit with transection of the neurovascular pedicle and retraction is recommended. Suture ligation in is not recommended by some experts, as this technique leads to pain, abnormal scarring, and painful neuroma formation.

- Macrodactyly is typically unilateral, with the index finger most commonly involved. Lipofibromatous hamartomas with generalized excess of adipose tissue throughout the involved digit is characteristic. Children with macrodactyly may be candidates for debulking or epiphysiodesis to arrest skeletal growth. More advanced cases or cases with delayed presentations may require distal amputations.

- Thumb hypoplasia may range from mild hypoplasia (small thumb with all structures intact) to total thumb aplasia. Reconstructive options range from preservation of hypoplastic thumb if the carpometacarpal joint is present to thumb remnant ablation and pollicization (i.e., transferring the index finger into the thumb position for prehensile function).

PHOTOGRAPHS OF SELECTED DIAGNOSES

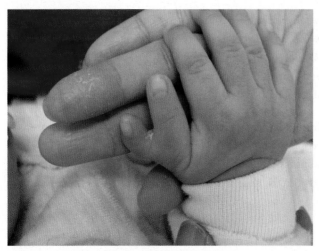

Figure 43-1 Polydactyly. An infant with a preaxial thumb duplication. (Courtesy of Esther K. Chung, MD, MPH.)

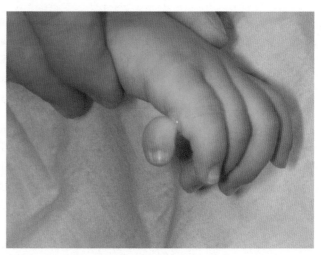

Figure 43-2 Postaxial polydactyly. An infant with postaxial fifth finger duplication on the right hand. (Courtesy of Paul S. Matz, MD.)

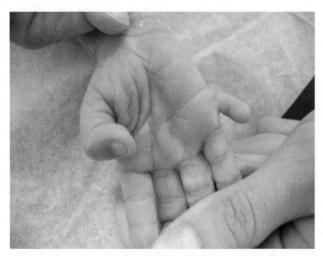

Figure 43-3 Postaxial polydactyly. A newborn with postaxial fifth finger duplication of the right hand. (Courtesy of Paul S. Matz, MD.)

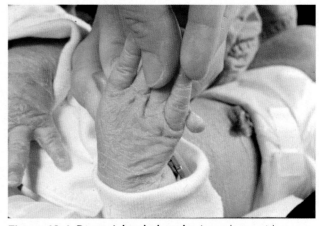

Figure 43-4 Postaxial polydactyly. A newborn with right fifth finger duplication. Note the partially formed digit is conceded by a thin band of tissue. (Courtesy of Kenneth Rosenbaum, MD.)

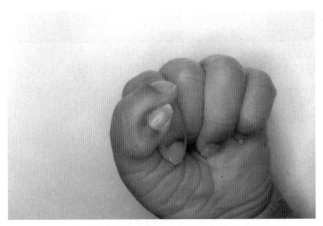

Figure 43-5 **Preaxial polydactyly.** A newborn with left preaxial duplication of the thumb. (Courtesy of Gerardo Cabrera-Meza, MD.)

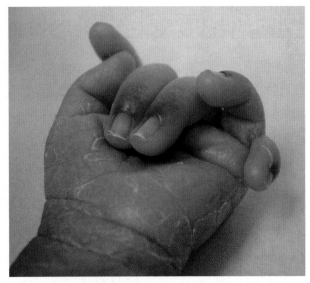

Figure 43-6 **Polydactyly.** A postaxial duplication of the left fifth finger in an African American infant. (Courtesy of Mary L. Brandt, MD.)

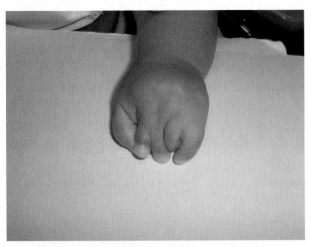

Figure 43-7 **Syndactyly/brachydactyly.** An infant with syndactyly and brachydactyly of the second, third, fourth, and fifth left fingers in a child with Poland syndrome. (Courtesy of Robert L. Zarr, MD, MPH, FAAP.)

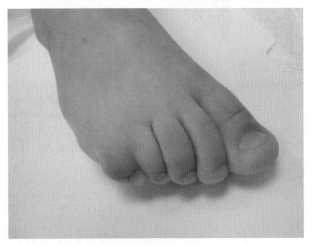

Figure 43-8 **Syndactyly.** A child with syndactyly of the right fourth and fifth toes. (Courtesy of Robert L. Zarr, MD, MPH, FAAP.)

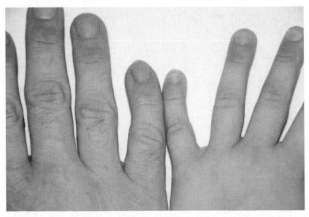

Figure 43-9 **Clinodactyly.** Inherited clinodactyly in a father (*left*) and son (*right*). (Courtesy of Julie A. Bloom, MD.)

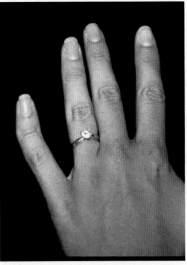

Figure 43-10 **Clinodactyly.** (Courtesy of George A. Datto, III, MD.)

DIFFERENTIAL DIAGNOSIS

DIAGNOSIS	ICD-10	DISTINGUISHING CHARACTERISTICS	DISTRIBUTION
Syndactyly	Q70.9	Soft tissue (simple) or skeletal connection (complex) between adjacent digits	Usually affects the third webspace (central syndactyly)
Clinodactyly	Q74.0	Curvature of digit in radioulnar (coronal) plane	Usually involves small finger, with middle phalanx (delta phalanx)
Camptodactyly	Q74.0	Painless flexion contracture of digit	Most commonly involves PIP joint of small finger
Polydactyly	Q69.9	Duplication of digit Radial—preaxial Ulnar—postaxial	Duplicated proximal and distal phalanges of thumb are the most common radial polydactyly. Ulnar polydactyly can be Type A, with well-formed digit, or Type B, with rudimentary, pedunculated digit on a soft tissue stalk.
Macrodactyly	Q74.0	Overgrowth of all digital structures Digital gigantism Lipofibromatous hamartoma	Single or multiple digits may be involved. Index finger is most frequently affected.
Thumb Hypoplasia	Q71.3	Small, abnormally shaped thumb Ranges from mild hypoplasia to complete absence (aplasia)	May be associated with broader radial deficiency
Congenital Constriction Band Anomaly	P02.8	Severity may range from simple constriction rings to intrauterine amputations.	Sporadic May affect any digit

ASSOCIATED FINDINGS	COMPLICATIONS	PREDISPOSING FACTORS	TREATMENT GUIDELINES
Apert syndrome—Complex Acrocephalosyndactyly (craniosynostosis, midface hypoplasia, hypertelorism) **Poland sequence**—unilateral hypoplasia or absence of pectoralis major muscle, breast, and nipple–areola complex; rib anomalies	Tethering and angular deformity if syndactyly involves digits of unequal length	80% of cases are sporadic. 10%–40% inherited in autosomal dominant mode with variable penetrance	Referral to a pediatric hand surgeon Syndactyly between digits of dissimilar length (border) digits and complex syndactyly is usually released by 6 months of age.
Down syndrome	No functional impairment	Autosomal dominant inheritance	Most do not require treatment.
Freeman–Sheldon syndrome (Whistling face syndrome)	Rigid, fixed contractures lead to a malformed joint with limited range of motion	Variable inheritance	Referral to Pediatric Hand Specialist Splinting during growth for mild, flexible deformity may be beneficial.
Ulnar (postaxial) polydactyly is more common in blacks. Down syndrome	With simple suture ligation pain, excessive scarring, or painful neuroma may develop	Mostly sporadic Postaxial polydactyly in Caucasian patients is often associated with chromosomal anomalies	May be ligated with simple suture in some instances Referral to Pediatric Hand Specialist Surgical treatment depends on type and severity of malformation
Proteus syndrome	Progressive overgrowth may lead to painful, disproportionate enlargement with age Decreased function and range of motion	Mostly sporadic	Referral to Pediatric Hand Specialist Debulking and epiphysiodesis may be considered in patients with mild enlargement. Distal amputations reserved for severe cases
Association with radial longitudinal deficiency: VACTERL syndrome TAR syndrome Fanconi anemia Holt–Oram syndrome	Loss of prehensile (grasp) function with severe forms	If associated with radial deficiency, the condition may be part of a syndrome.	Referral to Pediatric Hand Specialist
May be associated with syndactyly, club feet, or cleft lip and palate	Digital amputations	Most cases are sporadic and not hereditary.	Referral to Pediatric Hand Specialist Constriction bands may be released by Z-plasty

Other Diagnoses to Consider

- Kirner deformity

- Symphalangism

- Congenital clasped thumb

- Congenital trigger thumb

- Brachydactyly

When to Consider Further Evaluation or Treatment

- For most congenital hand and finger anomalies, referral to a Pediatric Hand Specialist for evaluation and possible surgical treatment is recommended.

- Radiographs of congenital hand and digital anomalies will aid in diagnosis and in delineating the degree of skeletal malformation.

- Simple suture ligation of Type B ulnar postaxial polydactyly should be reserved for most minor duplications. Suture ligation of supernumerary digit with a neurovascular stalk may lead to significant pain in the newborn, excessive scarring, or painful neuroma.

- A referral to a geneticist should be strongly considered in a patient with associated malformations.

SUGGESTED READINGS

Dobyns JH, Doyle JR, Von Gillern TL, et al. Congenital anomalies of the upper extremity. *Hand Clin.* 1989;5(3):321–342.
McCarroll HR. Congenital anomalies: a 25-year overview. *J Hand Surg Am.* 2000;25(6):1007–1037.
Netscher DT. Congenital hand problems. Terminology, etiology, and management. *Clin Plast Surg.* 1998;25(4):537–552.
Netscher DT, Baumholtz MA. Treatment of congenital upper extremity problems. *Plast Reconstr Surg.* 2007;119(5):101e–129e.
Van Heest AE. Congenital disorders of the hand and upper extremity. *Pediatr Clin North Am.* 1996;43(5):1113–1133.
Watson S. The principles of management of congenital anomalies of the upper limb. *Arch Dis Child.* 2000;83(1):10–17.

Fingertip Swelling

David Y. Khechoyan, Julieana Nichols,
and Larry H. Hollier, Jr

Approach to the Problem

Fingertip swelling in a child is usually a consequence of trauma or infection. Traumatic injuries with a crush mechanism (e.g., digit crushed between door and door frame) are common in toddlers. These injuries may damage the fingertip soft tissues (nail fold, pulp), distal phalanx, and nail bed. Infections of the distal digit may be precipitated by trauma (felon) or occur spontaneously (paronychia) and may be caused by bacteria, viruses, or fungi.

Key Points in the History

- Crush injury is the most common etiology of fingertip trauma.

- Penetrating injuries from splinters, shards of glass, or minor puncture wounds may lead to an abscess of the distal finger pulp (felon).

- Thumb sucking or nail biting habits may predispose to infections (paronychia).

- Herpetic whitlow may occur as a complication of oral lesions due to herpes simplex virus.

Key Points in the Physical Examination

- Severe pain and multiple clear vesicles on an erythematous base are suggestive of a herpetic whitlow.

- Pain, erythema, and globular swelling of the distal pulp are consistent with a felon.

- Angulation deformity of the distal phalanx because of a fracture may be best detected by examining the finger flexion cascade, or flexion of all the digits together.

PHOTOGRAPHS OF SELECTED DIAGNOSES

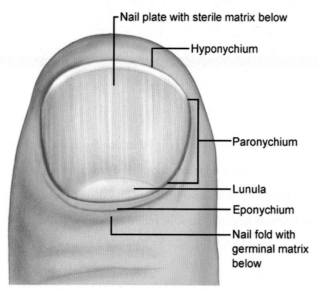

Figure 44-1 **The perionychium and its associated structures.** From Hunt TR, Wiesel SW. *Operative Techniques in Hand, Wrist, and Forearm Surgery.* 1st ed. Philadelphia, PA: Lippincott Williams & Wilkins; 2010.

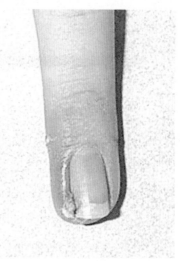

Figure 44-2 **Acute paronychia.** Visible swelling, erythema, and discharge along the nail fold, yet the nail itself is intact. (Courtesy of Mary L. Brandt, MD.)

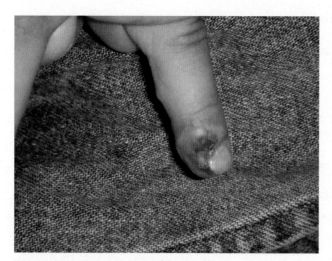

Figure 44-3 **Acute paronychia.** Swelling, erythema, and discharge along the lateral nail edge. (Courtesy of Larry H. Hollier, Jr, MD, FACS.)

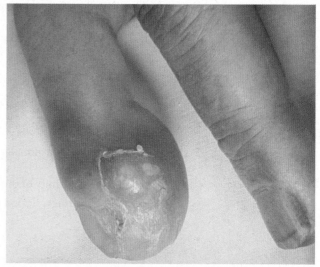

Figure 44-4 **Felon.** (Used with permission from Greenberg MI. *Greenberg's Atlas of Emergency Medicine.* Philadelphia, PA: Lippincott Williams & Wilkins; 2005:458.)

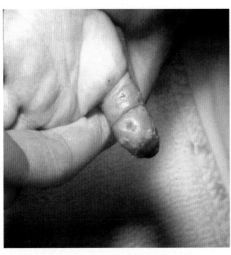

Figure 44-5 Herpetic whitlow. Ulcers where previously there were vesicles along the ventral thumb. (Courtesy of Mark A. Ward, MD.)

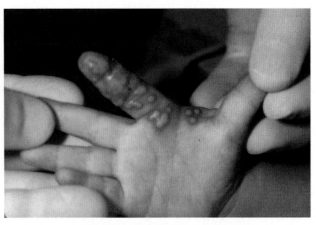

Figure 44-6 Herpetic whitlow. Grouped vesicles on an erythematous base along the ventral surface of the finger. (Courtesy of Mark A. Ward, MD.)

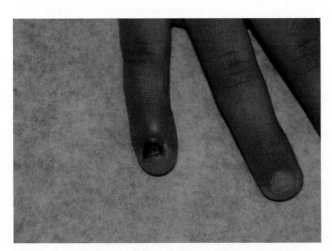

Figure 44-7 Subungual hematoma. A 2-year-old child with a subungual hematoma that resulted from a fall with a plate in his hand. (Courtesy of Julie A. Boom, MD.)

DIFFERENTIAL DIAGNOSIS

DIAGNOSIS		ICD-10	DISTINGUISHING CHARACTERISTICS	DURATION
Acute Paronychia		L03.0	Pain, edema, erythema about nail fold Lesion may be on one side of nail fold or horseshoe type	Acute onset
Chronic Paronychia		L03.0	Edema and bogginess along nail fold	Usually weeks to months (chronic)
Felon		L03.0	Edema, erythema, and severe pain of distal finger pulp Usually pain prevents patient from sleeping	Acute onset, usually 2–5 days after trauma
Viral Infections— Herpetic Whitlow		B00.8	Multiple painful vesicles on an erythematous base	Abrupt onset Spontaneous resolution in 2–3 weeks without treatment
Fracture		S62.2	Pain, edema, decreased range of motion, deformity (angulation)	Abrupt onset
Subungual Hematoma		S60.1	Discoloration (brown, black, purple) deep to the nail plate	Abrupt onset

ASSOCIATED FINDINGS	PREDISPOSING FACTORS	TREATMENT GUIDELINES
Subungual purulence Severe cases may extend into a finger pulp	Usually no specific history of exposure May be associated with trauma to the perionychium	Oral antibiotics Elevation, soap and water soaks, and finger range of motion exercises Incision and drainage for moderate and severe infections with partial removal of nail plate
Abnormal, thick nail plate with chronic colonization with fungus	Chronic dermatitis or frequent exposure to water *Candida albicans* is the most common pathogen	Oral or topical antifungal agents Minimize water exposure Refractory cases respond to complete removal of nail plate and marsupialization of the proximal nail fold (eponychium)
Loculated infection in the pulp space between septae May be associated with a foreign body	Puncture wound 5–7 days before onset of symptoms *Staphylococcus aureus* is the most common pathogen	Hand radiograph to rule out foreign body Incision and drainage of pulp space infection with a longitudinal incision Division of multiple septae to decompress all loculations Oral antibiotics
Vesicles may be present on dorsal and volar aspects of fingertip. Fever, malaise, and lymphadenopathy	Herpes simplex virus type I Usually transmitted by oral contact Immunosuppressed patients	Antiviral agents if infection is present for less than 48 hours Fluid from broken vesicle may be sent for Tzanck smear for confirmation Supportive care is mainstay of treatment. Surgical treatment may lead to secondary bacterial infection.
Distal phalanx fractures may be associated with nail bed injury or injury to the growth plate (physis).	Acute trauma to fingertip Crush injury is most common mechanism	Hand radiograph in three views to evaluate fracture Digital block and fracture reduction if significant displacement is noted Repair of nail bed laceration and replacement of nail plate Splint immobilization
May be associated with fracture of distal phalanx or nail bed laceration	Acute trauma Crush injury is the most common mechanism	Drainage of hematoma with nail plate trephination For suspected nail bed injuries, elevation of nail plate and repair of nail bed laceration

SECTION 12 • EXTREMITIES

Other Diagnoses to Consider

- Subungual melanoma

- Ligamentous injury (sprain) to the distal interphalangeal joint

- Atypical mycobacterial (*Mycobacterium marinum)* or fungal infections

- Flexor tendon sheath infections (tenosynovitis)

- Extensor tendon injury (mallet finger)

- Flexor tendon injury (jersey finger)

When to Consider Further Evaluation or Treatment

- Distal phalanx fractures that are associated with nail bed lacerations, suspected injury to the growth plate, extensor tendon injuries (mallet finger), or displacement should prompt a referral to a pediatric hand surgeon.

- Acute paronychia that does not resolve with a treatment course of oral antibiotics may require formal incision and drainage of the nail fold.

- Consider atypical organisms such as *M. marinum* for infections that do not resolve with standard surgical and antimicrobial treatments.

SUGGESTED READINGS

Clark DC. Common acute hand infections. *Am Fam Physician.* 2003;68(11):2167–2176.
Doraiswamy NV, Baig H. Isolated finger injuries in children—incidence and aetiology. *Injury.* 2000;31(8):571–573.
Hart RG, Kleinert HE. Fingertip and nail bed injuries. *Emerg Med Clin North Am.* 1993;11(3):755–765.
Ljungberg E, Rosberg HE, Dahlin LB. Hand injuries in young children. *J Hand Surg.* 2003;28B(4):376–380.
Rockwell PG. Acute and chronic paronychia. *Am Fam Physician.* 2001;63(6):1113–1116.
Shmerling RH. Finger pain. *Prim Care.* 1988;15(4):751–766.
Zitelli BJ, Davis HW. *Atlas of Pediatric Physical Diagnosis.* 4th ed. Philadelphia, PA: Mosby; 2002.

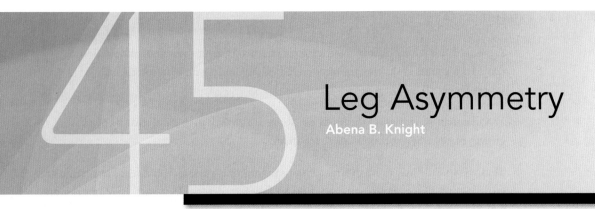

Leg Asymmetry

Abena B. Knight

Approach to the Problem

Lower extremity asymmetry includes inequalities in length and size. Leg length inequality may be structural from abnormalities in any of the bones, nerves, or vasculature in the pelvis or limb, or functional as a result of contractures. Discrepancies in extremity size can also occur from a wide array of congenital, developmental, or acquired conditions that speed or slow growth. A thorough clinical history and careful physical examination are crucial to determining where the abnormality originates and its potential etiologies. The underlying etiology typically will dictate the course and outcome of the limb inequality.

Key Points in the History

- Timing of limb asymmetry is important: limb aplasias, hypoplasias, hyperplasias, and clubfoot are congenital, whereas discrepancies that become more evident as the child grows are usually acquired. Developmental dysplasia of the hip, and hemihypertrophy or hemihypotrophy are exceptions, as they may not be noted at birth.

- Risk factors for developmental dysplasia of the hip include firstborn status, female gender, breech position, positive family history, and oligohydramnios.

- Family history of any bony anomalies is helpful in elucidating if there is an underlying dysplasia, hemangioma, or other anomalies in the bony matrix that would affect growth.

- Skin abnormalities overlying the spine or progressive asymmetric deformities in the limbs may indicate the presence of spinal dysraphism or a tethered cord.

- Inflammatory processes, such as rheumatoid arthritis and hemophilia, can be associated with bony overgrowth.

- Hypotonia, weakness, or paralysis of a limb occurring in those with cerebral palsy or other neurologic disorders often results in growth inhibition from actual discrepancies or apparent ones due to contractures and posturing.

- Disorders or events that cause diminished blood flow to the leg, such as vascular injury, can result in growth interference.

357

- A medical and family history significant for cutaneous, arteriovenous malformations (AVMs) warrants evaluation for internal AVMs and underlying syndromes, such as Osler–Weber–Rendu.

- Vascular malformations on the limbs can stimulate growth in the limb that involves all growth plates, not just those adjacent to them.

- Tumors typically may cause shortened limbs in multiple ways, such as direct destruction and growth inhibition or postirradiation therapy; however, certain ones, such as Wilms tumor, may accompany accelerated growth.

- Infection and trauma history are important to elicit as they can cause leg length discrepancies by either impeding growth through physeal disruption or increasing growth by stimulating blood flow to the limb.

Key Points in the Physical Examination

- Perform a careful and complete head-to-toe examination to determine whether the asymmetry is confined to the lower extremities or exists elsewhere, which may indicate an underlying syndrome.

- Utilize body proportions to determine which limb appears to be the affected one—the pathologic one may be smaller, shorter, larger, or longer depending on the etiology; then evaluate limb segments to ascertain the exact location of the anomaly.

- The true leg length is determined by using a tape measure to measure from the anterior superior iliac spine to the tip of the medial malleolus and the apparent leg length from the umbilicus to the medial malleolus, which can help determine whether the inequality is structural or functional, respectively.

- Blocks can be placed under the heel of the short leg to level the pelvis and measure length discrepancy; the block height needed should correspond to the difference in true leg length.

- Children alter their gait to compensate for significant length inequalities over 2 cm by flexing the knee, circumducting the hip, and/or springing over the long extremity or by walking on tiptoe on the short extremity.

- Anterior bowing of the tibia with or without a dimple at the apex is often associated with fibular hemimelia.

- A hip clunk found on the Barlow maneuver (displacing the femoral head out of socket) or Ortolani maneuver (relocating the femoral head back into the socket), and/or a positive Galeazzi (femoral height discrepancy with hips and knees flexed) sign indicate possible developmental dysplasia of the hip.

- Hemihypertrophy associated with cutaneous lesions or other anomalies may indicate an underlying condition. Café au lait spots may be seen in neurofibromatosis type 1, macroglossia in Beckwith–Wiedemann syndrome, and vascular malformations in Klippel–Trenaunay–Weber syndrome.

- If hemihypertrophy is present, perform a thorough abdominal examination to rule out tumors, including Wilms, adrenal carcinoma, and hepatoblastoma.

- Hemihypotrophy (or hemiatrophy of the leg) should increase suspicion for neurologic etiologies, such as cerebral palsy, and warrants a thorough neurologic assessment, including examination of the back for midline cutaneous lesions indicating possible spinal abnormalities.

PHOTOGRAPHS OF SELECTED DIAGNOSES

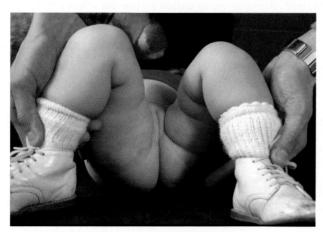

Figure 45-1 Positive Galeazzi sign. Note asymmetry in femoral heights. (Courtesy of Douglas A. Barnes, MD.)

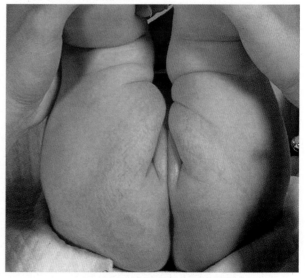

Figure 45-2 Developmental dysplasia of the hip. Note the asymmetry of this infant's thigh folds. (Courtesy of Texas Scottish Rite Hospital for Children, Dallas, Texas.)

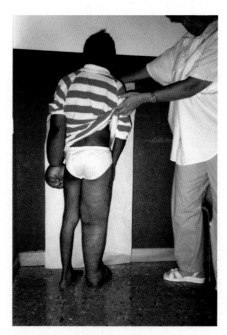

Figure 45-3 Hemihypertrophy secondary to Proteus syndrome. Note the hypertrophy of the right lower extremity and the left upper extremity. (Courtesy of Shriners Hospitals for Children, Houston, Texas.)

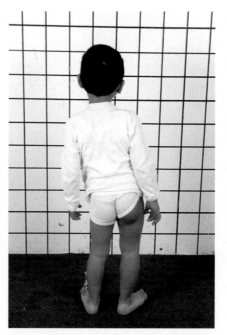

Figure 45-4 Isolated hemihypertrophy. Note the hypertrophy of the right lower extremity. (Courtesy of Shriners Hospitals for Children, Houston, Texas.)

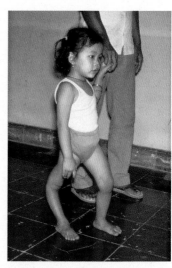

Figure 45-5 Polio. The deformed leg of this child is due to polio. (Photo courtesy of World Health Organization.)

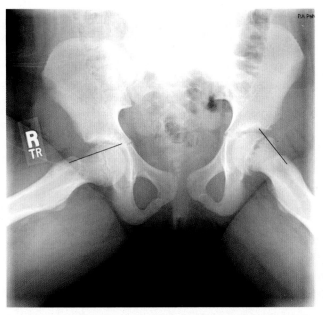

Figure 45-6 Slipped capital femoral epiphysis. Note how Klein line (drawn as an extension of a line drawn along the top border of the femoral neck) does not intersect any part of the femoral head of the abnormal left side. (Courtesy of Texas Scottish Rite Hospital for Children, Dallas, Texas.)

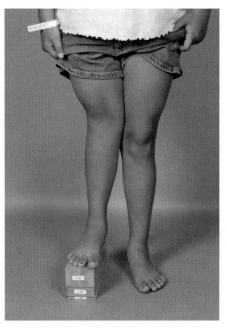

Figure 45-7 Proximal femoral focal deficiency. Note how the diagnosis of this child's congenital leg length discrepancy can be delineated to the right femur by having this child stand on blocks. (Courtesy of Texas Scottish Rite Hospital for Children, Dallas, Texas.)

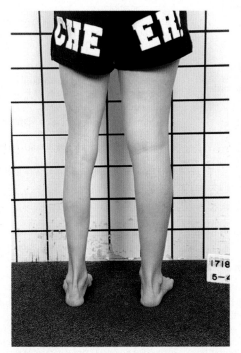

Figure 45-8 Hemi-atrophy from linear scleroderma. Note normal appearing size, muscle mass, and overall bulk of the normal right leg. (Courtesy of Shriners Hospitals for Children, Houston, Texas.)

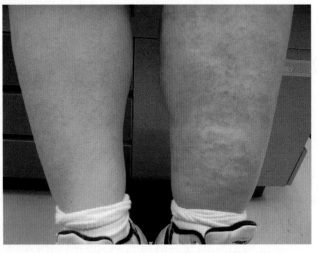

Figure 45-9 Klippel–Trenaunay–Weber syndrome: port-wine stain, varicose veins, and bony and soft-tissue hypertrophy. (Used with permission from image provided by Stedman's.)

DIFFERENTIAL DIAGNOSIS

DIAGNOSIS	ICD-10	DISTINGUISHING CHARACTERISTICS	ASSOCIATED FINDINGS
Congenital Amelia/Hemimelia	Q73.0, Q73.8	Absence of limb or portion of limb (fibular, tibial, or femoral) Fibular deficiency is the most common of all long bone deficiencies. Limb shortening may be terminal (portion distal to defect affected) or intercalary (portions proximal and distal to defect are present)	Craniofacial anomalies and other evidence of bands in amniotic band syndrome Valgus knee, rigid valgus foot with 1–2 missing postaxial rays, and anterior tibial bowing with skin dimple in fibular deficiency Fixed equinovarus-supinated foot, preaxial polydactyly, and other musculoskeletal anomalies in tibial deficiencies Abducted, flexed, and externally rotated femur with a bulbous thigh and knee and hip flexion contractures in femoral deficiencies
Developmental Dysplasia of the Hip	Q65	Relatively common (1:1000 live births) Range of abnormalities in the developing hip from laxity to frank dislocation Unilateral or bilateral (60% left, 20% right, 20% bilateral) Hip clunk on Barlow and/or Ortolani maneuvers Positive Galeazzi sign Asymmetric hip abduction May take repeated examinations to identify	Limited hip abduction of affected side(s) If unilateral, shortening of affected side and/or asymmetric skin folds Torticollis Metatarsus adductus Trendelenburg gait
Hemihypertrophy	Varies based on idiopathic (M89.3) vs syndromic etiologies	Often becomes more apparent as limb enlarges with growth Usually involves both skeleton and soft tissue May be idiopathic or syndromic (e.g., Beckwith–Wiedemann)	Vary with etiology Visceromegaly and other hypertrophic body parts, thicker skin, and thicker hair on head on affected side Cutaneous and vascular lesions seen in syndromic etiologies Functional spinal curvature (resolves with limb correction) and genitourinary anomalies seen in nonsyndromic etiologies
Hemihypotrophy (Also, Hemiatrophy)	M62.5 or specific to syndrome	Idiopathic, syndromic (e.g., Russell–Silver), or secondary to an asymmetric neurologic disorder	Vary with etiology Congenital scoliosis and genitourinary anomalies in idiopathic cases Short stature in Russell–Silver Functional leg length inequality from hip adduction or flexion contractures Structural leg length inequality and muscle atrophy from disuse Limb weakness with abnormal tone and reflexes
Legg–Calvé–Perthes Disease	M91.1	Idiopathic avascular necrosis of the femoral head Mostly unilateral; bilateral in 10% with more than 1-year interval between development Present with subtle onset of antalgic gait	Typically small with delayed skeletal maturation Knee, hip, and/or thigh pain with activity Limited hip medial rotation and abduction Mild atrophy of thigh, calf, and buttock
Slipped Capital Femoral Epiphysis	M93.0	Displacement of femoral head relative to femoral neck and shaft Bilateral in 20%–25% of cases Vague knee, thigh, groin, or hip pain, and/or limp on presentation	Limited medial rotation of hip and external rotation when hip flexed Out-toeing, antalgic, or Trendelenburg gait Hip flexion contracture with apparent length inequality or limb atrophy if chronic slip

COMPLICATIONS	PREDISPOSING FACTORS	TREATMENT GUIDELINES
Residual limb too short for prosthesis, requiring lengthening Bony overgrowth at end of amputated limb Hip, knee, and ankle instability Angular and rotational deformities Phantom pain Psychosocial issues	Usually unknown Amniotic band syndrome Dominant genetic transmission in some tibial hemimelias Thalidomide	Multifaceted management team, including an orthopedist, geneticist, physical/occupational therapist, prosthetist, social worker and/or mental health provider Amputation often performed immediately prior to walking to improve fit of prosthesis
Leg length inequality Degenerative hip findings by skeletal maturity Avascular necrosis of femoral head Painful osteoarthritis	Family history Breech presentation Multigestation Female gender Oligohydramnios Firstborn Neuromuscular disorder Postnatal positioning (hip swaddling in adduction and extension)	Ultrasound in infants from birth to 4 months Radiograph after bony ossification in infants after 4–6 months Orthopedic referral for medical (e.g., Pavlik harness) and/or surgical management
Accelerated bone age on affected side Variably increased risk of malignant abdominal tumors, especially Wilms, hepatoblastoma, and adrenal carcinoma	Variable—some syndromic etiologies appear to or have a genetic cause (e.g., neurofibromatosis type 1)	Varies widely with etiology Screening for abdominal tumor development Orthopedic referral for management of musculoskeletal issues
Vary with etiology Skeletal abnormalities (e.g., contractures, kyphoscoliosis, hip dislocation or subluxation, and osteoarthritis)	Poliomyelitis Spinal dysraphism Cerebral palsy Peripheral neuropathy Spinal cord trauma	Vary widely with etiology Orthopedic referral for management of musculoskeletal issues Neurologic and/o neurosurgical referral for management of neurologic concerns
Leg length inequality Osteoarthritis of the hip if growth arrest occurs in older children	Male gender (4:1) Ages 4–8 years	Radiographs are diagnostic Orthopedic referral for medical (observation and limited physical activity) and/or surgical management (rare)
Chondrolysis Avascular necrosis (from disease or treatment) Early hip osteoarthritis	Male gender Obesity Peak age of 13 years in males, 11 years in females Endocrine (e.g., hypothyroidism) or metabolic (e.g., rickets) disorders that affect physis	Radiographs are diagnostic Non-weight bearing Immediate orthopedic referral for surgical management

(continued)

SECTION 12 • EXTREMITIES

DIFFERENTIAL DIAGNOSIS *(continued)*

DIAGNOSIS	ICD-10	DISTINGUISHING CHARACTERISTICS	ASSOCIATED FINDINGS
Trauma/Infection	M21.7 Unequal limb length, acquired	Typically unilateral Lengthening develops from growth stimulation during healing of fracture, or during active infection Shortening develops from physeal injury or arrest or malunion	Abnormal gait to compensate for asymmetry Pain or refusal to bear weight or move limb Erythema, effusion, skin changes, or warmth in active infection
Vascular Anomalies	D18.0, D18.1, Q27.3 or specific to syndrome	May be isolated or part of a systemic condition (e.g., Klippel–Trenaunay) Vary widely—hemangiomas vs vascular malformations (dysplastic capillary, venous, arterial, and lymphatic vessels, or mixed) Lesions can be cutaneous, subcutaneous, intramuscular, skeletal, or visceral	Vary with location of anomaly and syndrome Limb hypertrophy from growth and/or edema (rare atrophy due to hemiplegia or disuse) Leg length discrepancies Pain

COMPLICATIONS	PREDISPOSING FACTORS	TREATMENT GUIDELINES
Joint damage or deformities Avascular necrosis Pathologic fractures (from infection)	History of trauma or malunion Infection in affected limb Overgrowth and shortening associated most with femur fracture	Orthopedic referral for trauma and limb discrepancy management Infectious disease and orthopedic consultations, joint aspiration/incision and drainage if applicable, and systemic antibiotic therapy in infection
Vary with etiology (e.g., cardiac overload in Klippel–Trenaunay, gastrointestinal bleeding in blue rubber bleb nevus, malignancies in Maffucci) Skeletal deformities and contractures Cellulitis and other infections due to poor hygiene	Unknown	Vary widely with etiology Ultrasound with Doppler examination and/or MRI to assess extent of anomaly Compressive garments for venous stasis Orthopedic referral for management of musculoskeletal issues

Other Diagnoses to Consider

- Clubfoot

- Congenital pseudarthrosis of the tibia, femur, or fibula

- Hemophilia

- Juvenile idiopathic arthritis

- Mosaic Turner syndrome

- Proteus syndrome

- Radiation therapy

- Scleroderma or scarring and fibrosis from other etiologies (e.g., severe burns)

- Skeletal dysplasias or dyostoses

- Thrombosis of iliac or femoral veins

- Tumors

When to Consider Further Evaluation or Treatment

- Leg length inequalities less than 2 cm are typically managed conservatively with shoe lifts, and discrepancies greater than 2 cm require orthopedic referral for possible surgical intervention.

- Consider radiographic evaluation in female infants with breech presentation, especially if firstborn, have a positive family history, or history of oligohydramnios.

- Legg–Calvé–Perthes disease rarely requires surgical intervention, but slipped capital femoral epiphysis almost always does.

- Children with hemihypertrophy should undergo evaluation for abdominal masses due to the increased incidence of malignancies.

- Limb asymmetry associated with vascular anomalies requires a thorough evaluation for an underlying syndrome and other vascular malformations in view of the life-threatening complications that can occur.

- Although the etiology of limb asymmetry is diverse, all patients benefit from orthopedic referrals to manage either orthopedic causes of the asymmetry, the musculoskeletal issues arising from the asymmetry, or both.

SUGGESTED READINGS

Ballock RT, Wiesner GL, Myers MT, et al. Hemihypertrophy. Concepts and controversies. *J Bone Joint Surg Am.* 1997;79(11):1731–1738.

Enjolras O, Chapot R, Merland JJ. Vascular anomalies and the growth of limbs: A review. *J Pediatr Orthop B.* 2004;13(6):349–357.

Herring JA, ed. *Tachdjian's Pediatric Orthopedics.* 4th ed. Philadelphia, PA: NB Saunders Company; 2008.

Morrissy RT, Weinstein SL, eds. *Lovell and Winter's Pediatric Orthopaedics.* 6th ed. Philadelphia, PA: Lippincott Williams & Wilkins; 2006.

Staheli LT, ed. *Practice of Pediatric Orthopedics.* 2nd ed. Philadelphia, PA: Lippincott Williams & Wilkins; 2006.

Storer SK, Skaggs DL. Developmental dysplasia of the hip. *Am Fam Physician.* 2006;74(8):1310–1316.

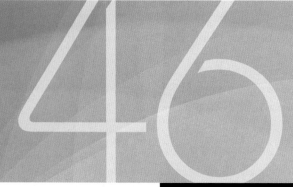

Leg Bowing and Knock-Knees

Abena B. Knight

Approach to the Problem

Angular deformities of the lower extremities, known as leg bowing (genu varum) and knock-knees (genu valgum), are common orthopedic diagnoses in early childhood. Leg bowing and knock-knees are most often physiologically normal, as the angle of the knee changes with age. Infants typically have bowlegs, which are often not noticed by parents until children begin to stand and walk. The varum angle declines until 3 years of age, when the majority of children appear knock-kneed. Valgus angulation lessens to the more neutral angle of adults by 6 to 7 years of age. Lack of gradual resolution, asymmetry of extremity findings, and progression of angulation are indications of a pathologic etiology, and require further evaluation and possible intervention.

Key Points in the History

- Deviation from the expected natural history or asymmetry of bowlegs and knock-knees are concerning for nonphysiologic etiologies.

- Growth history and timing of symptoms are essential to distinguishing between physiologic, systemic, and mechanical etiologies.

- Genu varum or valgum in infancy associated with a patient and family history of short stature could indicate skeletal dysplasia.

- Patients with hypophosphatemic rickets, also known as vitamin D-resistant rickets, often have a history of poor linear growth and a family history of genu varum.

- Nutritional rickets, also known as vitamin D-deficiency rickets, should be considered if the patient was breastfed without receiving vitamin D supplementation, has abnormal dietary habits, or has limited sun exposure.

- Infantile tibia vara, the more common form of Blount disease, is usually found in obese African American females younger than 3 years of age who walked before 11 months of age.

- Adolescent tibia vara is typically found in obese African American males older than 8 years of age who walked before 11 months of age.

- Asymmetric valgus or varus deformities can be found following lower-extremity fractures or infections.

- Worsening genu valgum during the ages of expected physiologic valgus, without a history of trauma or infection, is concerning for renal osteodystrophy.

- If the child is less than 2 years old with symmetric bowing and a tibiofemoral metaphyseal–diaphyseal angle falling within two standard deviations of the mean and otherwise has a normal history and physical examination, it is considered to be physiologic genu varum.

- Physiologic bowing is often characterized by the entire lower extremity appearing bowed, whereas greater apparent deformity in the proximal tibia can indicate a nonphysiologic cause.

- If the child is 2 to 8 years old with symmetric knock-knees and a tibiofemoral metaphyseal–diaphyseal angle falling within two standard deviations of the mean and otherwise has a normal history and physical examination, it is considered to be physiologic genu valgum.

- The differential diagnosis can be narrowed depending on whether or not physical findings are asymmetric, are isolated to the lower extremities, or are associated with other anomalies, such as short stature.

- A lateral thrust of the knee joint in stance while observing walking is characteristic of pathologic genu varum; however, its absence does not always indicate a physiologic process.

- Worsening genu valgum on examination after age 8 is highly suggestive of underlying pathology.

PHOTOGRAPHS OF SELECTED DIAGNOSES

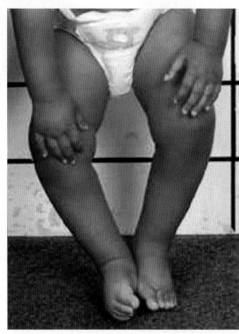

Figure 46-1 Infantile tibial bowing.
Outward angulation of the tibia bilaterally in an infant. (Courtesy of Shriners Hospitals for Children, Houston, Texas.)

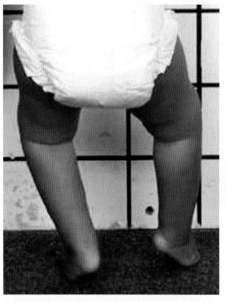

Figure 46-2 Infantile tibial bowing.
Outward angulation of the tibia is also notable in the posterior view of the infant with tibial bowing. (Courtesy of Shriners Hospitals for Children, Houston, Texas.)

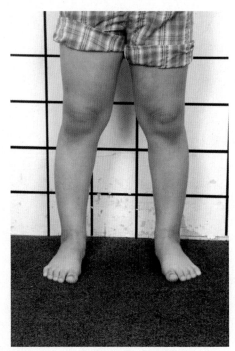

Figure 46-3 Genu varum. Outward angulation of the knees in a child. (Courtesy of Shriners Hospitals for Children, Houston, Texas.)

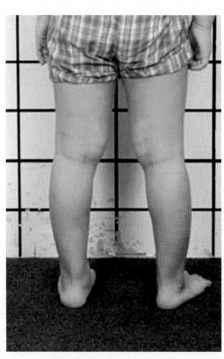

Figure 46-4 Genu varum. Posterior view of a child with genu varum. (Courtesy of Shriners Hospitals for Children, Houston, Texas.)

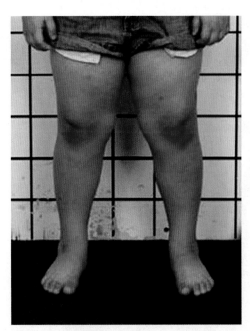

Figure 46-5 **Blount disease.** Genu varum deformity is seen in this obese male with Blount disease. (Courtesy of Shriners Hospitals for Children, Houston, Texas.)

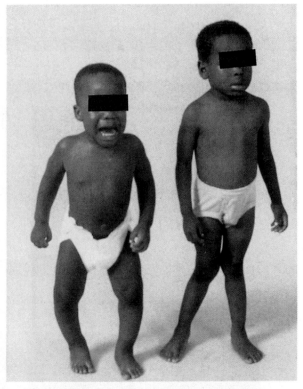

Figure 46-6 **Physiologic Genu Varum and Genu Valgum.** Physiologic genu varum (bowlegs) in a toddler (left) and genu valgum (knock-knees) in a toddler (right), which is often seen in children between 2 and 6 years of age. (Used with permission from Weinstein S.L., Buckwalter J.A. [1994]. Turek's orthopaedics [5th ed.] Philadelphia: J.B. Lippincott.)

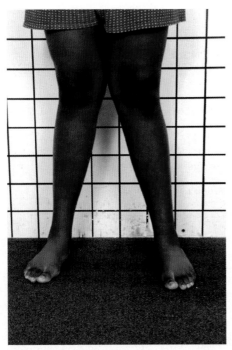

Figure 46-7 Genu valgum. Inward angulation of the knees seen in this child. (Courtesy of Shriners Hospitals for Children, Houston, Texas.)

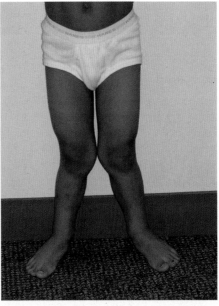

Figure 46-8 Genu valgum. A toddler with notable inward angulation of the knees. (Courtesy of Bettina Gyr, MD.)

DIFFERENTIAL DIAGNOSIS

DIAGNOSIS	ICD-10	DISTINGUISHING CHARACTERISTICS	ASSOCIATED FINDINGS
LEG BOWING (GENU VARUM)			
Physiologic Genu Varum	M21.1	Bilateral, involving both distal femur and tibia Usually symmetric Physis normal on radiograph Angle of varum greatest between 6 and 12 months Alignment neutral by 2 years of age	Internal tibial torsion with intoeing gait Varus foot Ligamentous laxity laterally in knee
Infantile Tibia Vara (Blount Disease)	M92.5	Progressive or persistent bowing beyond age 2 Usually bilateral (60%) Bowing prominent in proximal tibia Limp (lateral knee thrust during stance phase) Four key radiographic changes: 1. Varus angulation at junction of proximal metaphysis–epiphysis 2. Medial physeal line irregularity and widening 3. Epiphysis sloped medially and ossified unequally 4. Medial metaphysis with major beaking containing lucent cartilage areas	Internal tibial torsion with intoeing gait Physiologic bowing on contralateral side in unilateral cases
Adolescent Tibia Vara (Blount Disease)	M92.5	Often unilateral Onset after age 8 May present with medial knee pain or patellofemoral complaints Pain along palpation of medial joint line of knee Radiographic widening of the medial tibial growth plate	Leg length discrepancy if unilateral Distal femoral varus deformity Internal tibial torsion Slipped capital femoral epiphysis rarely
Focal Fibrocartilaginous Dysplasia	M85.0	Unilateral Rare cause in infants and toddlers Radiographic changes are diagnostic: 1. Fibrocartilaginous tissue metaphysis 2. No physeal or epiphyseal involvement	Knee hyperextension, if ambulatory
Posttraumatic/Postinfectious Genu Varum	M21.1	Unilateral Prior history of proximal tibia metaphyseal fracture or infectious event	N/A
Rickets	E64.3 Vitamin D-Deficient E83.3 X-linked Hypophosphatemic Rickets	Bilateral and symmetric Present with poor linear growth (<10th percentile) and delayed walking Radiographic findings include: 1. Metaphyseal widening/fraying/cupping 2. Physeal widening 3. Rachitic rosary—prominence of the costochondral junction 4. Osteopenia	Low-serum calcium, vitamin D, and phosphorus and high alkaline phosphatase

COMPLICATIONS	PREDISPOSING FACTORS	TREATMENT GUIDELINES
N/A	Early ambulation More common in Asians	Resolves spontaneously
Growth plate injury with growth retardation or arrest, extremity shortening, and joint deformity	Early ambulation Obesity African American race/ethnicity	Orthopedic referral for possible orthoses and/or surgical intervention based on age and staging
Knee instability, especially in the medial and lateral collateral ligaments Growth plate arrest	Early ambulation Morbid obesity African American race/ethnicity More common in males	Weight loss recommended but requires referral for orthopedic surgical intervention
N/A	Unknown	Orthopedic referral for observation and/or orthoses as often resolves spontaneously (may take 7 years) Surgical intervention if fails to resolve or progresses
Growth plate injury Partial physeal arrest causing leg length discrepancy	Insult in early childhood during physiologic varum	Orthopedic referral—deformity may resolve over time but may require surgery if persists
Deformities at sites of rapid growth (proximal humerus, distal radius, distal femur, and both ends of tibia) Stunted growth Fractures	Nutritional: 1. Exclusively breastfed without supplementation or atypical diet 2. Darker pigmented individuals 3. Limited sun exposure 4. Disorders of malabsorption Resistant: 1. Family history due to X-linked dominant inheritance 2. Metabolic bone disease most active during physiologic varum	Endocrinology, renal and/or gastroenterology referrals for medical management Orthopedic referral in late childhood/adolescence for surgery if needed

(continued)

SECTION 12 • EXTREMITIES

DIFFERENTIAL DIAGNOSIS *(continued)*

DIAGNOSIS	ICD-10	DISTINGUISHING CHARACTERISTICS	ASSOCIATED FINDINGS
KNOCK-KNEES (GENU VALGUM)			
Skeletal Dysplasias	Varies	Bilateral and symmetric Poor linear growth (<10th percentile) Varying radiographic changes specific to dysplasia, e.g., knee-centered varus deformity with elongated fibula in achondroplasia vs bilateral femur and tibial bowing in camptomelic dysplasia	Short stature Ligamentous laxity
Physiologic Genu Valgum	M21.0	Bilateral Symmetric Angle of valgus maximal between 3 and 5 years Alignment more neutral by 8 years Stance with one knee behind the other to align feet	Pes planus Valgus foot Ligamentous laxity of knee Occasional medial foot or knee pain
Postinfectious Genu Valgum	M21.0	Unilateral May have history of osteomyelitis, tuberculosis, poliomyelitis, or other chronic infection	May see leg muscle atrophy and tight iliotibial band
Posttraumatic Genu Valgum	M21.0	Unilateral Prior fracture history of proximal tibial metaphysis (Cozen fracture) or distal lateral femoral physis Valgus angulation due to tibial overgrowth, fracture malunion, interposition of soft tissue in fracture, or tethering of lateral physis Develops 12–18 months following event	N/A
Renal Osteodystrophy/Rickets	N25.0	Bilateral and symmetric Presents with poor linear growth (<10th percentile) Radiograph shows: 1. Physeal widening and fraying 2. Cortical subperiosteal erosion in long bones and phalanges 3. Osteopenia, osteoporosis, or osteosclerosis	Abnormal serum chemistries, especially calcium and phosphorus with secondary hyperparathyroidism Anemia Proteinuria
Bony (Spondyloepiphyseal and Metaphyseal) Dysplasias	Varies	Bilateral and symmetric Poor linear growth (<10th percentile) Varying radiographic changes specific to dysplasia	Short stature Marked joint laxity
Pathologic/Idiopathic Genu Valgum	M21.0	Typically develops in early adolescence, though may result from persistent or progressive childhood knock-knee Radiograph usually shows asymmetric growth of distal femur, occasional abnormality in proximal tibia	Medial knee or foot pain common Out-toed gait Awkward gait due to knees rubbing/hitting Ligamentous laxity of knee

COMPLICATIONS	PREDISPOSING FACTORS	TREATMENT GUIDELINES
Specific to type of dysplasia	Specific to type of dysplasia	Orthopedic referral for surgical management
N/A	More common in obese females	Resolves spontaneously
Growth plate injury with possible leg length discrepancy	Insult during physiologic valgum	Orthopedic referral—deformity may resolve over time but may require surgery if persists
Partial physeal arrest causing leg length discrepancy Lateral compartment arthritis	Insult to the proximal tibial metaphysis in early childhood during physiologic valgum No intervention (casting versus surgical reduction) has been shown to prevent or predispose to valgus development.	Orthopedic referral—deformity often resolves over time but may require surgery if valgus extreme or symptomatic
Poor linear growth/failure to thrive Bone pain Long bone deformities	Often acquired renal failure as typically at age of physiologic valgus at the height of active metabolic bone disease Anorexia/Malabsorption Family history if secondary to genetic renal or metabolic disease	Endocrinology and/or nephrology referrals for medical management Orthopedic referral in late childhood/adolescence for surgery if needed
Specific to type of dysplasia	Specific to type of dysplasia	Orthopedic referral for surgical management
Lateral patellar subluxation (uncommon)	Many are >90th percentile for weight and height	Orthopedic referral for surgical management (typically done after 10–11 years of age)

Other Diagnoses to Consider

- Bony tumors or malignancies

- Connective tissue disorders (e.g., Ehlers–Danlos syndrome, Marfan syndrome)

- Fluoride or lead intoxication

- Hemophilia

- Lysosomal storage disorders (e.g., Gaucher disease, Morquio syndrome)

- Neurofibromatosis

- Osteoarthritis

- Osteogenesis imperfecta

- Osteoporosis

- Rheumatoid arthritis

- Tibial or fibular hemimelia (congenital genu varum or genu valgum)

When to Consider Further Evaluation or Treatment

- Patients should be evaluated clinically every 3–6 months if findings appear consistent with physiologic genu varum or genu valgum. Obtain radiographs, and consider referral to an orthopedic specialist if individual deviates from expected natural history of physiologic genu varum or valgum, such as persistence or progression of angulation beyond expected ages.

- Clinical history that includes dietary anomalies, prior trauma or infection, or growth anomalies (large or small for age) should raise suspicion for possible pathologic etiologies and warrants radiographic evaluation and possible evaluation for metabolic bone disease. Results of further evaluation should guide specialist referrals.

- Physical examination showing asymmetry or unilateral involvement of extremities or other anomalies, such as short stature or dysmorphic features, should increase suspicion for nonphysiologic causes. Obtain radiographs, and consider metabolic bone disease and/or dysplasia assessment. Results of further evaluation should guide specialist referrals.

- Genu varum and genu valgum in metabolic bone disease are initially managed medically. Referral to the appropriate specialist—typically an endocrinologist and/or nephrologist—is essential. Involvement by an orthopedic surgeon may still be required for surgical management later.

- Genu varum and genu valgum in children with skeletal dysplasias typically require orthopedic surgical intervention.

SUGGESTED READINGS

Cheema JI, Grissom LE, Harcke HT. Radiographic characteristics of lower-extremity bowing in children. *Radiographics*. 2003;23(4):871–880.

Cozen L. Knock-knee deformity in children. Congenital and acquired. *Clin Orthop Relat Res*. 1990;(258):191–203.

Do TT. Clinical and radiographic evaluation of bowlegs. *Curr Opin Pediatr*. 2001;13(1):42–46.

Herring JA, ed. *Tachdjian's Pediatric Orthopedics*. 4th ed. Philadelphia, PA: NB Saunders Company; 2008:973–1004.

Morrissy RT, Weinstein SL, eds. *Lovell and Winter's Pediatric Orthopaedics*. 6th ed. Philadelphia, PA: Lippincott Williams & Wilkins; 2006:1165–1189.

Staheli LT, ed. *Practice of Pediatric Orthopedics*. 2nd ed. Philadelphia, PA: Lippincott Williams & Wilkins; 2006:81–85.

47

Intoeing

Kenya Maria Parks

Approach to the Problem

Intoeing is a lower extremity rotational abnormality. It is one of the most common reasons why children are referred to an orthopedic surgeon. Concerned parents perceive that their child will have lasting structural, cosmetic, and/or functional issues. Concomitantly, many pediatricians feel ill-equipped to deal with or address orthopedic issues. The pediatric practitioner can effectively address intoeing by knowing the normal lower extremity developmental process, normal variations, key historical red flags, and a few basic physical examination maneuvers. The vast majority of cases of intoeing resolve with time. It is only a minority of cases that will necessitate referral and/or surgical intervention.

Intoeing is the manifestation of one of three likely underlying processes: metatarsus adductus, internal tibial torsion, or femoral anteversion. Rotational variation is a more concise term to describe these processes. As a result of intrauterine crowding, many infants are born with varying degrees of femoral anteversion, internal tibial torsion, or angulation of the feet. The normal maturational process of the lower extremity involves external rotation of the tibia and femur as the child grows. The foot also rotates to assume the normal position. Thus, these counteracting forces result in the resolution of most cases of intoeing as the child grows.

Key Points in the History

- It is essential to obtain a thorough birth history, including prenatal complications, Apgar scores, gestational age, and the nursery or NICU course. Cerebral palsy should be part of the differential diagnosis for complicated births.

- Multiple gestation births, due to intrauterine crowding, have higher rates of rotational issues.

- Genetic disorders such as achondroplasia and vitamin D resistant rickets predispose children to lower extremity rotational and structural issues.

- Clubfoot is associated with syndromes such as arthrogryposis, Down syndrome, and myelodysplasia. Children with these syndromes will likely require corrective surgery.

- Pain, progression, and worsening of the disorder warrant further evaluation.

- Children with neuromuscular and/or developmental disorders warrant a more in-depth and encompassing assessment.

- Ascertain if there is a family history of lower extremity rotational disorders. There are familial and ethnic tendencies for rotational issues.

Key Points in the Physical Examination

- Assess the child for any sign of dysmorphism associated with an underlying genetic disorder that could predispose to rotational abnormalities.

- The child with disproportionate or severe short stature should be evaluated for skeletal dysplasia.

- In metatarsus adductus, the medial aspect of the foot is convex, and the lateral aspect is concave, giving the foot a "C" or kidney bean appearance. There might also be a medial foot crease.

- An outline or photocopy of the feet is helpful in assessing the resolution of metatarsus adductus.

- The heel bisector is a line drawn bisecting the heel and extending to the forefoot. The normal point of bisection is the second interspace. Metatarsus adductus is mild if the line intersects the third ray, moderate if it intersects the fourth ray, and severe if it bisects the fifth ray.

- Clubfoot is a rigid deformity of the foot.

- Children with femoral anteversion tend to sit in the "W" position and run with an "egg-beater" gait.

- Femoral anteversion is marked by medial thigh rotation greater than 60 to 65 degrees.

- Tibial torsion is assessed with the thigh-foot angle. The normal angle is 10 to 15 degrees; children with internal tibial torsion have negative thigh-foot angles.

PHOTOGRAPHS OF SELECTED DIAGNOSES

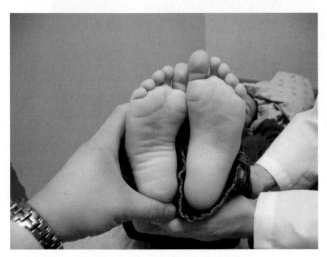

Figure 47-1 Metatarsus adductus. The convex ("C") shape of the child's right foot suggests metatarsus adductus. (Courtesy of Paul S. Matz, MD.)

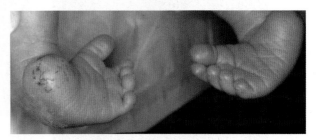

Figure 47-2 Clubfeet. Bilateral clubfeet in an infant with notable metatarsus adductus. (Courtesy of Gerardo Cabrera-Meza, MD.)

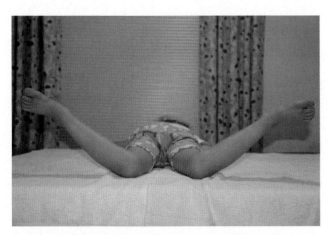

Figure 47-3 Femoral torsion. A 5-year-old girl with increased medial rotation of the hips because of femoral torsion. (Courtesy of Julie A. Boom, MD.)

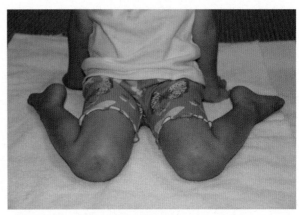

Figure 47-4 Femoral torsion. A 5-year-old girl comfortably "W" sitting. (Courtesy of Julie A. Boom, MD.)

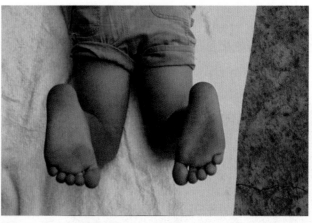

Figure 47-6 **Tibial torsion.** A 4-year-old child with a negative thigh-foot angle. (Courtesy of Julie A. Boom, MD.)

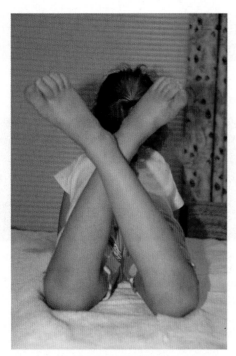

Figure 47-5 **Femoral torsion.** Limited lateral hip rotation in a 5-year-old girl with femoral torsion. (Courtesy of Julie A. Boom, MD.)

DIFFERENTIAL DIAGNOSIS

DIAGNOSIS	ICD-10	DISTINGUISHING CHARACTERISTICS	DURATION/ CHRONICITY	ASSOCIATED FINDINGS	COMPLICATIONS	PREDISPOSING FACTORS	TREATMENT GUIDELINES
Metatarsus Adductus Type I—mild Type II—moderate Type III—severe	Q66.2	Mild—the child can self-correct the foot to the neutral position Moderate—the child's foot can be passively moved to the neutral position Severe—the foot cannot be moved to the neutral position	Resolution for 80%–90% by 1 year of age	Medial instep crease	Usually none	Higher in males, twins, and preterm infants	Mild—none Moderate—lateral stretching exercises Severe—serial casting or Wheaton brace Surgery for recalcitrant cases
Clubfoot	Q66.8	There are components that must be present: cavus, metatarsus adductus, equinus, and hindfoot varus	N/A	Can be associated with hip dysplasia	Residual deformity	Arthrogryposis, dwarfism, neuromuscular disorders, myelodysplasia, genetic predisposition, male predominance	Serial casting is attempted up to 6–9 months Surgery, if there is no amelioration
Femoral Anteversion	Q65.89	Increased anterior rotation of the femoral neck	Resolution typically by 10–12 years of age	None	Usually none	Cerebral palsy, muscle tone abnormalities	Derotational osteotomy for persistent or severe cases
Tibial torsion	M21.80	Rotation of the tibia resulting in foot misalignment	Resolution typically by age 5–6 years	Infantile tibia vara in some cases	Usually none	Cerebral palsy, neuromuscular disorders, joint laxity	Derotational osteotomy for persistent or severe cases

SECTION 12 • EXTREMITIES

Other Diagnoses to Consider

- Metatarsus primus varus

- Skew foot

- Dynamic hallux abductus

- Neuromuscular disorders

- Genetic syndromes

- Skeletal dysplasia

When to Consider Further Evaluation or Treatment

- Severe or marked femoral anteversion or internal tibial torsion that results in functional issues and/or fails to resolve by the age of 8

- Patients with rigid metatarsus adductus or clubfoot

- Children with underlying genetic, developmental, or neuromuscular disorders

- Progression of the abnormality instead of the expected resolution

- Metatarsus adductus that persists beyond the ages of 4 to 5 years

SUGGESTED READINGS

Craig CL, Goldberg MJ. Foot and leg problems. *Pediatr Rev.* 1993;14:395–400.
Lincoln TL, Suen PW. Common rotational variation in children. *J Am Acad Orthop Surg.* 2003;11:312–320.
Sass P, Hassan G. Lower extremity abnormalities in children. *Am Fam Physician.* 2003;68:461–468.
Scherl SA. Common lower extremity problems in children. *Pediatr Rev.* 2004;25:52–61.
Smith BG. Lower extremity disorders in children and adolescents. *Pediatr Rev.* 2009;30:287–294.

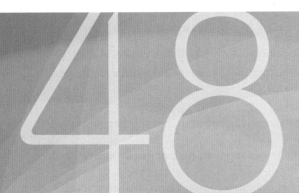

Knee Swelling

Anand Gourishankar and
Lisa E. De Ybarrondo

Approach to the Problem

Knee swelling in the pediatric patient suggests a broad differential diagnosis, including musculoskeletal, rheumatic, and infectious processes. Knees are large joints commonly involved in juvenile idiopathic arthritis (JIA) (previously known as juvenile rheumatoid arthritis). Because there are many soft-tissue structures within it, the knee may be injured in almost every type of sport. The knee is involved in approximately 90% of cases of joint swelling associated with Lyme disease. Knee swelling in children can be subtle or obvious. A thorough history and complete physical examination cannot be overemphasized. Knowing the age, ethnicity, gender, and geographic location of the affected individual is vital to narrowing the differential diagnosis. Specifically, gonococcal arthritis may be seen in an adolescent, Lyme disease should be considered in a patient from Connecticut, girls more than boys are diagnosed with pauciarticular arthritis, osteosarcoma is more predominant in whites than in African Americans, and sports injuries are common in young athletes.

Knee swelling can be approached by acuity of presentation and the presence or absence of pain, recurrence (as with tuberculosis), and localized or systemic disease. Identifying the etiology also depends on the history: recent or past trauma, symptoms of infection, presence of inflammation, a family history of rheumatic disease or cancer, recent travel, and so forth. A child with septic arthritis, osteomyelitis, systemic onset JIA, or acute leukemia may be ill-appearing. On the other hand, a child with exostosis may be well-appearing. Swelling of the knee joint may occur as a result of surrounding skin and soft-tissue infection, a knee effusion with blood (as with bone and growth plate fractures and an anterior cartilage ligament tear) or nonbloody fluid (as with a meniscal tear and ligament sprain), synovial thickening, a cyst, or bursitis.

Key Points in the History

- An acute onset of knee swelling suggests trauma, septic arthritis, rheumatic fever, or Lyme disease.

- Chronic knee swelling suggests JIA, tuberculosis, or malignancy.

- The mechanism of trauma may provide clues to the most likely structures injured. For example, a history of knee hyperextension may suggest an anterior cruciate ligament (ACL) injury.

- An audible pop may be concerning for a serious ligamentous injury or fracture.

- Knee instability or "giving way" may indicate a ruptured ACL or patellar instability.

- Knee locking with limited extension may indicate a torn meniscus, avulsed cruciate ligament, or bony fragment.

- Extremely painful migratory polyarthritis, involving the knees, elbows, wrists, and ankles, and a prior Group A streptococcal pharyngitis warrant the consideration of rheumatic fever.

- Antecedent diarrheal illness can be a clue for reactive arthritis.

- Pain in septic arthritis is constant and generally worsens over time.

- Morning joint stiffness is seen in JIA or systemic lupus erythematosus (SLE).

- Fever may be suggestive of an infectious or rheumatologic process; high intermittent fevers (≥39.5°C) that occur once or twice daily may indicate systemic onset JIA.

- An evanescent rash (small, pale red macules with central clearing) that occurs during periods of temperature elevation is suggestive of systemic onset JIA.

- Consider Lyme disease when knee arthritis with an erythema chronicum migrans rash follows a tick bite or an exposure to a Lyme-endemic area.

- Individuals with hemophilia are susceptible to hemarthrosis.

- A growing painless bony lump in the arm or leg of a 10- to 20-year-old could be exostosis.

- A painful soft-tissue mass growing over months may be osteosarcoma; fever, weight loss, and malaise are generally absent.

- Consider risk factors such as exposure to tuberculosis or sexually transmitted infections in monoarticular arthritis.

Key Points in the Physical Examination

- The site of bruising may provide a clue to the direction of force that caused the swelling.

- An effusion, indicated by asymmetry of the suprapatellar pouches, may indicate synovitis—the hallmark of late Lyme disease.

- Effusion immediately following trauma may suggest acute bleeding into the knee.

- Edema over the lower pole of the patella suggests a prepatellar bursitis.

- A mass palpated in the popliteal area that gets bigger upon standing suggests the presence of a popliteal cyst (Baker cyst).

- The discovery of a new heart murmur, especially one consistent with mitral or aortic insufficiency, may suggest acute rheumatic fever.

- Excruciating knee pain with bright erythema or dramatic warmth is characteristic of acute rheumatic fever or septic arthritis.

- Knee swelling accompanied by urticaria, erythematous maculopapules, or purpura involving primarily the lower extremities with gastrointestinal symptoms suggests Henoch–Schönlein purpura.

- A malar rash with painful knee swelling can be SLE.

- Pain with palpation over the tibial tuberosity suggests Osgood–Schlatter disease.

PHOTOGRAPHS OF SELECTED DIAGNOSES

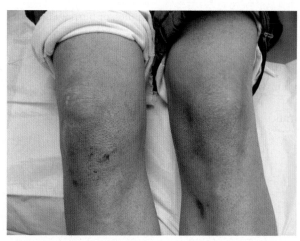

Figure 48-1 Knee effusion. Clinically obvious effusion of the right knee. (Used with permission from Fuchs MA. Hemarthrosis. In: Greenberg MI, ed. *Greenberg's Atlas of Emergency Medicine.* Philadelphia, PA: Lippincott Williams & Wilkins; 2005:525.)

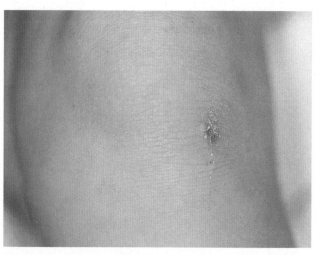

Figure 48-2 Knee cellulitis. Localized erythema suggestive of cellulitis overlying the knee. (Used with permission from Fleisher GR, Ludwig S, Baskin MN, eds. *Atlas of Pediatric Emergency Medicine.* Philadelphia, PA: Lippincott Williams & Wilkins; 2004:202.)

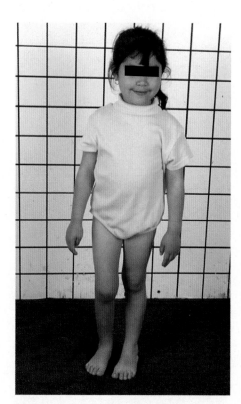

Figure 48-3 Juvenile idiopathic arthritis. Unilateral swelling of the right knee in a young girl with JIA. (Courtesy of Shriners Hospitals for Children, Houston, Texas.)

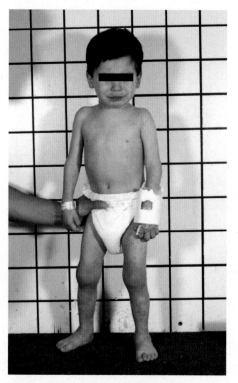

Figure 48-4 Juvenile idiopathic arthritis. A toddler with bilateral knee swelling due to JIA. (Courtesy of Shriners Hospitals for Children, Houston, Texas.)

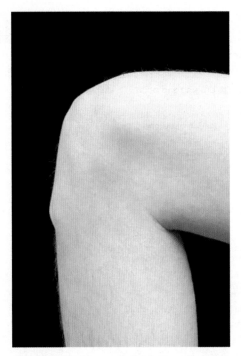

Figure 48-5 Osgood–Schlatter disease. Lateral view demonstrating prominence of the tibial tuberosity. (Courtesy of Julie A. Boom, MD.)

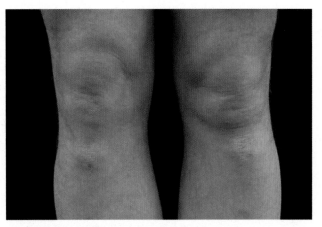

Figure 48-6 Osgood–Schlatter disease. Pain with palpation over the tibial tuberosity is suggestive of Osgood–Schlatter disease. (Courtesy of Julie A. Boom, MD.)

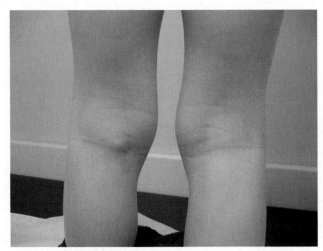

Figure 48-7 Baker cyst. Discrete swelling in the left popliteal fossa without overlying erythema. (Courtesy of Mary L. Brandt, MD.)

DIFFERENTIAL DIAGNOSIS

DIAGNOSIS	ICD-10	DISTINGUISHING CHARACTERISTICS	DISTRIBUTION
Trauma	S80 Superficial injury of knee and lower leg S83 Dislocation and sprain of joints and ligaments of knee M25.469 (knee effusion, unspecified)	Asymmetry with bruising and point tenderness Decreased range of motion (ROM) depending on location of trauma	Unilateral
Septic Arthritis	M00.861	Warmth, swelling, tenderness, or an effusion with decreased ROM in all directions Swelling after several days of decreased movement Limp or refusal to walk in a previously ambulatory child	Usually monoarticular
Acute Rheumatic Fever	I00-I02	Painful polyarthritis Arthritis presents early and lasts <4 weeks	Polyarticular (elbows, wrists, and ankles)
Juvenile Idiopathic Arthritis	M08	Autoimmune disorder Joint swelling lasting ≥ 6 weeks May limp or may refuse to walk Morning stiffness that improves later in the day	Ankle, wrist, and elbow swelling Polyarticular >5 joints Pauciarticular <4 joints
Lyme Disease	A69.20	Migratory, painful arthritis of sudden onset	Monoarticular or oligoarticular Usually large joints, but any may be affected

ASSOCIATED FINDINGS	COMPLICATIONS	PREDISPOSING FACTORS	TREATMENT GUIDELINES
Usually none	Intra-articular fractures, injury to more than one ligament, or neurovascular compromise require(s) immediate orthopedic or vascular surgical consultation	Fall or blow to the knee Hyperextension or twisting injury	Initiate PRICE within 24 hours of injury P—protection R—rest I—ice C—compression E—elevation Nonsteroidal anti-inflammatory medication for analgesia If a fracture is suspected or if there is a gross deformity (knee dislocation), immobilization and transfer to an emergency department for orthopedic consultation
Irritability Poor oral intake Fever in children >12–18 months Crying with passive movement Voluntary splinting to prevent movement (pseudoparalysis)	Permanent decreased ROM because of tissue destruction, scarring, or necrosis Impaired growth if epiphysis involved Bacteremia and septic embolization	Penetrating trauma causing direct inoculation Hematogenous spread from another location	Joint aspiration and examination of the synovial fluid; cell count, Gram stain, and culture IV antibiotics to cover methicillin-resistant *Staphylococcus aureus* and streptococcal infections, until culture results are obtained Antibiotics to cover Gram-negative bacteria until culture results available Imaging of the affected joint and bone if osteomyelitis is suspected In sexually active adolescents, consider treatment for gonococcal infection. Orthopedic consultation for possible open drainage and lavage
Carditis Erythema marginatum Subcutaneous nodules Sydenham chorea	Carditis Valvulitis (especially mitral) leading to vascular insufficiency Recurrence can occur unless secondary prophylaxis is instituted.	History of recent streptococcal infection	Anti-inflammatory agents until all symptoms are absent and the erythrocyte sedimentation rate and C-reactive protein are normal Evaluation by a cardiologist; consider corticosteroids for severe carditis. Antibiotic therapy during the acute illness; long-term antibiotic (benzathine penicillin G IM) prophylaxis every 4 weeks until age 18–20 years, if no relapse
Fatigue High regularly spiking fevers Pleuritis Pericarditis Anemia Leukocytosis Rash Lymphadenopathy Uveitis	Joint degeneration Contractures Leg length discrepancies Loss of vision because of chronic uveitis	HLA-B27 positivity ANA positivity Genetic predisposition; family history of rheumatoid arthritis Females > males	Nonsteroidal anti-inflammatory medications Corticosteroids Disease-modifying drugs
Most commonly, expanding skin rash, erythema chronicum migrans Malaise Fatigue Neck stiffness Arthralgia Low-grade fevers	Cardiovascular abnormalities including AV block, pericarditis, cardiomegaly, and left ventricular dysfunction Neurologic abnormalities, including meningitis, cranial neuropathy, and peripheral radiculopathy	Tick bite of the *Ixodes* genus, the deer tick that is infected with the spirochete *Borrelia burgdorferi* Lyme-endemic areas in the United States include the Northeast, Mid-Atlantic region, upper North-Central region, and northwestern California 92% of cases occur in the following states: CT, RI, NJ, NY, PA, DE, MD, MA, and WI	Disseminated disease treatment: oral or IV antibiotics depending on age of patient Lyme arthritis (joint swelling) treatment; initially oral antibiotics; if no improvements after 28 days, consider IV antibiotics.

Other Diagnoses to Consider

- Osteochondritis dissecans

- Osgood–Schlatter disease

- Pigmented villonodular synovitis (rare—painless chronic knee swelling in an adolescent)

- Serum sickness

- SLE

- Osteomyelitis

- Viral arthritis associated with parvovirus, adenovirus, Epstein–Barr virus, and rubella, mumps, varicella, and hepatitis B virus infection

- Malignancy including leukemia, neuroblastoma, lymphoma, Hodgkin disease, malignant histiocytosis, rhabdomyosarcoma, osteosarcoma, and Ewing sarcoma

- Immunodeficiency and inflammatory bowel disease-associated arthritis

- Rickets secondary to vitamin D deficiency

When to Consider Further Evaluation or Treatment

- Neurovascular injury to the popliteal artery and peroneal nerve occurs most commonly in knee dislocations and displaced fractures. Immediate vascular surgery consultation is warranted if popliteal artery compromise is suspected.

- According to the Ottawa Knee Rules, radiographs of the knee should be obtained after an acute injury in children who meet one of the following criteria: isolated tenderness of the patella, tenderness at the head of the fibula, inability to flex the knee to 90 degrees, inability to bear weight immediately and in the emergency department for four steps, regardless of limp.

- The most serious complication of pauciarticular JIA is the development of uveitis or iridocyclitis, which occurs most commonly in the subgroup of children below 6 years of age who are ANA positive. A prompt ophthalmology evaluation and routine screening are necessary.

- Bleeding disorders should be considered when hemarthrosis of the knee occurs with minimal or no recollected trauma. Initial laboratory tests include a complete blood count, prothrombin time, and activated partial thromboplastin time. Joint bleeding is typically seen in deficiencies in coagulation factors, such as hemophilia.

- Recurrent painful monoarticular hemarthrosis of the knee may be caused by a synovial hemangioma, which occurs more commonly in children. MRI is the preferred mode of imaging. Refer to orthopedic surgery for treatment, which includes embolization, local steroid injection, and surgical excision.

SUGGESTED READINGS

Baskin MN. Injury—knee. In: Fleisher GR, Ludwig S, Henretig FM, eds. *Textbook of Pediatric Emergency Medicine.* 6th ed. Philadelphia, PA: Lippincott Williams & Wilkins; 2010:345–352.

Fleisher GR, Ludwig S, Baskin MN, eds. *Atlas of Pediatric Emergency Medicine.* Philadelphia, PA: Lippincott Williams & Wilkins; 2004:202.

Greenberg MI, ed. *Greenberg's Atlas of Emergency Medicine.* Philadelphia, PA: Lippincott Williams & Wilkins; 2004:525.

Mirkinson L. The diagnosis of rheumatic fever. *Pediatr Rev.* 1998;19:310–311.

Schaller JG. Juvenile rheumatoid arthritis. *Pediatr Rev.* 1997;18:337–349.

Schwartz MW, Bell LM, Bingham P, et al., eds. *The 5-Minute Pediatric Consult.* 5th ed. Philadelphia, PA: Lippincott Williams & Wilkins; 2008:58–59, 724–725, 760–761.

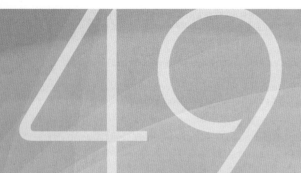

Foot Deformities

Laura. A. Monson and
Larry H. Hollier, Jr

Approach to the Problem

An understanding of the natural history; a careful physical examination including range of motion, neurovascular examination, visual inspection, and palpation; and serial measurements allow proper diagnosis for most pedal (foot) deformities. Most importantly, the timing of presentation is critical. Congenital pedal deformities include metatarsus adductus, metatarsus varus, calcaneovalgus foot, rocker-bottom foot (congenital vertical talus), and clubfoot (talipes equinovarus). Pes planus (flatfeet) may be of either the soft or the rigid variety, and both are typically noticed as the child begins to ambulate. Flat feet are common in children because arch development occurs primarily before 4 years of age, and because the development has a wide variation in the rate or onset in any given child. The treatment of these defects is overwhelmingly conservative, and surgery is reserved for older children with severe deformities that will not improve over time.

Key Points in the History

- Intoeing and outtoeing may result from more proximal, tibial, femoral, or hip defects, such as long bone torsion, bowlegs, or knock-knees.

- While the majority of clubfoot and pes planus deformities are sporadic, these deformities have also been linked to inherited defects.

- The timing of ambulation in children with metatarsus adductus and pes planus is not generally delayed.

- Metatarsus adductus is the most common congenital foot deformity. It occurs more frequently in women, is more common on the left side than on the right side, and typically improves with time.

- Metatarsus adductus, clubfoot, and flexible pes planus are infrequently associated with pain, whereas rigid pes planus may be associated with significant discomfort.

- Trauma, occult infection, a foreign body, tarsal coalition, bone tumors, or osteochondrosis of the tarsal navicular bone may cause a stiff and painful flat foot.

392

CHAPTER 49 • FOOT DEFORMITIES

- The presence of systemic symptoms, such as fever, may be suggestive of more serious foot disorders, such as infection or malignancy.

- When metatarsus adductus is also associated with hindfoot inversion, plantar flexion, a hypoplastic ipsilateral calf, or a slightly shortened tibia, a diagnosis of clubfoot should be considered.

Key Points in the Physical Examination

- With a clubfoot defect, there is extreme plantar flexion of the ankle (equinus). The heel is in varum (medial deviation), and the sole is kidney shaped (adducted and supinated) when viewed from the bottom. Also, callous and hyperpigmentation may be present on the dorsolateral clubfoot. The foot will have a deep medial skin furrow and, in bilateral cases, the soles of the feet will face each other. The Achilles tendon is tight, and there is limited dorsiflexion.

- In evaluation of metatarsus adductus, the forefoot has a convex, lateral border, and a crease over the medial midfoot is visible. The metatarsals are deviated medially. Also, the forefoot easily corrects to midline with gentle pressure.

- A calcaneovalgus foot appears flat, the heel is angled away from midline, and the ankle is in dorsiflexion so that the dorsal foot rests against the tibia. The ankle typically has limited dorsiflexion.

- Congenital vertical talus appears similar to calcaneovalgus, but is a rigid deformity.

- Flexible pes planus (flatfoot) is identified by appearance of the pedal arch when the child stands on his or her toes. Upon standing, however, the arch disappears.

- Rigid pes planus (flatfoot) is indicated by the lack of pedal arching while standing normally and standing on one's toes.

- A compensatory flatfoot may occur as the result of a tight heel cord.

- Substantial pain upon gentle palpation, erythema, or localized firmness may be suggestive of more significant underlying pathology, such as cellulitis, osteomyelitis, joint infection, or malignancy.

SECTION 12 • EXTREMITIES

PHOTOGRAPHS OF SELECTED DIAGNOSES

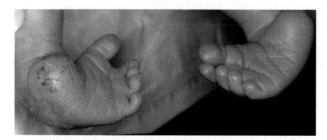

Figure 49-1 Clubfeet. Bilateral clubfeet in an infant with notable metatarsus adductus. (Courtesy of Gerardo Cabrera-Meza, MD.)

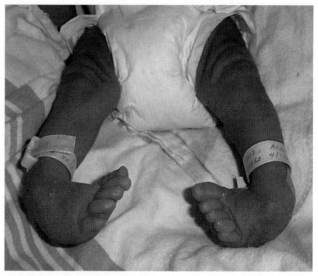

Figure 49-2 Clubfeet. Dorsal view of clubfeet in an infant with plantar flexion and foot inversion. (Courtesy of Gerardo Cabrera-Meza, MD.)

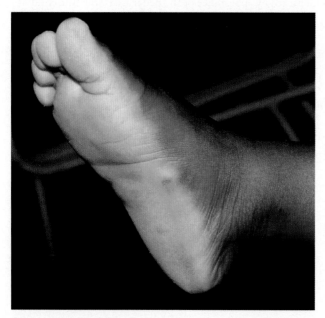

Figure 49-3 Pes planus. Arch absent in non weight-bearing position in this child with rigid pes planus. (Courtesy of Tom Thacher, MD.)

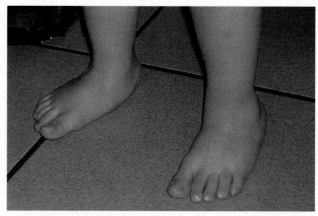

Figure 49-4 Pes planus. Mild pronation noted in this child with pes planus. (Courtesy of Sujata R. Tipnis, MD.)

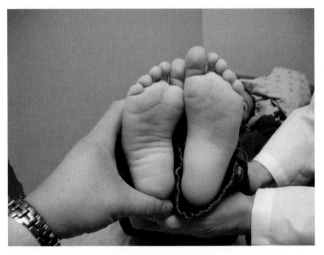

Figure 49-5 Metatarsus adductus. The convex ("C") shape of the child's right foot suggests metatarsus adductus. (Courtesy of Paul S. Matz, MD.)

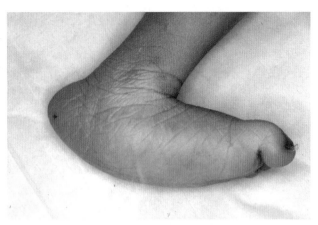

Figure 49-6 Rocker-bottom feet. Gentle curvature to the bottom of this infant's feet is typical of rocker-bottom feet and may be associated with Patau syndrome or Edward syndrome. (Courtesy of Gerardo Cabrera-Meza, MD.)

DIFFERENTIAL DIAGNOSIS

DIAGNOSIS	ICD-10	DISTINGUISHING CHARACTERISTICS	DISTRIBUTION	DURATION/ CHRONICITY	ASSOCIATED FINDINGS	COMPLICATIONS	PREDISPOSING FACTORS	TREATMENT GUIDELINES
Clubfoot	Q66.89	Adduction of midfoot and forefoot Varus deformity of hindfoot Cavus deformity of midfoot	May be bilateral in ~50% of cases	May be diagnosed in utero Chronic, unless treated	Associated syndromes: Prune belly syndrome Mobius syndrome Arthrogryposis Constriction bands Pierre Robin sequence Diastrophic dwarfism Larson syndrome Opitz syndrome Meningo-myelocele	If untreated, significant gait abnormalities may result If treated, gastrocsoleus weakness and difficulty with push-off may occur	Multiple genetic models proposed First-degree relatives have 17 times higher occurrence Maternal smoking may increase risk. Boys more commonly affected than girls	Referral to an orthopedic surgeon for bracing, casting, and possible surgical correction
Flexible Pes Planus	M21.40	Arch present in sitting (non weight bearing) and in toe standing positions Arch absent when standing (weight bearing)	Typically bilateral	Ubiquitous in newborns Usually resolves by school age without therapy	Occasionally associated with a tight Achilles tendon	If fails to resolve with age, foot pain and lower extremity stress injuries may occur	Incidence decreases with increasing age May be more common in boys Valgus knees, joint laxity, and obesity may increase incidence	None indicated
Rigid Pes Planus	M21.40	Arch absent in weight-bearing and non weight-bearing positions Subtalar joint rigid	May be bilateral in ~50% of cases	Persists into school age and adolescence	Tarsal coalition Heel cord contracture	Pain Abnormal gait	Cerebral palsy Bone abnormalities	Referral to an orthopedic surgeon
Meta-tarsus Adductus	Q66.2	Medial deviation of forefoot Deep medial crease Prominent proximal fifth metatarsal	Typically bilateral	Usually resolves by 3–4 years of age	Intoeing	None	Increased incidence, if positive family history Increased incidence in twins	Mild forms resolve spontane-ously over time

Other Diagnoses to Consider

- Trauma

- Infection

- Cavus foot (high-arched foot)

- Trauma (sprains, strains, or fractures)

- Infection

- Cavus foot (high-arched foot)

- Neoplasm

When to Consider Further Evaluation or Treatment

- Clubfoot deformity should be referred to an orthopedic surgeon for bracing, casting, and possible surgical correction.

- Flexible pes planus and metatarsus adductus should be simply observed as treatment is generally not indicated.

- A stiff or painful flat foot should be referred to an orthopedic surgeon.

- A tight heel cord should be further evaluated by an orthopedic surgeon and/or by a neurologist if hypertonicity is present.

SUGGESTED READINGS

Dietz FR. Intoeing—fact, fiction and opinion. *Am Fam Physician.* 1994;50(6):1249–1259.

Horn BD, Davidson RS. Current treatment of clubfoot in infancy and childhood. *Foot Ankle Clin.* 2010;15(2):235–243.

Kasser JR. The foot. In: Morrissy RT, Weinstein SL, eds. *Lovell and Winter's Pediatric Orthopaedics.* 6th ed. Philadelphia, PA: Lippincott Williams & Wilkins; 2006:1258–1328.

McCrea JD. *Pediatric Orthopedics of the Lower Extremity: An Instructional Handbook.* Mount Kisco, NY: Futura Publishing Company, Inc.; 1985.

Roye BD, Hyman J, Roye DP Jr. Congenital idiopathic talipes equinovarus. *Pediatr Rev.* 2004;25(4):124–130.

Sass P, Hassan G. Lower extremity abnormalities in children. *Am Fam Physician.* 2003;68(3):461–468.

Scherl SA. Common lower extremity problems in children. *Pediatr Rev.* 2004;25(2):52–62.

Yagerman SE, Cross MB, Positano R, et al. Evaluation and treatment of symptomatic pes planus. *Curr Opin Pediatr.* 2011;23(1):60–67.

Foot Swelling

Lisa E. De Ybarrondo
and Mark Jason Sanders

Approach to the Problem

Foot swelling or edema is a common manifestation of many disease states. It may be part of a localized or generalized process. Unilateral foot swelling may develop from a variety of causes, including trauma (e.g., sprains, fractures), infection (e.g., cellulitis, osteomyelitis, abscess), angioedema (i.e., allergic reaction vs hereditary), vasculitis (e.g., Henoch–Schönlein purpura, Kawasaki disease), insect bites, snake bites with envenomation, lymphedema (i.e., hereditary, acquired), soft-tissue tumors (e.g., benign—fibromas, malignant—rhabdomyosarcoma, other sarcomas), or bone tumors (e.g., benign—exostosis and unicameral bone cyst, malignant—osteosarcoma and Ewing sarcoma). Pain may be a significant complaint with all of these etiologies except for angioedema, lymphedema, and benign tumors. Historical factors such as chronicity of symptoms (recurrent vs acute onset), environmental exposures, systemic symptoms, a family history of angioedema or lymphedema, underlying renal/cardiac/hepatic disease, medications, and a thorough physical examination will help determine the etiology of foot swelling. Bilateral painless foot swelling is more likely due to an underlying systemic condition such as nephrotic syndrome, heart failure, cardiomyopathy, cirrhosis, malnutrition, hypoproteinemia, renal failure, or pregnancy.

Key Points in the History

- The typical ankle sprain is an inversion injury that occurs in the plantar-flexed position. The lateral stabilizing ligaments are most commonly affected in this type of injury.

- Ankle sprains in children are less common than fractures because the ligaments of a preadolescent are much stronger than the growth plate or bone. Associated avulsion fractures are typically present if a ligamentous injury occurs.

- Most foot fractures in children result from direct trauma, such as crush injuries from a falling object or the child falling from a height.

- Acute traumatic compartment syndrome of the foot is the result of a serious injury such as a fracture, dislocation, and/or crush injury. Vascular injuries and coagulopathies are risk factors for the development of this condition.

- Acute, painful, unilateral foot swelling is often associated with infection or trauma. Chronic unilateral painful foot swelling over a period of weeks to months may indicate a malignant neoplasm of the soft or bony tissue.

- Recurring paroxysms of subcutaneous angioedema in the extremities, face, trunk, genitals, or the intestinal and laryngeal submucosae are the characteristics of hereditary angioneurotic edema. Family history is positive in 75% of patients.

- Unilateral or bilateral, neonatal pedal edema suggests a diagnostic evaluation for Turner syndrome, Noonan syndrome, or Milroy disease (hereditary lymphedema with autosomal dominant inheritance).

- Medications such as calcium channel blockers and vasodilators may cause peripheral edema. Oral contraceptives may predispose a female teenager to deep venous thrombosis/thrombophlebitis with lower extremity swelling.

Key Points in the Physical Examination

- Findings associated with severe ankle sprains include swelling, bruising, pain on palpation, and a positive anterior drawer test of the ankle. Patients with all four of these findings are likely to have a lateral ligament rupture.

- Angioedema secondary to cutaneous vessel damage in Henoch–Schönlein purpura may be significant. It may precede the palpable purpura, and it is most prominent over the dorsal hands and feet, and the periorbital regions.

- Snake bites with envenomation cause edema and erythema at the location of the bite and in adjacent tissues, usually within 30 to 60 minutes. Oozing from the wound suggests envenomation. Edema progresses rapidly and may involve the entire extremity. Ecchymosis is common and may appear within 3 to 6 hours.

- Subcutaneous angioedema in hereditary angioedema is nonpruritic, nonerythematous, and well circumscribed. It is not accompanied by urticaria and is most commonly seen on the extremities.

- Edema, typically pitting edema, is the major clinical manifestation of nephrotic syndrome. It is more noticeable in the face in the morning upon arising and predominately in the lower extremities later in the day.

- Infants with beriberi have muscle wasting, upper and lower extremity edema, pallor, restlessness, and diarrhea. Infants who are breastfed by a thiamine-deficient mother are at risk for developing beriberi.

PHOTOGRAPHS OF SELECTED DIAGNOSES

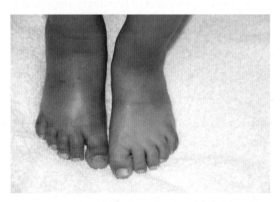

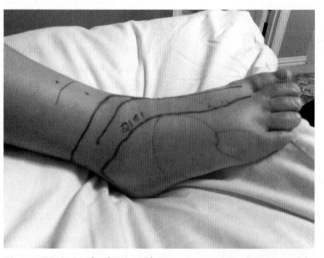

Figure 50-1 Insect bite. A 2-year-old child with swelling and erythema of the right foot and ankle because of an insect bite. A pustule and vesicles are noted over the dorsum of the foot. (Courtesy of Julie A. Boom, MD.)

Figure 50-2 Snake bite with envenomation. A 9-year-old with swelling, erythema, and ecchymosis of the right foot and ankle 2 days after a Southern Copperhead bite. The fang marks are visible on the lateral aspect of the foot, and the area of swelling and erythema has been marked with a pen. (Courtesy of Lisa E. De Ybarrondo, MD.)

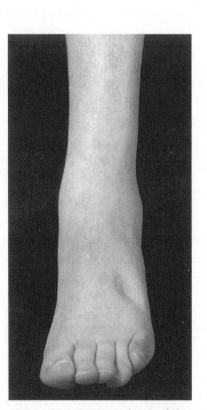

Figure 50-3 Pitting edema of the foot. An edematous foot with evidence of pitting following firm pressure. (Used with permission from Bickley LS, Szilagyi P, eds. *Bates Guide to Physical Examination and History Taking.* 8th ed. Philadelphia, PA: Lippincott Williams & Wilkins; 2003:455.)

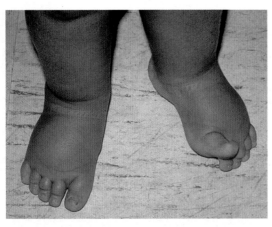

Figure 50-4 Lower extremity and foot edema.
Clinical picture of lower extremities showing
marked edema. (Used with permission from Gold
DH, Weingeist TA. *Color Atlas of the Eye in Systemic Disease*. Baltimore, MD: Lippincott Williams
& Wilkins; 2001:643.)

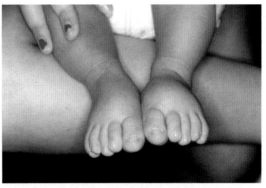

Figure 50-5 Congenital lymphedema. Bilateral
foot swelling noted by the mother of a newborn,
4 days following hospital discharge. (Courtesy of
Jan Edwin Drutz, MD.)

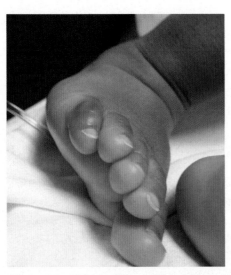

**Figure 50-6 Foot edema and erythema
in a child with Kawasaki disease.**
(Courtesy of Esther K. Chung, MD, MPH.)

DIFFERENTIAL DIAGNOSISS

DIAGNOSIS	ICD-10	DISTINGUISHING CHARACTERISTICS	DISTRIBUTION	DURATION/ CHRONICITY
Insect Bite	S90.869D	Pruritic, erythematous, urticarial papules, central punctum	Unilateral or bilateral local reaction May have multiple lesions on exposed areas of skin	Swelling may not be apparent until the next day.
Ankle or Foot Sprain	S93.40 (ankle) S93.6 (foot)	Acute onset Inversion injury, most common Minimal to severe pain Swelling Ecchymosis	Unilateral swelling localized to the injured ligaments	Swelling subsides within 48–72 hours Recovery depends on severity and location: mild ankle sprain, within 2 weeks; severe sprain, 6 weeks
Ankle Fracture	S82	Acute onset Inversion injury, in the preadolescent most commonly causes a Salter type I fracture of the distal fibula	Unilateral swelling localized to the injured bone or more diffuse swelling	Depends on the type of fracture, usually between 3 and 6 weeks
Foot Fracture	S92	Acute onset Metatarsal and toe fractures are the most common in children. Most frequently fractured metatarsal in older children is the fifth. Stress fractures present with progressive worsening of pain. Mid- and hindfoot fractures have the greatest potential for causing permanent disability and deformity.	Unilateral swelling can be diffuse or localized	Depends on the fracture location, usually between 3 and 6 weeks
Cellulitis and/or Abscess	L03.11	Acute onset Pain Erythema Warmth Induration	Unilateral Localized or diffuse swelling	Symptomatic improvement within 24–48 hours after initiating antimicrobial therapy Visible improvement within 72 hours

ASSOCIATED FINDINGS	COMPLICATIONS	PRDISOPOSING FACTORS	TREATMENT GUIDELINES
Pain associated with hymenoptera stings, spider bites, and biting flies	Infection: impetigo, cellulitis, abscess Central necrosis/eschar (Brown recluse spider)	Warm months of the year, moist environment	Oral antihistamines Topical corticosteroids Insect control measures including repellants
Loss of functional ability Difficulty bearing weight with moderate to severe sprains Point tenderness over the affected ligaments	Chronic ankle instability Residual pain Recurrent sprains Stiffness Recurrent swelling	History of previous ankle sprain Sports such as basketball, ice skating, and soccer have highest prevalence of ankle injuries. Limited dorsiflexion may increase risk.	Initiate PRICE within 24 hours of injury: P—protection R—rest (up to 72 hours) I—ice C—compression E—elevation Exercises to restore motion and strength within 48–72 hours Lace-up or semirigid supports are more effective than tape or elastic bandages Nonsteroidal anti-inflammatory medication
Pain, swelling, and ecchymosis observed over the lateral malleolus with the Salter type I distal fibula injury Inability to bear weight immediately after injury	Compartment syndrome Arthritis Chronic pain Gait disturbances Infection, if open fracture Chronic instability Nonunion Stiffness	Sports injury Crush injury Motor vehicle and auto-pedestrian accidents Bone tumors may predispose to pathological fractures.	Depends on the type of fracture: Salter type I distal fibula fracture—a below-the-knee walking cast is applied for 3 weeks Salter type II requires closed reduction and a long-leg cast. Salter–Harris type III (Tillaux fracture) requires open reduction with internal fixation.
Pain, swelling, ecchymosis, and point tenderness over the affected bone Difficulty bearing weight or unable to walk Fifth metatarsal fractures often difficult to differentiate from an ankle injury because of swelling at the lateral malleolus	Compartment syndrome Arthritis Nonunion Malunion Reflex sympathetic dystrophy Chronic pain Talar (neck fracture): avascular necrosis Tarsometatarsal fracture (Lisfranc fracture): forefoot ischemia, skin necrosis	Motor vehicle collision Falls from a height or at a level surface Sports injury Crush injury Machine (e.g., lawn mower) related injury Stress fractures from repetitive stress: high incidence in military recruits but also common in ballet dancers, gymnasts, and athletes	Displaced foot fractures warrant urgent orthopedic consultation. Stress fractures: rest for 3–4 weeks, use of crutches or a walking boot, physical therapy Metatarsal shaft fractures: short-leg non weight-bearing cast 4–12 weeks Jones fractures of the fifth metatarsal may need closed reduction and internal fixation, if severe Talar neck fracture (minimally displaced): long-leg cast, 6–8 weeks Calcaneal fracture: non weight-bearing short-leg cast, 5–6 weeks Lisfranc fracture: short-leg cast 3–4 weeks
For puncture wounds on the plantar surface of the foot, look for evidence of a foreign body Systemic symptoms; fever, chills, malaise, headache	Lymphangitis Osteomyelitis Septic arthritis Tissue necrosis Septic emboli	Diabetes mellitus Immunocompromise Burns Trauma Crush and penetrating injuries Foreign bodies Lacerations Degloving injuries Tinea pedis/onychomycosis, lymphedema, venous insufficiency	Depends on the type of infection Treatment for *Pseudomonas aeruginosa* if puncture wound occurs through sneakers or tennis shoes Cellulitis (mild/superficial): systemic antibiotics directed toward *Staphylococcus aureus* and Group A streptococci, 7–10 days, rest, elevation Surgical I&D or debridement for abscesses or deep infections

SECTION 12 • EXTREMITIES

(continued)

DIFFERENTIAL DIAGNOSIS *(continued)*

DIAGNOSIS	ICD-10	DISTINGUISHING CHARACTERISTICS	DISTRIBUTION	DURATION/ CHRONICITY
Dactylitis	D57.00	Acute onset Painful swelling of the hands and feet Occurs typically between 6 months and 3 years	Bilateral	Lasts 1–2 weeks Rarely occurs after age 5
Angioedema	T78.3	Rapid onset over minutes to hours Skin may be normal in color or erythematous Painful Warm to palpation	Asymmetrical pattern Face, genitalia, bowel wall, and mucosal tissues commonly involved	Resolves in 24–48 hours
Orthostatic Edema	T67.7	Painless, pitting edema in postpubertal females	Bilateral, primarily in lower legs, ankle, and feet	Duration variable, weeks to months after therapy initiated
Nephrotic Syndrome	N04	Painless, progressive swelling Pitting edema Peak incidence 2–3 years Male-to-female ratio 2:1 Minimal change nephritic syndrome is most common	Bilateral	Duration variable Edema improves after initiation of treatment: 90% of steroid-sensitive nephrotic syndrome respond to steroids with 4 weeks Few develop renal failure or renal insufficiency

ASSOCIATED FINDINGS	COMPLICATIONS	PRDISOPOSING FACTORS	TREATMENT GUIDELINES
Low-grade fever Leukocytosis Warmth and tenderness around the affected bones Infarction of bone marrow in the metacarpals, metatarsals, and proximal phalanges	Permanent shortening of the involved digits Osteomyelitis Septic arthritis	Sickle cell disease Sickle cell/hemoglobin C disease Sickle cell/beta thalassemia disease More common during colder months	Hydration Analgesics for pain relief Nonsteroidal anti-inflammatory medications Hot packs Hydroxyuria

Urticaria with intense pruritus
 	
Respiratory compromise; dyspnea, wheeze, stridor, chest or throat tightness
 	
Hypotension, tachycardia, syncope
 	
Gastrointestinal symptoms
	Life threatening if laryngeal edema with anaphylaxis or hereditary angioedema
	
	Secondary to asphyxia and respiratory compromise
	
	Cardiovascular collapse
		Mast cell-mediated: exposure to common allergens from food, drugs, stinging insects, latex, inhalants, and food additives
		
		Hereditary angioedema: following trauma, infection, emotional stress, puberty
			Immediate stabilization of anaphylaxis using:
			
			  Epinephrine IM
			
			  Antihistamines
			
			  Corticosteroids
			
			  H_2 antihistamines
			
			  Bronchodilators
			
			Hereditary angioedema: Intravenous C1-inhibitor if severe laryngeal attacks or severe abdominal attacks

Weight gain during the day May present with fatigue, dizziness, syncope, headache, abdominal swelling, breast swelling, breast discomfort, pruritus Symptoms worse in hot weather	Susceptible to bacterial infections and poor healing if trauma Associated psychological symptoms	Postpubertal females Genetic predisposition	Sodium intake reduction Avoidance of excessive fluid intake unless orthostatic hypotension is present Exercise Compression stockings Dextroamphetamine, ephedrine, and pseudoephedrine are agents that have been used
Edema usually appears first in the periorbital, scrotal, and labial regions Weight gain Hypertension Hypoalbuminemia/ hypoproteinemia Hyperlipidemia Proteinuria Ascites Hematuria	Chronic renal failure Infections Atherosclerosis, thrombotic complications Congestive heart failure Malnutrition Long-term immunosuppression may cause osteoporosis, nephrolithiasis, obesity, diabetes mellitus	Congenital nephrotic syndrome Infection Collagen vascular disease Sickle cell disease Toxins Medications Diabetes mellitus Henoch–Schönlein purpura	Glucocorticoid therapy, high dose then maintenance Diuretics Antihypertensives Dietary salt restriction Alkylating agents

SECTION 12 • EXTREMITIES

<table>
<tr><td>

Other Diagnoses to Consider

</td><td>

- Juvenile idiopathic arthritis

- Deep venous thrombosis

- Glomerulonephritis, renal failure

- Burns

- Myxedema

- Kawasaki disease

- Primary lymphedema (Turner syndrome, Noonan syndrome, or Milroy disease)

- Secondary lymphedema (filariasis, lymphatic obstruction)

- Köhler disease (osteonecrosis of the navicular bone)

- Acute hemorrhagic edema of infancy

- Malnutrition (kwashiorkor, scurvy, beriberi)

- Hypoalbuminemia

</td></tr>
<tr><td>

When to Consider Further Evaluation or Treatment

</td><td>

- It is important to reexamine an ankle sprain 3 to 5 days following the injury to assess the extent of ligamentous injury (partial tear vs rupture). Consider referral to orthopedic surgery for a severe sprain that includes a ligament rupture.

- Compartment syndrome presents with tense swelling of the foot and pain out of proportion to the degree of injury. Palor, paresthesias, and pulselessness are late signs. If there is a suspicion of compartment syndrome, then a prompt surgical evaluation is required with intracompartmental pressure monitoring.

- Indications for referral to an orthopedic surgeon include fracture, dislocation, subluxation, tendon rupture, wound penetrating into the joint, soft-tissue tumors, or bone tumors (benign or malignant). Foot fractures involving the talar neck, tarsometatarsal or intra articular calcaneus warrant urgent orthopedic consultation.

- If cellulitis has not visibly improved within 72 hours and/or symptomatic improvement has not occurred within 24 to 48 hours after starting oral antibiotics, consider resistant pathogens or alternative diagnoses such as abscess, osteomyelitis, or other.

- Evaluation for a deeper soft-tissue infection should be considered in patients with underlying conditions such as diabetes or lymphedema, and in patients who are systemically ill.

- According to the Ottawa Ankle Rules, radiographs of the ankle should be obtained after an acute ankle injury in children (>5 years old) if there is any pain in the malleolar zone accompanied by any one of the following findings: bone tenderness along the distal 6 cm of the posterior edge of the tibia or tip of the medial malleolus, bone tenderness along the distal 6 cm of the posterior edge of the fibula or tip of the lateral malleolus, or an inability to bear weight both immediately and in the emergency department for four steps.

</td></tr>
</table>

- According to the Ottawa Foot Rules, radiographs of the ankle should be obtained after an acute foot injury in children (>5 years old) if there is any pain in the midfoot zone and any one of the following findings: bone tenderness at the base of the fifth metatarsal, bone tenderness at the navicular bone, or inability to bear weight immediately and in the emergency department for four steps.

SUGGESTED READINGS

Barillas-Arias L, Adams A, Lehman A. Pediatric vasculitic syndrome: Henoch-Schönlein purpura. *Consult. Pediatr.* 2008;7(9):361–367.

Bibbo C, Lin SS, Cunningham FJ. Acute traumatic compartment syndrome of the foot in children. *Pediatr Emerg Care.* 2000;16(4):244–248.

Dowling S, Spooner CH, Liang Y, et al. Accuracy of Ottawa Ankle Rules to exclude fractures of the ankle and midfoot in children: a meta-analysis. *Acad Emerg Med.* 2009;16(4):277–287.

Fleisher GR, Ludwig S, eds. *Textbook of Pediatric Emergency Medicine.* 6th ed. Baltimore, MD: Williams & Wilkins; 2010:233–234.

Jarvis JG, Moroz PJ. Fractures and dislocations of the foot. In: Beaty JH, Kasser JR, eds. *Fractures in Children.* 6th ed. Philadelphia, PA: Lippincott Williams & Wilkins; 2006:1129.

Sardana N, Craig TJ. Recent advances in management and treatment of hereditary angioedema. *Pediatrics.* 2011;128(6):1173–1180.

Tiemstra JD. Update on acute ankle sprains. *Am Fam Physicians.* 2012;85(12):1170–1176.

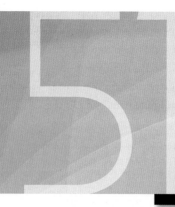

Foot Rashes
and Lumps

Mark Jason Sanders
and Lisa E. De Ybarrondo

Approach to the Problem

Often resulting from stressors placed on them by normal weight-bearing activities and the restrictive setting of everyday footwear, the feet are prone to dermatologic conditions. Developing within the enclosed environment of a warm and moist shoe, a rash can easily spread or worsen. For example, allergic dermatitis on an excoriated toe can evolve readily into an extensive foot cellulitis. A foot lump, whether related to infection or an underlying bony abnormality, may continue to grow, potentially compromise normal foot dynamics, and readily recur if not properly diagnosed and treated. Therefore, a good understanding of common pediatric foot ailments is important.

Key Points in the History

- Origin (between toes or overlying pressure points), natural course (timing or spread from a specific focus), and symptomatology (itching, burning, pain, redness, or swelling) may aid in differentiation of a foot rash or lump as reactive or infectious (dyshidrotic eczema vs tinea pedis; callus vs plantar wart).

- Seasonality may be an important clue, with tinea pedis and dyshidrotic eczema more common in the warm, summer months, and juvenile plantar dermatosis more common during colder months.

- A correlation with new or overly restrictive footwear may support the diagnosis of a corn or callus.

- Communal bathing has been associated with infections, including tinea pedis and plantar warts.

- Epidemiology may also provide clues: infantile acropustulosis occurs between birth and 2 years, juvenile plantar dermatosis occurs more commonly among prepubertal children, and tinea pedis and plantar warts are present in older children and adolescents.

- Delineation of dermatitis from an infectious rash may be based on appearance and distribution (warmth, tenderness, vesiculation, or crusting in a localized interdigital or global distribution).

- Juvenile plantar dermatosis tends to affect the balls of the feet bilaterally with a shiny, smooth appearance ("glazed doughnut"). The involvement of the interdigital spaces is more often seen in tinea pedis.

- Allergic contact dermatitis usually affects the dorsum of the feet, sparing the toe webs and soles.

- Dyshidrotic eczema tends to favor the lateral aspects of digits, palms, and soles.

- Plantar corns are more sensitive to direct pressure, whereas plantar warts are more sensitive to lateral compression or pinching.

- Plantar warts usually disrupt skin lines, with lines usually maintained in calluses.

- After paring, plantar warts will often show pinpoint black dots, which are thrombosed capillaries. Calluses will have a smooth, glassy, and homogenous surface.

- Infantile acropustulosis is characterized by pruritic, recurrent vesiculopustular lesions that are concentrated on the palms and soles, extending to the dorsum of the hands, feet, and ankles.

PHOTOGRAPHS OF SELECTED DIAGNOSES

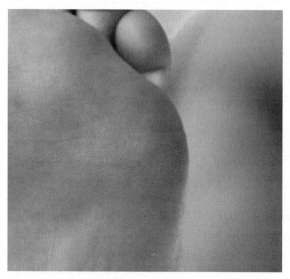

Figure 51-1 Callus. The skin over the head of the fifth metatarsal is thickened and slightly yellow, with skin lines maintained. (Courtesy of Julie A. Boom, MD.)

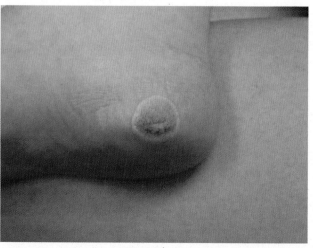

Figure 51-2 Plantar wart. Plantar wart on the medial surface of the heel. (Courtesy of Denise W. Metry, MD.)

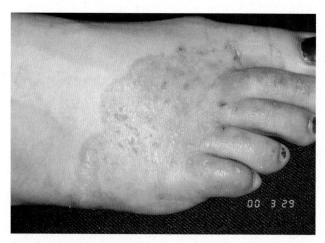

Figure 51-3 Tinea pedis. The interdigital pattern of tinea pedis is common. Note the spread onto the dorsum of the foot. (Courtesy of Denise W. Metry, MD.)

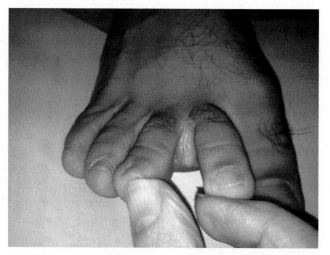

Figure 51-4 Tinea pedis. The interdigital pattern of tinea pedis is common. (Courtesy of Lisa E. De Ybarrondo, MD.)

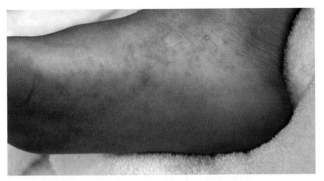

Figure 51-5 **Dyshidrotic eczema.** Multiple clear vesicles on the medial surface of the foot. (Courtesy of Julie A. Boom, MD.)

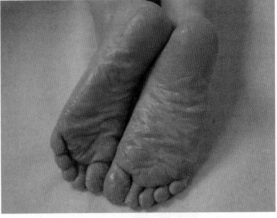

Figure 51-6 **Juvenile plantar dermatosis.** The skin on the soles has a smooth, shiny appearance with multiple fissures and cracks. (Courtesy of Denise W. Metry, MD.)

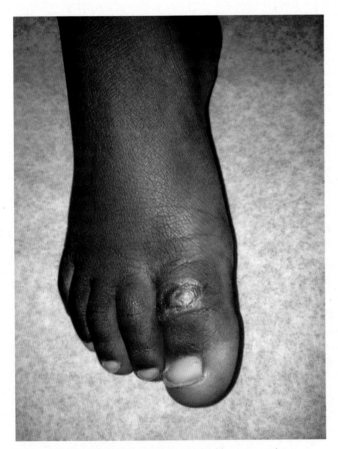

Figure 51-7 **Impetigo.** Classic crusted lesion on the great toe of a toddler with a history of eczema and similar lesions on her face and back. (Courtesy of Lisa E. De Ybarrondo, MD.)

DIFFERENTIAL DIAGNOSIS

DIAGNOSIS		ICD-10	DISTINGUISHING CHARACTERISTICS	DISTRIBUTION
Corn or Callus		M25.70	Corn: hyperkeratotic, well-circumscribed lesion with central conical core (hard) or ill-defined and macerated (soft) Callus: hyperkeratotic plaque with relatively even skin thickness, and skin lines maintained	Hard corns more common on dorsal fifth toe Soft corns more common between fourth and fifth toes Callus more common on ball of foot, margins of heel, and under metatarsal heads
Plantar Wart		B07.8	Papule, nodule, or plaque, with a rough surface that disrupts skin lines Solitary or multiple "Black dot" pattern related to thrombosed capillaries Common in young children and adolescents	Weight-bearing areas of soles
Tinea Pedis		B35.3	Interdigital pattern (most common) with erythema, peeling, fissuring, and/or maceration between toes Moccasin pattern (more chronic) with dry, scaly patches or hyperkeratotic papules surrounded by mild erythema Vesicular pattern Uncommon before puberty, and more common in male adolescents	Toe webs and soles usually may have a sharp border with uninvolved skin Interdigital pattern prominent in fourth digit web space, with possible spread to toes and dorsal foot Moccasin pattern diffusely involves plantar and lateral foot surfaces Vesicular pattern usually involves instep
Dyshidrotic Eczema		L30.1	Primary vesicular stage, with deep-set, clear vesicles that may coalesce to form bullae; intense pruritus over a few days to weeks Secondary desquamating stage, with dry skin peeling, cracking and crusting over a few weeks Relapses with disease-free intervals common Uncommon before school age, and more common in females aged 20–40 years	Lateral edges of toes and soles Usually bilateral and symmetric May involve fingers and palms
Juvenile Plantar Dermatosis		L98.9 (disorder of skin and subcutaneous tissue)	Erythema, scaling and/or fissuring, with shiny, and smooth skin ("glazed doughnut" appearance) Pruritus Pain with fissuring More common in prepubertal children	Usually bilateral and symmetric Anterior third of the sole, heel, or toes (especially great toe) Sparing of interdigital space

ASSOCIATED FINDINGS	PREDISPOSING FACTORS	TREATMENT GUIDELINES
Hammer toe deformity may promote a corn Callus may be painful	Abnormal foot mechanics/stress, promoting pressure, friction, or irritation (bony prominence abutting tight shoe)	Less restrictive footwear and/or padding Salicylic acid application Soaking and abrasive reduction Careful paring Specialiy referral (Podiatry or Orthopedics) for possible correction of underlying bony abnormalities
May be painful, especially with application of lateral pressure	Person-to-person spread, or indirect autoinoculation of foot via contaminated surfaces Trauma may facilitate spread through minor skin abrasions	Salicylic acid application Careful paring Duct tape has been used to successfully treat warts.
Onychomycosis	Communal bathing Physical exertion with foot sweating Restrictive and/or damp shoes Warm weather Household member with tinea pedis	Topical antifungal
N/A	Associated with hyperhidrosis May worsen during warm weather and with emotional stress Possible association with primary irritants, (soaps, detergents) May be an "id" reaction to candidal or other infection	Emollient Topical corticosteroid or immunomodulator
N/A	Associated with hyperhidrosis Exacerbated by occlusive, synthetic footwear and rapid drying without moisturizing May worsen during cold weather and in atopic children	Frequent changing of cotton socks Emollient Topical corticosteroid or immunomodulator

SECTION 12 • EXTREMITIES

Other Diagnoses to Consider

- Allergic contact dermatitis

- Infantile acropustulosis

- Pustular psoriasis

- Cellulitis

- Pitted keratolysis

When to Consider Further Evaluation or Treatment

- Specialty referral for alternative medical or surgical approaches should be considered for painful or progressive warts, and corns or calluses that do not respond to traditional therapies such as topical salicylate.

- Severe tinea pedis may require treatment with a systemic antifungal agent if refractory to a topical approach or associated with onychomycosis.

- Severe dyshidrotic eczema or juvenile plantar dermatosis rarely may require systemic immunosuppressive therapy.

- Cellulitis due to a deep penetrating injury of the foot may require orthopedic evaluation for wound exploration if bone or joint infection or a retained foreign body is suspected.

SUGGESTED READINGS

Buescher ES. Infections associated with pediatric sport participation. *Pediatr Clin North Am.* 2002;49(4):743–751.
Freeman DB. Corns and calluses resulting from mechanical hyperkeratosis. *Am Fam Physician.* 2002;65(11):2277–2280.
Guenst BJ. Common pediatric foot dermatoses. *J Pediatr Health Care.* 1999;13(2):68–71.
Morelli JG. Principles of therapy. In: Kliegman RM, Stanton BF, Schor NF, St. Geme JW, Behrman RE, eds. *Nelson Textbook of Pediatrics.* 19th ed. Philadelphia, PA: Elsevier Saunders; 2011:2215–2218.
Omura EF, Rye B. Dermatologic disorders of the foot. *Clin Sports Med.* 1994;13(4):825–841.

GENITAL AND PERINEAL REGION

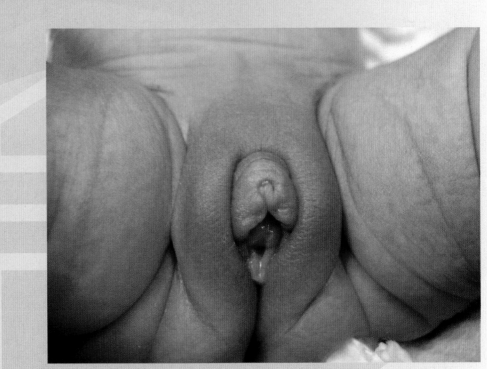

(Courtesy of Philip T. Siu, MD.)

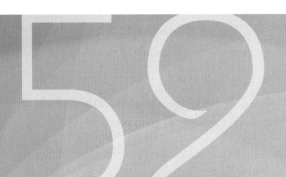

Female Genitalia—Variations

Colette C. Mull

Approach to the Problem

Variations in the physical appearance of female genitalia encompass findings within the spectrum of normal, ambiguous genitalia, and abnormalities—congenital or acquired. Although most variations represent isolated external findings, some are associated with variations in the structure and/or function of other organ systems. In the category of acquired abnormalities, it is crucial for pediatric clinicians to have a heightened sense of awareness for accidental and inflicted genital trauma, including female genital mutilation (FGM). Identifying variations in the appearance of female genitalia depends on the physical characteristics, the stage of the child's genital development, the presence of associated symptoms, ongoing parental involvement in the child's genital care, and the primary care provider's consistent inclusion of a careful genital examination at every health maintenance visit. Early detection may be imperative as with ambiguous genitalia, preferred as with imperforate hymen, or inconsequential as with normal hymenal variants. In addition, any complaints of abdominal pain, urinary symptoms, perineal/vaginal symptoms, change in bowel habits, and/or sexual maltreatment should prompt the clinician to carefully examine the perineum.

Key Points in the History

- A patient's age and Tanner stage are key to establishing whether a particular external genital finding is within the limits of normal.

- Imperforate hymen or a vaginal web may present with complaints of abdominal or lower back pain, pain with defecation, diarrhea, extremity pain, urinary retention, and nausea and vomiting.

- There may be a genetic predisposition to imperforate hymen.

- Congenital adrenal hyperplasia (CAH) occurs with higher frequency in Ashkenazi Jewish, Hispanic, Slavic, and Italian populations.

- A family history of neonatal death may represent a missed diagnosis of CAH.

- A family history of ambiguous genitalia, consanguinity, infertility, or amenorrhea suggests a genetic basis for ambiguous genitalia.

- Maternal history of certain ovarian tumors, drug ingestion, or teratogen exposure during pregnancy may contribute to the development of ambiguous genitalia.

- Labial adhesions are common and may result from vulvar exposure to irritants, including residual feces between the labia, bubble baths, harsh soaps, detergents, accidental trauma as with vigorous cleaning, or nonaccidental trauma as with child sexual abuse and FGM.

- Inquire about genital trauma with history of recurrent urinary tract infections (UTIs), chronic vaginitis, dysuria, dysmenorrhea, or adolescent dyspareunia.

- A report from an obstetrician or a birth history may reveal FGM in a patient's mother. Daughters of these mothers are at increased risk of FGM.

- Countries practicing FGM are found in Africa, Asia, and the Middle East. FGM practice continues in immigrant populations in countries including the United States.

- Subtle clues suggesting that a planned FGM may be upcoming include the following: upcoming cultural holidays, special ceremonies centered on the child, and requests for travel immunizations or prescriptions for antimalarial medications.

- Clues that FGM has recently occurred in a child include the following: genitourinary pain and bleeding, lengthy visits to the school bathroom, avoidance of physical activity (e.g., participation in physical education), and sudden change in behavior after a holiday.

Key Points in the Physical Examination

- The physiological red coloring of the prepubertal child's genital mucosa may be mistaken for child maltreatment.

- In a newborn with ambiguous genitalia, gonadal material palpable in the inguinal canal or labioscrotal folds is most commonly testicular material and rarely a herniated ovary or ovotestis in a hermaphrodite; its presence eliminates the diagnoses of Turner syndrome and pure gonadal dysgenesis.

- Varying degrees of labial adhesion typically create a fused segment, posteriorly to anteriorly.

- Imperforate hymen may be detected when yellow/white tissue as with mucohydrocolpos, or red/blue tissue, as with hematocolpos, is seen protruding from a child's vagina upon straining or crying.

- Genital trauma, accidental (e.g., motor vehicle accident), third party-inflicted (e.g., FGM), and self-inflicted (e.g., battery or cosmetic product burns) may present acutely as hemorrhagic shock, local infection, genital burns, human and animal bites, crush injuries, vulvar hematomas, or partial or complete excision of the external female genitalia.

- Consider FGM in a child or adolescent who has genital scars or perineal keloid formation, whose perineum has the classic appearance of FGM, or whose parent refuses genital examination.

PHOTOGRAPHS OF SELECTED DIAGNOSES

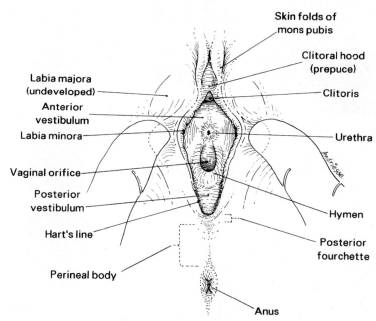

Figure 52-1 Prepubertal child genitalia. Undeveloped labia majora and other external structures are notable. (Used with permission from Emans SJ, Laufer MR, Goldstein DR, eds. *Pediatric and Adolescent Gynecology.* 5th ed. Philadelphia, PA: Lippincott Williams & Wilkins; 2005:3.)

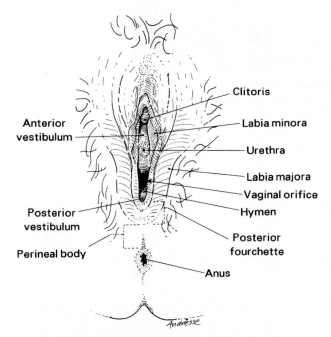

Figure 52-2 Pubertal child genitalia. Evidence of maturation of the external genitalia is prominent. (Used with permission from Emans SJ, Laufer MR, Goldstein DP, eds. *Pediatric and Adolescent Gynecology.* 5th ed. Philadelphia, PA: Lippincott Williams & Wilkins; 2005:28.)

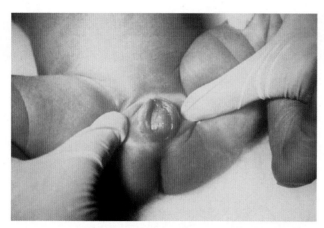

Figure 52-3 Imperforate hymen. Opening of the labia minora is not visualized. (Used with permission from Emans SJ, Laufer MR, Goldstein DP, eds. *Pediatric and Adolescent Gynecology.* 5th ed. Philadelphia, PA: Lippincott Williams & Wilkins; 2005:plate 21.)

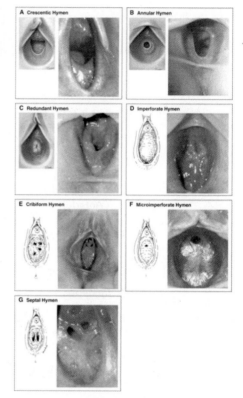

Figure 52-4 Hymen variations.
(A) Crescentic hymen. **(B)** Annular hymen. **(C)** Redundant hymen. **(D)** Imperforate hymen. **(E)** Cribriform hymen. **(F)** Microperforate hymen. **(G)** Septate hymen. (Used with permission from Dudek RW. *BRS Embryology.* 5th ed. Philadelphia, PA: Lippincott Williams & Wilkins; 2010.)

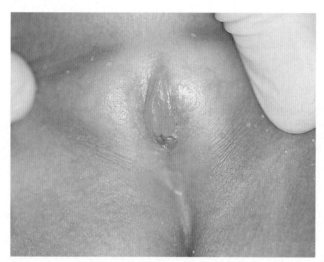

Figure 52-5 Labial adhesions. Fused labia majora in a prepubertal child. (Used with permission from Fleisher GR, Ludwig S, Baskin MN, eds. *Atlas of Pediatric Emergency Medicine.* Philadelphia, PA:Lippincott Williams & Wilkins; 2004:146.)

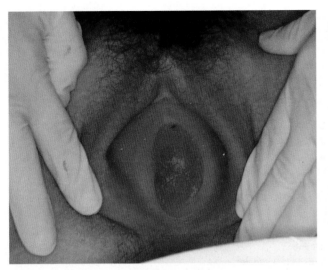

Figure 52-6 Hematocolpos. Bluish bulging membrane in a child with primary amenorrhea and lower abdominal pain. (Used with permission from Fleisher GR, Ludwig S, Baskin MN, eds. *Atlas of Pediatric Emergency Medicine.* Philadelphia, PA: Lippincott Williams & Wilkins; 2004:145.)

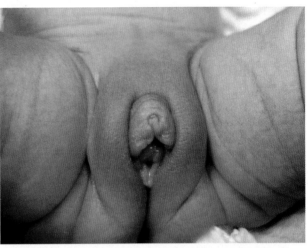

Figure 52-7 Ambiguous genitalia in a child with CAH. Note the prominent clitoris. (Courtesy of Philip Siu, MD.)

DIFFERENTIAL DIAGNOSIS

DIAGNOSIS		ICD-10	DISTINGUISHING CHARACTERISTICS	DURATION/CHRONICITY
Normal Genitalia		Newborn genitalia Z76.9	Findings are related to maternal estrogen effects: • Prominent labia majora • Thick labia minora • Pale pink and moist mucosa • Annular or redundant hymen May see variations (septate, microperforate, cribriform hymen)	Continuum between newborn and prepubertal periods
		Prepubertal genitalia Z76.9	Larger labia Labia minora exposed Crescentic or posterior rim hymen is common Mucosa pink-red, less moist Redundant or fimbriated hymen and annular hymen may be seen.	
		Pubertal genitalia Z76.9	Labia larger Hymen thick, elastic, and redundant Mucosa pale pink and moist	Puberty
Labial Adhesions		Q52.5	Pale, smooth, avascular line of fusion between labia minora	3 months to 6 years
Imperforate Hymen		Q52.3	Shiny membrane between labia Membrane yellow/white or red/blue and bulging	May present in the newborn period Less commonly detected in early infancy as hydrocolpos, mucocolpos, or hematocolpos Often detected in adolescents with menarche as hematocolpos
Ambiguous Genitalia		Q56.2 Female pseudohermaphroditism E25.0 Congenital Adrenal Hyperplasia	Variable virilization Ranges from mild clitoral gland enlargement to "male" phallus and scrotum	Diagnosed at birth
		Q56.1 Male pseudohermaphroditism E25.0 Congenital Adrenal Hyperplasia	Inadequate virilization Microphallus, variable hypospadias, chordee, bilateral cryptorchidism, female external genitalia	

ASSOCIATED FINDINGS	COMPLICATIONS	PREDISPOSING FACTORS	TREATMENT GUIDELINES
Physiological leukorrhea Pseudomenses	N/A	N/A	N/A
N/A	N/A	Onset of puberty with unopposed estrogen production	N/A
Physiological leukorrhea Onset of menses	N/A	N/A	N/A

N/A	Variable genitourinary outflow obstruction
	Urinary tract infections
		Vulvar inflammation or irritation	Typically self-limited
			When treatment requested or required for symptoms:
			   Estrogen cream to line of fusion once to twice per day for 2 weeks
			   May need longer course or larger volume of application to maintain labial separation
			   Irritant avoidance/removal
			   Meticulous perineal hygiene
			   Manual labial separation discouraged
			   Endocrinology evaluation (gender differentiation or androgen production abnormalities) required in cases of labial fusion present at 1–3 months of age or labial adhesions resistant to outlined treatment

Primary amenorrhea Lower abdominal mass Soft, tender, fluctuant mass on rectal exam Abdominal distension	Urinary retention Constipation Hydronephrosis	N/A	Surgical repair under anesthesia with membrane incision and drainage, excess tissue excision, and vaginal mucosa repair Best performed during newborn, premenarchal, and postpubertal periods, after tissue has undergone estrogen stimulation
Salt loss Salt retention/hypertension Testicular and ovarian tissue present: true hermaphroditism	Vascular collapse and death from salt-wasting nephropathy Gender mis-assignment	N/A	Immediate medical and psychosocial issue stabilization Evaluate and treat as salt-wasting form of CAH until proven otherwise Careful evaluation of patient and family by a multidisciplinary team, including specialists from pediatric endocrinology, genetics, pediatric surgery/urology, and psychology or social work Perform the following laboratory blood tests: electrolytes, adrenal steroid levels, and karyotype Obtain pelvic and abdominal ultrasound Correct hypovolemia, hypoglycemia, hyponatremia, and hyperkalemia Administer stress doses of glucocorticoids after adrenal steroid levels are obtained Provide mineralocorticoid replacement therapy Careful gender identity assignment and consideration for early genital surgery Long-term support for psychosexual issues
Salt loss Salt retention, hypertension Hypokalemia			

SECTION 13 • GENITAL AND PERINEAL REGION

Other Diagnoses to Consider

- Incomplete hymenal fenestration: microperforate, septate, and cribriform hymens

- Obstructive anomalies of the vagina

- Vulvar lichen sclerosis

- Vulvar hemangioma

- Genital trauma

- Urethral prolapse

- Rectal prolapse

- Child sexual abuse

When to Consider Further Evaluation or Treatment

- Surgery for imperforate hymen should be performed immediately in symptomatic patients and during the newborn, premenarchal, or postpubertal periods in asymptomatic patients.

- Evaluate and treat ambiguous genitalia immediately upon detection.

- Treat ambiguous genitalia as the salt-wasting form of CAH until proven otherwise.

- Gender assignment and genital surgery for ambiguous genitalia should be undertaken after careful research and deliberation by family and multidisciplinary team of specialists.

- Medical treatment of labial adhesions should be considered if patient is symptomatic, if process involves a large portion of the labia, if the urinary stream is affected, and/or if the adhesions have not resolved after puberty.

- Surgical treatment of labial adhesions should be performed only if patient is anuric, when parent/patient objects to or is noncompliant with medical treatment, and/or in cases of medical treatment failure.

- Further evaluation by endocrinology should be considered in cases of labial fusion present at 1 to 3 months of age or labial adhesions resistant to outlined treatment.

- If FGM is suspected, confirmed, or planned, the pediatric clinician should compassionately educate the parent and family on the physical and mental consequences of the procedure on the affected child. Every effort should be made to dissuade the practice of FGM.

SUGGESTED READINGS

Abu-Ghanem S, Novoa R, Kaneti J, et al. Recurrent urinary retention due to imperforate hymen after hymenotomy failure: a rare case report and review of the literature. *Urology.* 2011;78:180–182.

American Academy of Pediatrics Committee on Bioethics. Female genital mutilation. *Pediatrics.* 1998;102:153–156.

Merritt DF. Genital trauma in prepubertal girls and adolescents. *Curr Opin Obstet Gynecol.* 2011;23:307–314.

Romao RL, Salle JL, Wherrett DK. Update on the management of disorders of sex development. *Pediatr Clin North Am.* 2012;59:853–869.

Rome ES. Vulvovaginitis and other common vulvar disorders in children. *Endocr Dev.* 2012;22:72–83.

Simpson J. Female genital mutilation: the role of health professionals in prevention, assessment, and management. *BMJ.* 2012;344:e1361.

Tebruegge M, Misra I, Nerminathan V. Is the topical application of oestrogen cream an effective intervention in girls suffering from labial adhesions? *Arch Dis Child.* 2007;92:268–271.

WHO. Female genital mutilation. Fact sheet no 241, 2014. http://www.who.int/mediacentre/factsheets/fs241/en/. Accessed July 8, 2014.

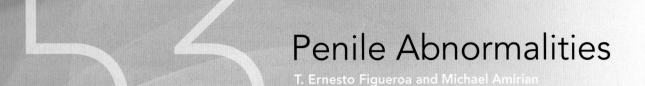

Penile Abnormalities

T. Ernesto Figueroa and Michael Amirian

Approach to the Problem

Abnormalities of the penis occur frequently. The recognition and accurate identification of these conditions are important because some of these abnormalities carry significant consequences for the patient and family. Genital anomalies are often isolated problems, although they may occur as a component of a congenital syndrome, such as Noonan, Opitz, Prader–Willi, Robinow, Beckwith–Wiedemann, or Trisomy 18 syndrome.

Evaluation for genital anomalies begins in the neonatal period with a careful examination of the genitalia. Systematically, the examination of the genitalia should assess the appearance of the prepuce (i.e., normal or incomplete), the location of the urethral meatus if visible, the size and appearance of the penis, the presence of penile chordee or torsion, the appearance of the scrotum, and the location and the size of the testes. Palpation of the scrotum or inguinal area to assess for two testes in the male and assessment of the corporal integrity of the penis are two important diagnostic maneuvers.

Key Points in the History

- Phimosis is a condition in which the prepuce cannot be retracted. It is considered a normal condition in infancy and childhood; hence, it is often referred to as "physiological phimosis." The timing for natural retraction of the prepuce varies, but most uncircumcised boys will have a retractile prepuce by 5 years of age. A "pathological phimosis" occurs when the distal portion of the prepuce is injured, either by forceful retraction or by infection, which leads to the development of a scar. The constricting cicatrix prevents retraction of the prepuce. A pathological phimosis always warrants treatment.

425

- Penile adhesions are extremely common. They are universally present in uncircumcised boys prior to natural retraction of the prepuce, and may develop secondarily in up to 60% of boys after undergoing a neonatal circumcision. The adhesions occur between the glans and the adjacent inner mucosal surface of the prepuce, and most are expected to separate naturally with time. The two physiological processes that aid in the natural separation of adhesions are penile erections and formation of smegma between the inner mucosal surface of the prepuce and the glans. Penile erections stretch the glans away from the inner prepuce, eventually promoting separation of these two surfaces. Smegma, though often mistaken as purulent drainage, is a normal physiological process of shedding of skin and oils or sebaceous substance. This cheesy material accumulates between the surfaces of the inner prepuce and adjacent glans, and cause separation of these surfaces. Most mucosal adhesions do not warrant intervention, and education of the family on the normal occurrence of these benign attachments is very important to avoid unnecessary anxiety or forceful separation.

- A hidden penis refers to a phallus that does not protrude beyond the surface of the abdominal wall. This is mainly due to subcutaneous fat displacing the penile skin away from the shaft, causing the penis to slide away from the body surface. In contrast, a concealed penis is buried by a cicatrix of the prepuce. This can occur following neonatal circumcision in males who have limited penile skin, or when an excessive amount of penile skin is removed during circumcision. If the glans recedes behind the healing preputial wound, then the scar will contract and bury the penis. In some patients, the concealed penis may be managed non-surgically by the application of topical corticosteroids; however, many of these patients will require a surgical release with revision of the circumcision.

- Hypospadias is a frequent anomaly, occurring in 1/300 live male births. Elements of hypospadias include a hooded prepuce, a ventral urethral meatus, and ventral penile skin hypoplasia that contributes to chordee, or a ventral curvature. The severity is variable, with most boys (75%) having a distal abnormality—glanular, coronal, or distal shaft. In more severe cases, profound androgenic failure may be evident, with the findings of a microphallus, bifid scrotum, and penoscrotal transposition.

- Chordee, present with or without hypospadias, is a ventral curvature of the penis. Most patients with hypospadias have chordee, partially because of the asymmetry between the normal dorsal penile skin and the hypoplastic ventral penile skin. This is referred to as cutaneous chordee. In more severe cases, as with fibrous chordee, the curvature may involve the ventral surface of the penis, including the corpus spongiosum and corpora cavernosa in addition to the cutaneous abnormality.

- Penile torsion is a lateral rotation of the penis in reference to the midline penoscrotal raphe. In approximately 5% to 10% of boys, the raphe may be directed laterally, causing the lateral rotation of the penile shaft.

- A micropenis is a phallus more than two standard deviations below the mean length for expected age. These are often visually abnormal penises, appearing small in context to the rest of the child's body habitus. The prepuce is normally formed. If the testes also are abnormally small or if other findings suggest an endocrine disorder, the patient should be evaluated by an endocrinologist. It is important to differentiate between a micropenis and a hidden penis, as the former will always require a thorough evaluation, and the latter is a common condition, which may not require intervention.

- Ambiguous genitalia refers to incomplete or abnormal genital development, preventing accurate definition of gender based on the appearance of the genitalia. Awareness of the possibility of sexual and genital ambiguity is critical to its recognition. These children may suffer from extremely variable conditions. These range from excessive androgen production in the female with congenital adrenal hyperplasia causing virilization of the genitalia to underdevelopment of the genitalia in a male with 5-alpha reductase insufficiency.

Key Points in the Physical Examination

- Phimosis refers to a conical protrusion of prepuce that cannot be retracted proximally. Contrast this with a secondary phimosis, a cicatrix in a flat distal prepuce that prevents retraction of the prepuce.

- Penile adhesions are soft attachments between inner (mucosal) prepuce and any part of the glans and will eventually separate on their own. Contrast this with skin bridging, where a band of skin becomes fused to the corona or glans following circumcision. The latter requires surgical repair.

- Paraphimosis refers to the condition in which a phimotic prepuce is retracted behind the corona of the glans. Due to the constricting effect of the phimosis, edema and swelling of the glans occur distally to the preputial orifice.

- Hidden penis refers to the appearance of a small penile shaft and excess penile skin. Retracting the prepubic fat pad usually reveals a normal-sized and circumcised penis.

- Micropenis refers to a small but normally formed penis.

- Chordee refers to abnormal ventral curvature, producing a curved penis.

- Hypospadias refers to a hooded prepuce and a ventral meatus in the area of the corona, shaft, or scrotum, accompanied by a chordee.

- Penile torsion refers to clockwise or counterclockwise rotation of the penile shaft and meatus with a laterally displaced penile raphe.

- Ambiguous genitalia refers to the appearance of phallus (penis or clitoris), bifid scrotum or labia, or ventral orifice that could represent hypospadias or a urogenital sinus.

PHOTOGRAPHS OF SELECTED DIAGNOSES

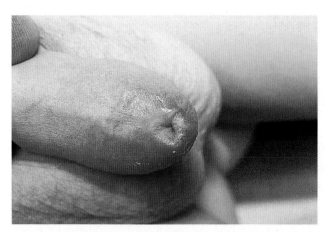

Figure 53-1 **Phimosis.** Notice the nonretractile prepuce consistent with this diagnosis. (Courtesy of T. Ernesto Figueroa, MD, FAAP, FACS.)

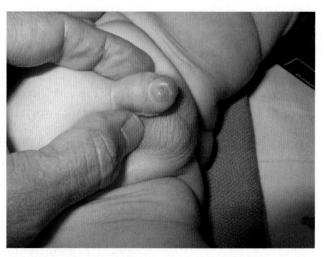

Figure 53-2 **Penile adhesion.** Whitish yellow mucosal attachments are noted between the prepuce and shaft of the penis. (Courtesy of T. Ernesto Figueroa, MD, FAAP, FACS.)

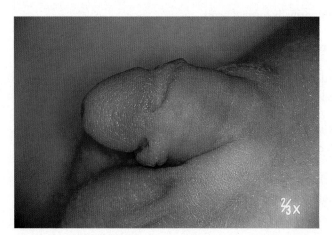

Figure 53-3 **Skin bridging.** Note the band of skin fused with the glans. (Courtesy of T. Ernesto Figueroa, MD, FAAP, FACS.)

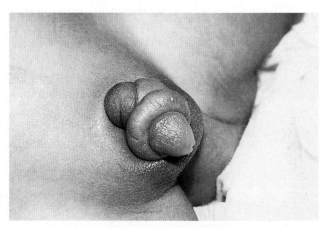

Figure 53-4 **Paraphimosis.** The glans appears edematous after becoming retracted behind the corona. (Courtesy of T. Ernesto Figueroa, MD, FAAP, FACS.)

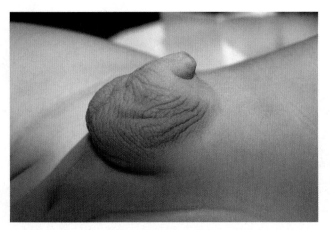

Figure 53-5 **Concealed penis.** Notice how the penis is buried by part of the prepuce. (Courtesy of T. Ernesto Figueroa, MD, FAAP, FACS.)

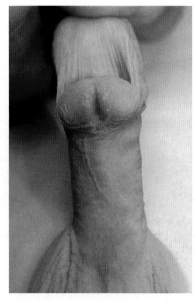

Figure 53-6 **Coronal hypospadias.** Note the ventral meatus and associated hooded prepuce. (Courtesy of T. Ernesto Figueroa, MD, FAAP, FACS.)

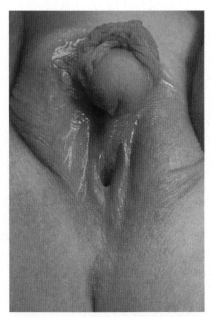

Figure 53-7 **Perineal hypospadias.** (Courtesy of T. Ernesto Figueroa, MD, FAAP, FACS.)

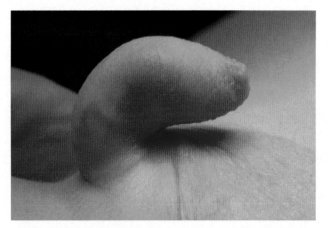

Figure 53-8 **Chordee.** A ventral curvature of the penis is evident. (Courtesy of T. Ernesto Figueroa, MD, FAAP, FACS.)

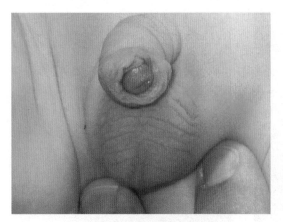

Figure 53-9 **Penile torsion.** Note the counterclockwise rotation of the penile meatus and shaft. (Courtesy of T. Ernesto Figueroa, MD, FAAP, FACS.)

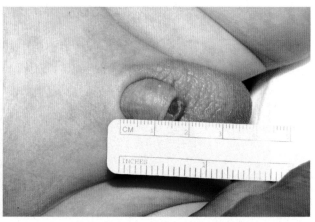

Figure 53-10 **Micropenis.** The penis measures less than 2 cm. (Courtesy of T. Ernesto Figueroa, MD, FAAP, FACS.)

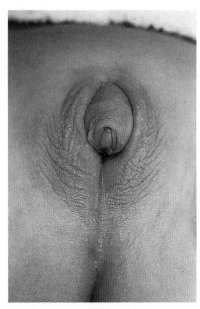

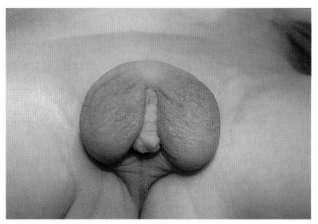

Figure 53-12 **Penoscrotal transposition.** (Courtesy of T. Ernesto Figueroa, MD, FAAP, FACS.)

Figure 53-11 **Ambiguous genitalia.** The scrotum appears to be absent. (Courtesy of T. Ernesto Figueroa, MD, FAAP, FACS.)

DIFFERENTIAL DIAGNOSIS

DIAGNOSIS		ICD-10	DISTINGUISHING CHARACTERISTICS	DISTRIBUTION	DURATION/ CHRONICITY
Phimosis		N41.7	Nonretractile prepuce	Universal at birth	Resolves by 5 years of age
Penile Adhesion		N47.5 Adhesions of prepuce and glans penis	Retractile prepuce with mucosal attachments Distinct from skin bridging	100% of newborn uncircumcised boys, Up to 60% of circumcised infants may develop secondary adhesions after the circumcision.	Resolves by 5 years of age
Paraphimosis		N47.2	Entrapment of the glans by constrictive preputial annulus causing edema of glans and prepuce	Rare	Acute event
Hidden Penis		Q55.64	Apparently small size, abundant prepubic fat Distinct from concealed penis Normal size penis	Very common in infancy	Resolves by 2–3 years of life
Hypospadias		Q54.1 hypospadias, penile	Ventral meatus, hooded prepuce, ventral penile hypoplasia	1/300 live male births	Lifelong consequences in more severe cases
Chordee		Q54.4 congenital chordee	Bent penis, or penile curvature because of abnormal skin (cutaneous chordee) Abnormal corporal bodies (fibrous chordee)	Similar to hypospadias	Correctable in most cases
Penile Torsion		Q55.63 congenital torsion of penis	Abnormal axis of meatus and lateral rotation of shaft Most are rotated counterclockwise.	5%–10% of boys	Correctable in most cases
Micropenis		Q55.62 hypoplasia of penis	Abnormally small penis, must distinguish between primary end organ or secondary hypogonadism	Rare	May be lifelong condition
Ambiguous Genitalia (Disorder of Sexual Differentiation)		Q56.4 indeterminate sex	Abnormal genitalia of uncertain gender	Uncommon	Lifelong condition

ASSOCIATED FINDINGS	COMPLICATIONS	PREDISPOSING FACTORS	TREATMENT GUIDELINES
Normal penis	Inability to retract prepuce, poor hygiene, urinary tract infection	Congenital, normal Secondary to injury to preputial annulus either by circumcision or by forceful retraction of prepuce	Reassurance Surgical correction, if secondary
Normal penis, either circumcised or uncircumcised	Tearing of adhesions Penile deviation	May occur after circumcision Common in uncircumcised males	Reassurance as they typically will resolve on their own After circumcisions parents can gently pull the skin covering the head of the penis down and apply some lubricating material like Vaseline, with diaper changes
Tight proximal preputial ring	Glanular ischemia	Tight preputial annulus, retracting the prepuce proximally without returning the prepuce to its normal position	Attempt at manual decompression of the glans and prepuce to reduce it through the tight band Severe cases may require surgery where the phimotic band is split open.
Prepubic fat pad	Skin irritation secondary to urine pooling in the area	Obesity, small penis, excessive or incomplete circumcision	Reassurance Penis size is usually normal when measured with the fat pad pressed down.
Chordee, micropenis	If meatus is stenotic, difficulty urinating Abnormal penile appearance	Abnormal production/timing of androgens in utero Genetic predisposition	Surgical repair before age 1 The infant should not be circumcised in the newborn period. Thorough examination to check for other congenital anomalies as further workup, such as a karyotype, may by warranted
Hypoplastic ventral penile surface Possible hypospadias	May interfere with quality of sexual intercourse	Abnormal corpus spongiosum	Surgical correction between 6 and 18 months of age
Abnormal symmetry of penile skin	Deviated urine stream	N/A	Surgical correction
Hypogonadism Prader–Willi syndrome—infant will also have poor feeding and hypotonia	Endocrinopathy Sexual intercourse may be difficult.	Endocrinopathy	Evaluation for a cause with treatment based on the etiology Some labs to obtain are comprehensive metabolic panel, karyotype, FSH, LH, HCG, and testosterone levels
Male pseudohermaphroditism associated with infertile aunts Congenital adrenal hyperplasia—excessive scrotal pigmentation, growth delay, hyponatremia, and hyperkalemia	Related to etiology Multiple complications, including need for surgery Psychological adjustment Infant may present in shock due to mineralocorticoid deficiency in congenital adrenal hyperplasia	Depends on underlying etiology Congenital adrenal hyperplasia—absence of enzymes needed for cholesterol synthesis 21-Alpha hydroxylase deficiency is most common. 5-Alpha reductase deficiency in male pseudohermaphroditism	Dependent on etiology Congenital adrenal hyperplasia—treat with mineralocorticoid and glucocorticoid replacement in consultation with a pediatric endocrinologist.

Other Diagnoses to Consider

- Secondary phimosis

- Concealed penis

- Penile skin bridging

- Idiopathic penile edema

- Epispadias

- Congenital buried penis

When to Consider Further Evaluation or Treatment

- A micropenis, which is defined as a penis less than 3 cm in length, should prompt endocrinologic and genetic evaluations.

- All patients with incompletely developed or ambiguous genitalia warrant a comprehensive evaluation, including genetic, endocrinologic, and urologic input.

- Features of Beckwith–Wiedemann syndrome include hypospadias, macroglossia, macrosomia, and hypoglycemia.

- Hypospadias with undescended testes warrants a genetic workup, including a karyotype.

- A boy with poor feeding, hypotonia, and micropenis raises suspicion for Prader–Willi syndrome.

- Evaluation of sex hormones and a karyotype are required prior to assigning gender in cases of ambiguous genitalia.

SUGGESTED READINGS

Figueroa TE. Congenital adrenal hyperplasia. In: Siedmon EJ, Hanno PM, Kaufman JJ, eds. *Current Urological Therapy.* 3rd ed. Philadelphia, PA: WB Saunders; 1994:2–6.

Figueroa TE, Casale P. Circumcision. In: Mattei P, ed. *Surgical Directives: Pediatric Surgery.* New York, NY: Lippincott Williams & Wilkins; 2002:709–712.

Kennedy AP, Figueroa TE. Common urological problems in the fetus and neonate. In: Spitzer A, ed. *Intensive Care of the Neonate and Fetus.* 2nd ed. Philadelphia, PA: Hanley & Belfus Press; 2003:1369–1383.

Palmer JS. Abnormalities of the external genitalia in boys. In: Walsh, ed. *Campbell's Urology.* 10th ed. Philadelphia, PA: WB Saunders; 2012:3257–3556.

Perovic S. *Atlas of Congenital Anomalies of the External Genitalia.* Yugoslavia: Refot-Arka; 1999:15–33.

Penile Swelling

T. Ernesto Figueroa and Michael Amirian

Approach to the Problem

Penile swelling is often a sudden condition which is alarming to the patient and parents, invariably prompting a visit to the emergency room or clinical office. Its presence can cause embarrassment and fear of difficulty with urination or sexual dysfunction. Pain may or may not be associated with the development of penile swelling. The penile skin and prepuce are unique tissues in their ability to stretch and tolerate trauma. The elastic and nonrigid nature of these tissues allow for interstitial fluid to accumulate readily and cause edema. The penile skin normally has a subtle, rugated appearance, and edema produces a tight and stretched appearance.

The causes of penile swelling can be determined by a thorough history and physical examination. Laboratory tests and/or radiological studies are rarely necessary to evaluate penile swelling. With careful assessment and implementation of appropriate treatment, the physician caring for a child with penile swelling can rapidly affect clinical improvement and emotional reassurance for the child and the family.

Penile swelling may be a primary (localized to the penis) or secondary (systemic) process, and it may occur in the circumcised or uncircumcised penis. If penile swelling is a secondary process, underlying causes may include renal, cardiac, hepatic, or gastrointestinal problems. Penile swelling is almost always present in anasarca, and may also occur as dependent edema in bedridden patients or patients postoperatively. On rare occasions, penile swelling may be the first sign of a systemic allergic reaction to certain medications. In these patients, the term angioedema is used to describe diffuse swelling of the loose subcutaneous tissues in addition to the dermis. This reaction can occur with or without urticaria. Lymphedema of the penis may be the first manifestation of Crohn disease. Congenital genital lymphedema is recognized in infancy by the thickened and leathery appearance of the penile skin and scrotum, particularly the prominent scrotal raphe, in the absence of erythema. This condition is secondary to abnormal lymphatic drainage and may occur with or without lower extremity involvement.

Primary causes of penile swelling, whether from infection, inflammation, or trauma, will present acutely, and tend to be more anxiety-provoking for the family. Many of the primary causes of penile swelling occur in association with edema, erythema, pain, and, in some cases, suppuration. Certain types of penile swelling, such as paraphimosis and posthitis, occur only in the uncircumcised male. The assessment of symptom duration, pain, erythema, and, importantly, the ability to urinate are the first steps in the assessment of penile swelling.

<table>
<tr>
<td>

Key Points in the History

</td>
<td>

- There may not be a clear history of trauma in infants or toddlers.

- The toilet seat can fall on the penis of the young child who is trying to hang the penis over the edge of the toilet, causing trauma to the penis.

- Traumatic penile injuries are likely to be painful causes of penile swelling. Patients may report bruising along the shaft, scrotum, and perineum.

- Traumatic injury may be associated with difficulty urinating.

- Patients may not have a known history of an insect bite, which can result in penile swelling.

- Surgery in the pelvic area may result in painless dependent edema.

- Paraphimosis and phimosis are problems related to the foreskin. Paraphimosis occurs when the foreskin is retracted behind the glans by the patient or caregiver for cleaning. Subsequent swelling of the foreskin prevents it from being returned to the normal position. This leads to further venous congestion, exacerbating the condition. Phimosis occurs when the foreskin cannot be retracted due to scarred adhesions and excessive foreskin tightness. If the phimosis is severe enough to make the foreskin opening stenotic, the foreskin may balloon during urination.

- Posthitis or balanoposthitis, infection and inflammation of the foreskin and foreskin/glans, respectively, does not occur in circumcised males.

- The presence of a prolonged, painful erection should raise the suspicion for priapism due to a vaso-occlusive crisis related to sickle cell disease. There have also been reports of priapism in boys who have accidentally ingested medication for erectile dysfunction.

</td>
</tr>
<tr>
<td>

Key Points in the Physical Examination

</td>
<td>

- Erythema usually represents a primary penile process.

- Any child with a traumatic genital injury that is not readily apparent as accidental (e.g., recent history of bicycle or playground straddle injury) may be a victim of child sexual abuse. Further examination is warranted to look for other evidence of abuse.

- A tourniquet with a constricting ring of hair or thread may be concealed in the edematous penis; therefore, it is important to do careful inspection of the penis for a transition point.

</td>
</tr>
</table>

- Dependent edema that is nonerythematous and nontender may occur after pelvic surgery, in allergic reactions, and with systemic disease processes associated with hypoalbuminemia and other conditions characterized by low oncotic pressure.

- An infection of the penis will present with swelling, erythema, and discharge or drainage. These findings may extend up the shaft to the perineum.

- A palpably distended bladder may be evident in a child with obstructive uropathy in association with penile swelling.

PHOTOGRAPHS OF SELECTED DIAGNOSES

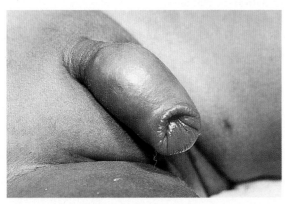

Figure 54-1 **Penile edema after reduction of paraphimosis.** (Courtesy of T. Ernesto Figueroa, MD, FAAP, FACS.)

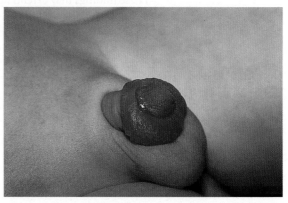

Figure 54-2 **Idiopathic penile edema.** (Courtesy of T. Ernesto Figueroa, MD, FAAP, FACS.)

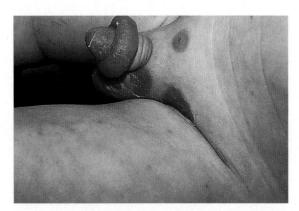

Figure 54-3 **Penile edema in association with varicella.** (Courtesy of T. Ernesto Figueroa, MD, FAAP, FACS.)

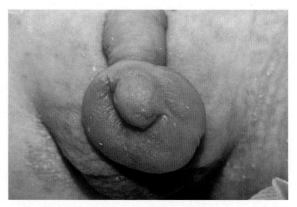

Figure 54-4 **Dependent penile edema.** (Courtesy of T. Ernesto Figueroa, MD, FAAP, FACS.)

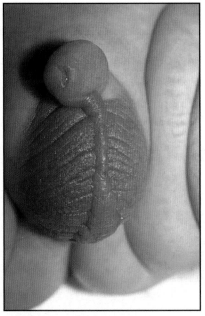

Figure 54-5 **Lymphedema in newborn.** (Courtesy of T. Ernesto Figueroa, MD, FAAP, FACS.)

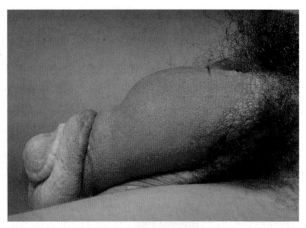

Figure 54-6 **Chronic penile lymphedema.** (Courtesy of T. Ernesto Figueroa, MD, FAAP, FACS.)

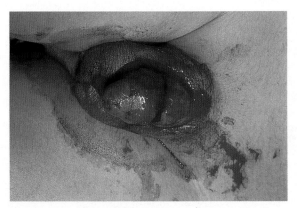

Figure 54-7 **Penile trauma.** (Courtesy of T. Ernesto Figueroa, MD, FAAP, FACS.)

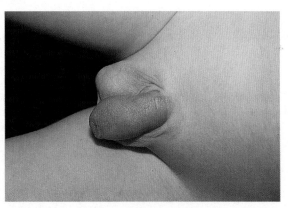

Figure 54-8 **Balanoposthitis.** (Courtesy of T. Ernesto Figueroa, MD, FAAP, FACS.)

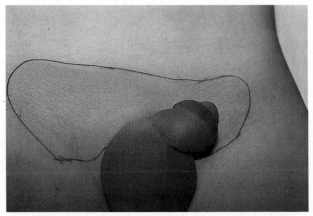

Figure 54-9 **Balanitis with cellulitis.** (Courtesy of T. Ernesto Figueroa, MD, FAAP, FACS.)

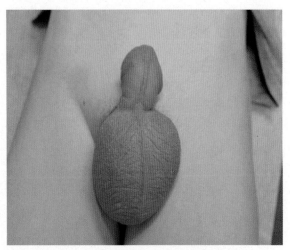

Figure 54-10 **Penile and scrotal inflammation in patient with Crohn disease.** (Courtesy of T. Ernesto Figueroa, MD, FAAP, FACS.)

SECTION 13 • GENITAL AND PERINEAL REGION

DIFFERENTIAL DIAGNOSIS

DIAGNOSIS	ICD-10	DISTINGUISHING CHARACTERISTICS	DISTRIBUTION
Penile Edema	N48.89	Diffuse edema of the penis, often painless. Erythema may be present • May occur as dependent edema • May occur as angioedema in association to allergic reactions • May be seen as a local response to penile cutaneous lesions seen with generalized rashes, such as varicella	All ages
Genital Lymphedema	N50.8	Painless, often asymmetrical swelling of penile skin and foreskin, sparing the glans Leathery and progressive May occur in isolation as genital lymphedema, as a manifestation of Milroy disease, or in association with lower trunk or extremity lymphedema. May be primary or secondary as in Crohn disease or filariasis	May be present in neonatal period, though most become evident in late childhood or adolescence
Penile Trauma	N48	History of trauma Ecchymoses Broken skin Bleeding Localized edema Bite mark	All ages
Paraphimosis	N47.2	Noncircumcised patient who develops acute swelling of prepuce and exposed glans	Young children, but can occur at any age Uncircumcised penis
Penile Infection • **Balanitis** • **Balanoposthitis** • **Posthitis** • **Fournier Gangrene**	N47.7 N48.1 N47.6 N47.8 N49.3	Inflammation of the glans and prepuce Penile edema, pain, erythema, purulent discharge from preputial space	Patients of all ages
Priapism	N48.3	Persistent, painful erection	Older children and young adults

DURATION/ CHRONICITY	ASSOCIATED FINDINGS	COMPLICATIONS	PREDISPOSING FACTORS	TREATMENT GUIDELINES
Acute condition when associated with acute inflammation Chronic as in congenital lymphedema or lymphedema praecox	Related to primary cause of edema Erythema and associated physical findings will distinguish primary inflammation from secondary causes.	Breakdown of skin Cosmetic deformity causing concern or embarrassment Secondary infections, bacterial or fungal Aggressive use of antibiotics may lead to monilial dermatitis.	Phimosis, trauma, spontaneous separation of prepuce from the glans, forceful retraction of prepuce, pelvic surgery, anasarca, or nephrotic syndrome	For acute inflammation, local care with topical antibiotics or steroids, and possibly systemic antibiotics Preventive care to minimize loss of tissue or abrasions
Chronic and in many instances progressive	Related to underlying disease Lower extremity involvement in Milroy disease Scrotal involvement: Hydrocele formation in addition to scrotal wall edema	Secondary infections, cosmetic deformity, difficulty with sexual activity	Primary lymphatic abnormality in children unless related to Crohn disease or filariasis In adults, it may be secondary to cancer, radiation, or infection of lymph nodes	Compression, prevention of secondary infections Surgical excision of abnormal lymphatic tissue and chronically indurated tissue
Acute condition	Erythema, pain, bleeding	Loss of penile skin Secondary infection Injury to urethra	Child sexual abuse Accidental injury Self-exploration	Local wound care Tetanus prophylaxis Consider referral to urology and child protective services. Keep NPO until assessed by urology.
Acute condition	Pain, difficulty with urination, progressive swelling	Difficulty with urination Secondary phimosis Loss of penile skin or glans necrosis due to vascular compromise	Forceful retraction of a phimotic prepuce causing proximal compression of distal penile shaft	Referral to emergency room or urologist for emergent reduction Keep NPO until seen by specialist
Acute condition	Erythema Pain and tenderness Phimosis Loss of penile skin	Urinary retention Secondary phimosis from scarring Progression to cellulitis Progression to Fournier gangrene	Phimosis and separation of prepuce from glans	Acute management with oral antibiotics for skin flora and topical care If purulent discharge is present, obtain bacterial culture. Suggestion of skin necrosis must raise concern for necrotizing fasciitis, a medical and surgical emergency
Acute condition	Secondary priapism: systemic symptoms if associated with sickle cell disease or leukemia Primary priapism if related to medications, trauma, or if idiopathic	Impotence Urinary retention Recurrent episodes	Sickle cell disease Leukemia Ingestion of PDE5 inhibitor (e.g., sildenafil, tadalafil, vardenafil) Perineal trauma	Consult hematology and urology.

Other Diagnoses to Consider

- Scrotal swelling (see Chapter 58: **Scrotal Swelling**)

- Nephrotic syndrome

- Lymphedema praecox

- Crohn disease

When to Consider Further Evaluation or Treatment

- Paraphimosis is painful and requires emergency treatment to prevent ischemic injury to the glans. Application of ice and gentle constant manual pressure to the foreskin to reduce the swelling may be implemented. A local anesthetic dorsal penile block may be helpful. Surgical division of the foreskin is rarely necessary to permit reduction. Circumcision may be considered on an elective basis after recurrent episodes.

- Erythema that extends proximal to the shaft of the penis into the prepubic area may be the result of a more extensive inflammatory condition requiring immediate referral to a urologist.

- Priapism warrants emergent consultation with a hematologist if the suspected etiology is sickle cell disease. If the cause of priapism is unclear, a urologist should be consulted.

- Any penile swelling accompanied by urinary retention requires emergent urologic evaluation and bladder decompression.

SUGGESTED READINGS

Harrison BP. Pediatric penile swelling. *Acad Emerg Med.* 1996;3(4):384, 387, 388.
Leslie JA, Cain MP. Pediatric urologic emergencies and urgencies. *Pediatr Clin North Am.* 2006;53:513–527.
MacDonald MF, Barthold JS, Kass EJ. Abnormalities of the penis and scrotum. In: Docimo SG, Canning D, Khoury A, eds. *The Kelalis-King-Belman Textbook of Clinical Pediatric Urology.* 5th ed. London: Informa Healthcare; 2007:1239–1270.
Synder HM. Urologic emergencies. In: Fleisher GR, Ludwig S, eds. *Textbook of Pediatric Emergency Medicine.* 6th ed. Philadelphia, PA: Williams & Wilkins; 2010:1560–1567.

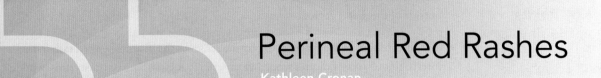

Perineal Red Rashes

Kathleen Cronan

Approach to the Problem

Rashes in the perineal (diaper) area, some of the most common skin disorders in infants and toddlers, peak at age 9 to 12 months. A variety of acute inflammatory skin reactions in the diaper area may occur. Chafing or frictional dermatitis is the most prevalent cause of diaper rash, followed in frequency by irritant contact dermatitis. Older children and adolescents with groin rashes present with lesions predominantly caused by fungal infections, such as vulvovaginitis and tinea cruris. In most cases, frequent diaper changes and the application of topical barrier agents are the mainstays of therapy. Groin rashes that indicate the presence of infection require topical antifungal or antibiotic agents. It is crucial to perform an entire body examination when evaluating rashes in the perineal area.

Key Points in the History

- A rash elsewhere on the skin suggests the possibility of seborrhea, psoriasis, or, less likely, Langerhans histiocytosis.

- A history of recent antibiotic use often precedes a *Candida albicans* diaper rash or vulvovaginitis in an adolescent female.

- Extremes of moisture or heat in the groin area may lead to contact dermatitis, candidal diaper dermatitis, or tinea cruris.

- Seborrheic, atopic, and contact dermatitis disrupt the integrity of the skin and place the patient at risk for infection with *C. albicans*.

- A family history of psoriasis may provide a clue regarding the etiology of a persistent diaper rash.

- Chafing diaper dermatitis waxes and wanes quickly.

- Persistent diarrhea may contribute to contact diaper dermatitis.

- A diaper rash that does not respond to typical treatment may indicate psoriasis or Langerhans histiocytosis.

- Genital herpes presenting in prepubertal children should warrant an investigation for child sexual abuse.

- Seborrhea, psoriasis, scarlet fever, and Langerhans histiocytosis are associated with rashes outside of the diaper region.

- The distribution of the diaper rash provides clues to the diagnosis: a red rash in the intertriginous areas indicates seborrhea, intertrigo, *C. albicans*, or tinea cruris, while a rash on the exposed convex surfaces is suggestive of contact dermatitis.

- Evaluation of the margins of the rash assists in making the diagnosis. Satellite lesions are seen with candidal dermatitis, and sharp borders are seen with tinea cruris.

- The color may help to distinguish one rash from another. Red beefy lesions indicate candidal diaper dermatitis, salmon yellow lesions suggest seborrhea, silvery scales overlying red bases indicate psoriasis, and yellow-to-reddish brown papules may suggest Langerhans histiocytosis.

- Henoch–Schönlein purpura may present with palpable purpura in the buttocks and thighs of young children.

- An ulcerative rash in the perineal area of an adolescent suggests herpes simplex virus infection.

- Pustules and bullae formation are indicative of impetigo due to *Staphylococcus* or *Streptococcus*.

- Associated perineal desquamation may be seen with scarlet fever, other streptococcal or staphylococcal toxin-mediated disease, or Kawasaki disease.

PHOTOGRAPHS OF SELECTED DIAGNOSES

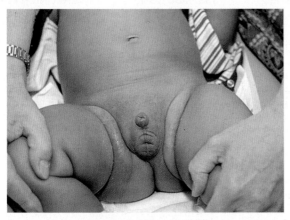

Figure 55-1 Contact dermatitis. Erythematous diaper dermatitis distributed primarily on convex surfaces with sparing of the intertriginous folds in an infant. (Courtesy of George A. Datto, III, MD.)

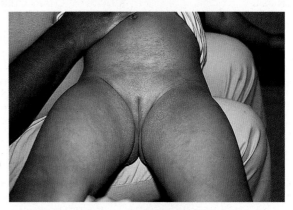

Figure 55-2 Contact dermatitis. Older child with contact dermatitis from a bathing suit. (Courtesy of George A. Datto, III, MD.)

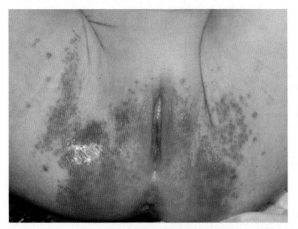

Figure 55-3 Candidal diaper dermatitis. The shiny, glazed appearance of buttocks, and the coalescing satellite papules and pustules are characteristic of candidal diaper dermatitis. This is confirmed by microscopic examination or culture. (Used with permission from Edwards L. Pediatric genital disease. In: Edwards L, Lynch PJ. *Genital Dermatology Atlas.* 2nd ed. Philadelphia, PA: Lippincott Williams & Wilkins; 2011.)

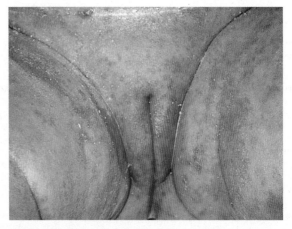

Figure 55-4 Seborrhea. Note the greasy intertriginous dermatitis with yellowish scale. (Used with permission from the Benjamin Barankin Dermatology Collection.)

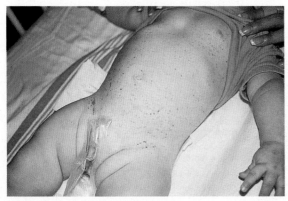

Figure 55-5 Histiocytosis. Clusters of hemorrhagic papules in groin and on abdomen. (Courtesy of George A. Datto, III, MD.)

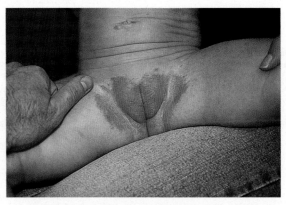

Figure 55-6 Psoriasis. Erythematous plaque with scale in diaper area; also note smaller lesions on abdomen. (Courtesy of George A. Datto, III, MD.)

DIFFERENTIAL DIAGNOSIS

DIAGNOSIS		ICD-10	DISTINGUISHING CHARACTERISTICS	DISTRIBUTION	DURATION/ CHRONICITY
Chafing Dermatitis		L22	Due to friction Mild redness and scaling Waxes and wanes quickly	Inner thighs Genitalia Buttocks Lower abdomen	Acute, but can recur often
Irritant Contact Dermatitis		L25.9	Spares intertriginous areas Located on convex surfaces Erosions occur occasionally	Buttocks Vulva Perineum Lower abdomen Upper thighs	Acute, but can recur often
Candidal Diaper Dermatitis		B37.49	Vivid beefy red color Raised edges with sharp margination White scales at the border Pinpoint satellite lesions	Buttocks Lower abdomen Inner thighs Intertriginous areas Occasionally generalized with an "id" reaction	Acute
Impetigo		L01.03	Pustules filled with exudate and bullae with straw-colored fluid	Can occur in any location, often not limited by diaper margin	Acute
Genital Herpes Simplex Virus Infection		A60.9	Vesicles and ulcerated lesions involving the skin and mucous membranes	Usually clustered around vaginal area or penis	Acute
Intertrigo		L30.4	Typical in hot weather Intense erythema in skin folds Often with white or yellow exudate	Inguinal creases Intergluteal area Thigh creases	Acute, but can recur
Seborrhea		L21.1	Salmon-colored, greasy lesions—yellowish scale	Intertriginous areas Spares convex areas	Chronic
Tinea Cruris		B35.6	Symmetrical, scaly, erythematous plaques with tiny pustules or vesicles on borders Sharply demarcated Most common in male adolescents	Intertriginous folds near the scrotum and upper inner thighs Occasionally on buttocks, perineum Spares penis Often symmetric	
Cutaneous Candidiasis (in Adolescent Female)		B37.3	Redness and swelling White patches on red bases on mucosal surfaces Cheesy exudate Itching, burning, dysuria	Labia Perineum Perianal area Gluteal folds	Acute
Langerhans Histiocytosis		C96.0	Clusters of yellow-to-reddish brown papules with purpuric qualities Hemorrhagic, seborrhea-like eruption	Groin Axilla Retroauricular areas of scalp Palms and soles	Chronic
Psoriasis		L40.0	Erythematous plaques with a scaling eruption; sharp demarcation of lesions Remissions and exacerbations typical Fails to respond to usual diaper dermatitis therapies	Girls—clitoral hood to upper gluteal cleft Boys—base of penis, inner thighs, gluteal cleft	Chronic

ASSOCIATED FINDINGS	COMPLICATIONS	PREDISPOSING FACTORS	TREATMENT GUIDELINES
N/A	None	Friction	Frequent diaper changes and careful diaper hygiene
N/A	Bacterial superinfection	Contact with proteolytic enzymes and irritant chemicals Alkaline pH Excessive heat and moisture Moderate to severe diarrhea Infrequent diaper changes	Reduce moisture Frequent diaper changes Use of absorbent gelling materials in diapers
Oral thrush	None	Systemic antibiotic therapy Warm, moist, occluded skin	Topical antifungal agent Avoid topical steroids, which are likely to make the rash worse. Oral nystatin if unresponsive to topical agents If severe, oral fluconazole
	Can progress to systemic infection in immunocompromised or in young infants	Break in skin integrity	Topical antibacterial agent If severe, oral, or parenteral antibacterial agent
	Bacterial superinfection Pain	Exposure to herpes simplex virus	Acyclovir begun in the first 72 hours may shorten duration of outbreak.
Same findings in neck folds and axillae	Candidal superinfection	Hot weather Overdressing of infant	Open wet compresses Cautious use of dusting powders
Involvement of the scalp, face, neck, postauricular areas, and flexural areas	Secondary candidal or bacterial infection	High sebaceous gland density	Low-dose topical steroids Antifungal agents or antibiotics, if superinfected
Pruritus Tinea pedis	Bacterial superinfection	Hot, humid weather Vigorous exercise Tight-fitting clothing Obesity	Topical antifungal agents for 3–4 weeks Avoid tight clothes; use loose fitting cotton underwear Weight loss Thorough drying of area
Leukorrhea Burning Painful urination Pruritus	None	Antibiotics Diabetes mellitus Pregnancy Oral contraceptives	Antifungal vaginal tablets, cream, or suppositories
Involvement of bone, liver, lungs, mucosa Premature tooth eruption Lymphadenopathy	Varies with extent of disease	Abnormal proliferation/accumulation of cells of the monocyte-macrophage system	Observation alone if restricted to skin
Dark red plaques with silvery scales on the trunk, face, scalp, axillae Nail involvement	None	Genetic predisposition	Topical corticosteroids

Other Diagnoses to Consider

- Acrodermatitis enteropathica (disorder due to zinc deficiency)

- Jacquet dermatitis

- Granuloma gluteale infantum

- Scarlet fever

- Henoch–Schönlein purpura

- Herpes simplex virus infection

When to Consider Further Evaluation or Treatment

- Diaper dermatitis is often recurrent, and recurrence does not always indicate treatment failure.

- Prior to initiating therapy, the etiology of the perineal rash must be determined.

- If secondary bacterial infection of the dermatitis is suspected, topical or systemic antibiotics are indicated.

- Genital herpes presenting in prepubertal children should warrant an investigation for child sexual abuse. If available and feasible, consider a local or regional center with expertise with these examinations.

- When a diaper rash is determined to be resistant to standard therapies, consider other diagnoses, such as psoriasis or Langerhans histiocytosis, and seek further evaluation.

- If the infant with a diaper rash is febrile and appears ill, a complete evaluation is warranted.

- Newborns with diffuse impetigo in the groin area should be given systemic (oral or parenteral) antibiotics. Evaluate for a systemic infection if the child presents with symptoms such as fever, ill appearance, or constitutional symptoms.

SUGGESTED READINGS

Centers for Disease Control and Prevention. Sexually transmitted diseases treatment guidelines. *MMWR* 2010;59(No. RR-12):1–110.
Long S, Pickering L, Prober C, eds. *Principles and Practice of Pediatric Infectious Diseases.* 4th ed. Philadelphia, PA: WB Saunders; 2012:353–363.
Nield LS, Kamat D. Prevention, diagnosis, and management of diaper dermatitis. *Clin Pediatr.* 2007;46:480–486.
Paller AS, Mancini AJ, eds. *Hurwitz Clinical Pediatric Dermatology: A Textbook of Skin Disorders of Childhood and Adolescence.* 4th ed. Philadelphia, PA: Elsevier; 2011:20–23.
Ravanfar P, Wallace JS, Pace NC. Diaper dermatitis: a review and update. *Curr Opin Pediatr.* 2012;24:472–479.
Zsolway K, Harrison A, Honig P. Diaper rash in a young infant. *Pediatr Case Rev.* 2002;2(4):220–225.

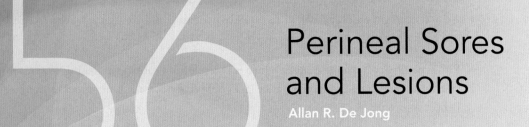

Perineal Sores and Lesions

Allan R. De Jong

Approach to the Problem

The most common cause of genital irritation and bleeding in a prepubertal girl beyond the neonatal period is vulvovaginitis, and hygiene-related problems are often implicated. Other causes of postneonatal genital bleeding include genital warts, trauma, vaginal foreign body, hemangioma, tumors, and urethral prolapse. Dermatologic conditions—psoriasis; lichen sclerosis; impetigo; and seborrheic, contact, and atopic dermatitis—commonly cause rashes, pain, itching, bleeding, and fissures in the anogenital area. The distribution of the individual lesions is important for differentiating a generalized dermatitis from localized infections, trauma, and congenital lesions. The differential diagnosis of perineal sores and lesions includes child sexual abuse, which must be addressed by an experienced clinician.

Key Points in the History

- When approaching child sexual abuse, most of the medical history, review of systems, and context and content of the child's disclosure can be obtained from adults who accompany the child without the child present. The child should be interviewed without the caretakers' presence, if necessary for medical management. Questioning should be nonleading, open-ended, and carefully documented.

- The key to diagnosis of sexual abuse is the clear history of sexual contact provided by the child, whereas the diagnosis of straddle injury is supported by a clear history of blunt genital impact particularly during a fall onto an object.

- Midline fusion defects and hemangiomas should be recognized within the first few months of life if not detected at birth.

- The history of painful oral plus genital lesions suggests herpes simplex virus infection or Behçet syndrome.

- The history of dermatologic or allergic conditions involving other body sites should be considered because the anogenital rash, itching, pain, bleeding, or lesions may be the result of the same generalized condition.

- A history of maternal, congenital, or acquired syphilis with inadequate treatment precedes the condyloma lata of secondary syphilis.

- Genital itching typically accompanies candidal dermatitis and/or vaginitis, lichen sclerosis, and genital warts.

- Pain typically accompanies trauma (which may result from rubbing or itching), lesions from viral infections (caused by herpes, varicella, Epstein–Barr, coxsackie, or influenza), and Behçet syndrome.

Key Points in the Physical Examination

- The evaluation of a child who presents with a chief complaint of sexual abuse is often done best at a local or regional sexual abuse center. Clinicians should explain the examination in advance to the child who should be reassured that examination of the genital area by a physician is all right and that it will not be painful. A gentle, deliberate manner is appropriate, and physical force should not be used.

- The most common physical findings in cases of sexual abuse are normal or nonspecific anogenital examinations. When sexual abuse injuries are found, they are typically near the posterior midline within the vaginal vestibule and involve the hymen.

- Injuries from straddle trauma are typically unilateral or asymmetrical and anterior or anterolateral in location.

- Lesions associated with bleeding include acute straddle or sexual abuse injuries, hemangiomas, lichen sclerosis, and genital warts. Unlike most of the other lesions, hemangiomas and failure of midline fusion should be completely unchanged when reexamined 2 to 4 weeks later.

- Oral ulcerations with genital ulcerations suggest herpes simplex virus infection or Behçet syndrome.

- Lesions in nongenital areas may be found in some individuals with perineal hemangiomas, genital warts, or both.

- Molluscum contagiosum does not involve mucous membranes or palms and soles, but a rash of the palms and soles may accompany condyloma lata.

- Bilateral, diffuse labial redness is usually from vulvovaginitis, but it may also accompany lichen sclerosis.

- Hemangiomas typically blanch with pressure, but most other lesions do not.

PHOTOGRAPHS OF SELECTED DIAGNOSES

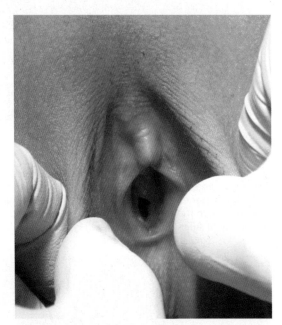

Figure 56-1 Sexual abuse, acute. Acute laceration in posterior wall of the vaginal vestibule extending to hymenal membrane found in a 7-year-old girl who reported penile vaginal penetration by an 11-year-old stepbrother occurring a few hours ago. (Courtesy of Allan R. De Jong, MD.)

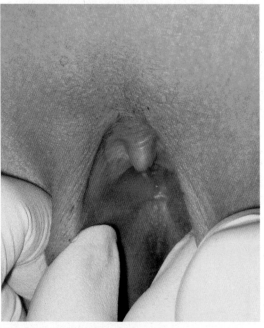

Figure 56-2 Sexual abuse, acute. Same child as in Figure 56-1 demonstrating the acute laceration. (Courtesy of Allan R. De Jong, MD.)

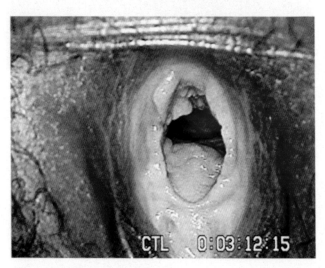

Figure 56-3 Sexual abuse, nonacute. Deep, wide posterior midline hymenal cleft extending to the vaginal wall (examined in prone knee chest position). Cleft represents healed complete hymenal tear or transection in a 15-year-old girl who disclosed multiple acts of penile vaginal penetration. (Courtesy of Allan R. De Jong, MD.)

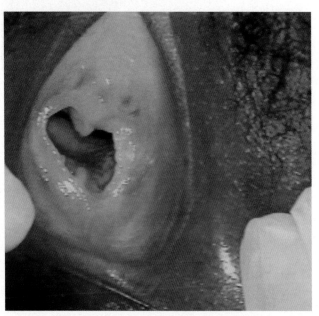

Figure 56-4 Sexual abuse, nonacute. Two deep, posterior midline hymenal clefts extending to the vaginal wall. Clefts represent healed complete hymenal tears or transections in an 11-year-old girl who described a single act of penile vaginal penetration accompanied by pain and bleeding 2 weeks previously. (Courtesy of Allan R. De Jong, MD.)

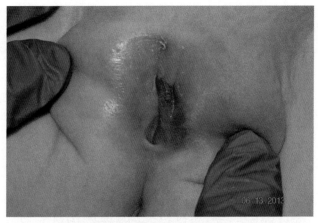

Figure 56-5 Straddle injury. Crush or blunt impact injury with typical asymmetric pattern to the left labia minora with marked swelling and labia majora with both external blue bruising and red bruising of medial surface in a 2-year-old girl who fell straddling the edge of a sandbox. (Courtesy of Allan R. De Jong, MD.)

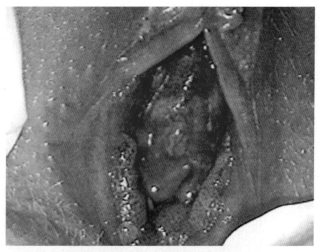

Figure 56-6 Genital warts. Multiple genital warts are seen in vaginal vestibule of 6-year-old girl who disclosed only digital penetration. Blood vessels in the irregular masses create the red stippling of the wart surface. (Courtesy of Allan R. De Jong, MD.)

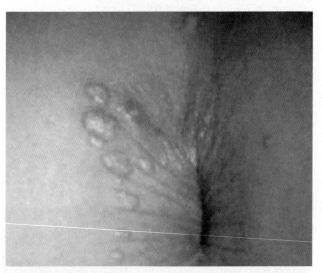

Figure 56-7 Molluscum contagiosum. Dome-shaped individual lesions and clustered lesions with shiny or pearly surface on perineum of 5-year-old girl referred for "genital warts." She had similar lesions on arms and trunk. (Courtesy of Allan R. De Jong, MD.)

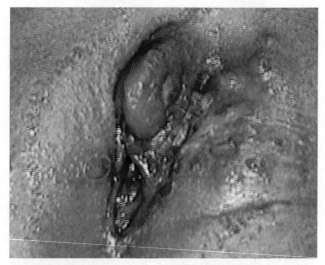

Figure 56-8 Herpes simplex virus infection. Multiple, painful, erythematous ulcerations on the labia of a 4-year-old girl who reported penile genital contact with an adult relative. Culture was positive for herpes simplex virus type II. (Courtesy of Allan R. De Jong, MD.)

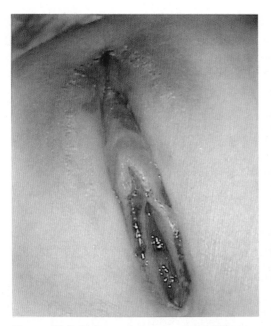

Figure 56-9 Lichen sclerosus et atrophicus. Characteristic subepidermal hemorrhages in a 4-year-old girl with a 3-week history of genital itching and intermittent dysuria. Note lesions extend over clitoral prepuce with fissuring due to friability in midline superior to clitoris. Lesions showed only slight improvement at follow-up weeks later. (Courtesy of Allan R. De Jong, MD.)

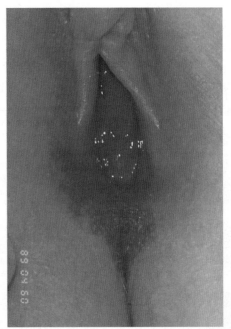

Figure 56-10 Hemangioma. Superficial, red capillary hemangioma of the posterior commissure and perineal body. Initially mistaken as an abrasion, it blanched with pressure. (Used with permission from Bays J. Conditions mistaken for child sexual abuse. In: Reece R, Ludwig S, eds. *Child Abuse: Medical Diagnosis and Management.* 2nd ed. Philadelphia, PA: Lippincott Williams & Wilkins; 2001:290.)

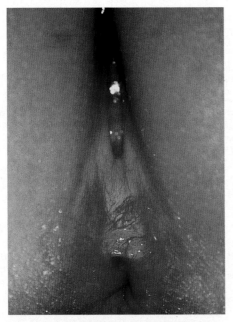

Figure 56-11 Failure of midline fusion. Midline, pale indented defect with prominent vascularity and the appearance of mucosa that was initially mistaken for trauma. (Used with permission from Bays J. Conditions mistaken for child sexual abuse. In: Reece R, Ludwig S, eds. *Child Abuse: Medical Diagnosis and Management.* 2nd ed. Philadelphia, PA: Lippincott Williams & Wilkins; 2001:292.)

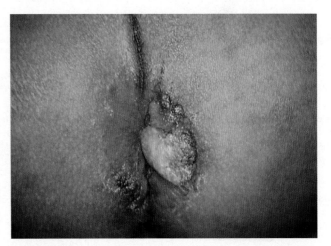

Figure 56-12 Condyloma lata. Pale hypertrophic plaque of condyloma lata in a 2-year-old girl with previously untreated primary syphilis. (Used with permission from De Jong AR, Finkel MA. Medical findings in child sexual abuse. In: Reece R, Ludwig S, eds. *Child Abuse: Medical Diagnosis and Management.* 2nd ed. Philadelphia, PA: Lippincott Williams & Wilkins; 2001:259.)

DIFFERENTIAL DIAGNOSIS

DIAGNOSIS		ICD-10	DISTINGUISHING CHARACTERISTICS	DISTRIBUTION
Sexual Abuse		T74.22XA (confirmed) T76.22XA (suspected)	Acute—laceration or bruising of hymen Nonacute—hymenal transection or healed tear (cleft) extending to the base of hymen or vaginal wall	Injuries when present typically involve posterior one-third of hymen and vestibule.
Straddle Injury		S38.002A	Asymmetrical bruising, swelling, or laceration accompanied by acute pain Has clear history of blunt impact or straddle event	Typically involves anterior two-thirds of vulva, especially the labia, periclitoral folds, or folds between labia majora and labia minora
Genital Warts		A63.0	On mucosal surfaces, flesh-colored to pink, raised lesions with red stippling On moist skin surfaces, usually multiple irregular papules, filiform, and multidigited lesions	Usually multifocal Can involve skin and mucosal surfaces
Molluscum Contagiosum		B08.1	Dome-shaped, skin-colored papules on nonerythematous base Often umbilicated with white center	Any body surface except palms and soles
Herpes Simplex Virus Infection		A60.04	Multiple vesicular and ulcerative lesions Associated with pain and erythema	Often involves both skin and mucosa May be clustered or scattered individual lesions
Lichen Sclerosus et Atrophicus		L90.4	White, wrinkled plaques with fissures producing "parchment-like" skin Subepidermal bruising or bullae and bleeding with minor trauma	Sharp demarcation from normal skin Symmetrical "figure 8" or "hour glass" depigmentation and involvement of vulva and perianal area
Hemangioma		D18.09	Reddish-to-bluish flat or elevated lesion that often blanches with pressure Appearance depends on type and size of blood vessels	Often asymmetrical Lesions, multiple or single
Failure of Midline Fusion		Q89.9	Painless indented midline lesion Pale tissue centrally at base of lesion with normal vascularity and smooth edges bordering lesion	Midline and symmetrical lesion extending posteriorly from posterior commissure
Condyloma Lata		A51.53	Large, moist, pale, hypertrophic plaques	Moist, warm areas, including labia and perianal tissues
Behçet Syndrome		M35.2	Painful, persisting ulcerations of vagina, vulva, and cervix associated with simultaneous oral ulcers	Genital area but not involving genitocrural folds or interlabial sulci

DURATION/ CHRONICITY	ASSOCIATED FINDINGS	PREDISPOSING FACTORS	TREATMENT GUIDELINES
Acute or nonacute Single episode or multiple episodes (chronic)	Sexually transmitted infections occasionally present Most victims show no specific injuries or infections.	Multiple psychosocial risk factors, such as poor parental attachment, nonbiologically related males in household, parental drug/alcohol abuse, child with unmet emotional needs, adolescent risk-taking	Acute injury treated with proper hygiene, sitz baths, topical emollient, or antibiotic ointments Reporting of suspected abuse to police and child protective service agencies is required.
Acute onset Resolving completely in days to weeks	Rarely involves injury to hymen	Activities involving boys' bicycles, monkey bars, balance beams, and falls onto other objects or being kicked in the genital area	Acute injury treated with proper hygiene, sitz baths, topical emollient, or antibiotic ointments
Variable duration, can grow very slowly and spontaneously Regress after months or years	Occasionally, warts present on hands or feet or around lips	Sexual contact Autoinoculation Perinatal transmission Vertical transmission	Consider waiting for spontaneous resolution Patient-applied therapy with topical podofilox or imiquimod can be considered.
Chronic, variable duration	Can appear inflamed or pustular when resolving	Exposure to individual infected with viral agent (5% of all children infected)	Consider waiting for spontaneous resolution Curettage, cryotherapy, or topical cantharidin, trichloroacetic acid or imiquimod can be considered.
Acute lesions resolve within 2–3 weeks. Can be recurrent	Primary infection often associated with fever and inguinal adenopathy Pain may precede rash.	Caretaker or child with oral herpes lesions (cold sores) Perinatal transmission Primary herpes gingivostomatitis Sexual contact	Oral or topical acyclovir Alternative treatment with famciclovir, or valacyclovir in adolescents and adults only
Chronic but variable course; many cases improve with puberty	Peak at 6–8 years of age Itching and burning are frequent symptoms.	Predilection for areas of mechanical or thermal skin injury	Proper perineal hygiene practices Avoid tight fitting clothing. Topical mid- to high-potency steroids
Chronic, with typically unchanging appearance	Can ulcerate and bleed or change slowly with involution Other nongenital lesions are common.	None (congenital)	No treatment required If involuting lesions become ulcerative, consider topical antibiotic ointments.
Chronic (congenital)	Mucosal appearance Often associated with anterior placement of anal opening	None (congenital)	No treatment required
Chronic	Secondary syphilis lesions, including maculopapular or papulosquamous rash, especially on palms, soles	Untreated congenital syphilis or primary syphilis	Single intramuscular dose of penicillin G benzathine (50,000 units/kg, to maximum of 2.4 million units)
Chronic, relapsing pattern	Triad of recurrent oral ulcers, genital ulcers, and eye lesions Skin lesions and positive pathergy test (induration and erythema produced at the site of a sterile needle stick)	None	Topical anesthetics Topical or intralesional steroids In severe disease, systemic treatment with immunosuppressant or immunomodulatory agents

Other Diagnoses to Consider	• Poor hygiene
	• Seborrheic, psoriatic, atopic, or contact dermatitis
	• Impetigo, streptococcal vulvovaginitis
	• Labial adhesions or agglutination
	• Ulcerations from varicella, herpes zoster, influenza, Epstein–Barr, or coxsackievirus infection
	• Stevens–Johnson syndrome
	• Crohn disease

When to Consider Further Evaluation or Treatment	• Sexual abuse requires a multidisciplinary approach. Medical care providers should initiate medical evaluation and treatment, including counseling, but suspected cases should be reported to the state child protective services agency and to local police departments for further investigation.
	• The general treatment of genital injuries, infections, and inflammation includes excellent perineal hygiene, sitz baths with warm water only, and topical lubricant ointments.
	• Avoidance of irritants including soaps, application of topical aluminum acetate solution, and several days of low-dose topical steroids are helpful for specific and nonspecific vulvovaginitis.
	• The diagnosis of genital warts, genital infections with herpes virus, and genital syphilis should result in evaluation for other sexually transmitted infections and consideration of possible sexual abuse.

SUGGESTED READINGS

Baldwin DD, Landa HM. Common problems in pediatric gynecology. *Urol Clin North Am.* 1995;22:161–176.

De Jong AR, Finkel MA. Medical findings in child sexual abuse. In: Reece R, Ludwig S, eds. *Child Abuse: Medical Diagnosis and Management.* 2nd ed. Philadelphia, PA: Lippincott Williams & Wilkins; 2001:207–286.

Emans SJH, Laufer MR, Goldstein DP, eds. *Pediatric and Adolescent Gynecology.* 5th ed. Philadelphia, PA: Lippincott-Raven Publishers; 2005:565–684, 939–975, 1024–1036.

Frasier L. Medical conditions that mimic sexual abuse. In: Kaplan R, Adams JA, Starling SP, Giardino AP, eds. *Medical Response to Child Sexual Abuse.* St. Louis, MO: STM Learning, Inc.; 2011:145–166.

Quint EH, Smith YR. Vulvar disorders in adolescent patients. *Pediatr Clin North Am.* 1999;46:593–606.

Vulvar Swelling and Masses

Allan R. De Jong

Approach to the Problem

Swelling and masses found in the female external genitalia include acquired and congenital lesions. Acquired lesions typically present with symptoms including masses, pain, urinary symptoms, and/or bleeding, but may be found as incidental findings on examination. Congenital lesions are often recognized as masses in the perinatal period, but they may go unrecognized until later childhood. The presence or absence of symptoms and the location of the mass are essential pieces of information when considering the differential diagnosis. Some benign lesions may require surgical intervention. Malignant tumors are rare in childhood.

Key Points in the History

- Neonatal onset of swelling is common in paraurethral (Skene) duct cysts, mucocolpos or hematocolpos, and inguinal hernias, but these lesions may also appear later in life. Other masses are rarely present in the neonatal period.

- Painless genital bleeding or spotting is the presenting symptom in most cases of urethral prolapse and in some cases of genital tumors.

- Labial abscesses, incarcerated or strangulated hernias, or secondarily infected cysts are accompanied by acute pain, whereas other genital masses usually are not.

- Typically, a history of urinary tract infections (UTIs), incontinence, or voiding difficulties accompanies prolapsed ureteroceles, and occasionally accompanies Gartner duct cysts and urethral prolapse. They are rarely associated with other genital masses.

- A history of intermittent swelling, particularly increasing with crying or Valsalva maneuvers, is only typical for masses caused by hernias.

- Abdominal pain, lower abdominal mass or increasing abdominal girth, and amenorrhea are common symptoms of hematocolpos or hematometrocolpos.

- A positive family history is present in 10% of children with hernias.

- Masses that originate or are present in the midline include urethral caruncle, urethral prolapse, prolapsed ureterocele, sarcoma botryoides, mucocolpos, and hematocolpos.

- Asymmetrical or nonmidline masses include most inguinal hernias; labial abscesses; and Bartholin, Gartner, and paraurethral duct cysts.

- Paraurethral duct cysts usually displace the urethral opening from the midline, whereas all other common genital masses do not.

- Urethral prolapse is the only vulvar or urogenital lesion producing a circular mass surrounding the urethral opening.

- Most urogenital masses are nontender to palpation except for labial abscesses, incarcerated or strangulated hernias, or secondarily infected cysts.

- If painful, enlarged inguinal nodes accompany the mass, the mass is either a labial abscess or a secondarily infected cyst.

- The presence of blood with the mass is most indicative of a urethral prolapse, but occasionally blood will accompany a sarcoma botryoides.

- Lower abdominal masses may accompany mucocolpos and hematocolpos because retained mucus and/or blood causes distention of the uterus.

PHOTOGRAPHS OF SELECTED DIAGNOSES

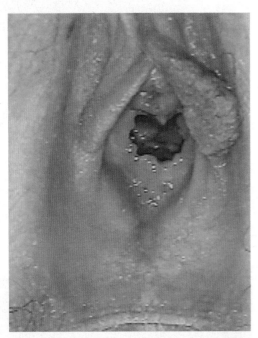

Figure 57-1 Labial hypertrophy. Unilateral hypertrophy of the left labia minor in a 14-year-old girl evaluated for sexual abuse. (Courtesy of Allan R. De Jong, MD.)

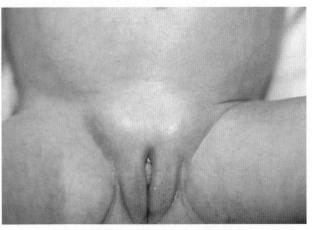

Figure 57-2 Inguinal hernia. One-month-old girl with bilateral inguinal hernias. Normal ovaries were found in the hernia sacs. (Courtesy of Allan R. De Jong, MD.)

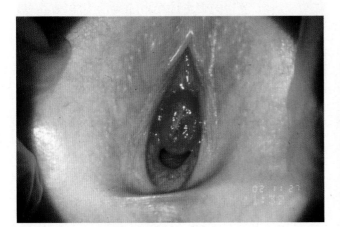

Figure 57-3 Urethral prolapse. Circular, reddish mass in the anterior midline, with the urethral opening in the center of the mass and a portion of the crescentic hymen and hymenal opening seen inferior to the mass. This 4-year-old girl presented with painless genital bleeding. (Courtesy of Tony Olsen, MD.)

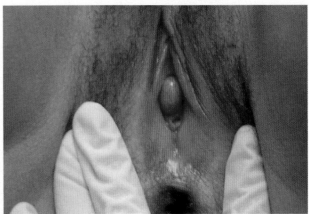

Figure 57-4 Paraurethral duct cyst. Yellowish, smooth mass in a 12-year-old with dysuria. Urethral opening is obscured, but hymenal opening is clearly visible below mass. (Courtesy of Joyce Adams, MD.)

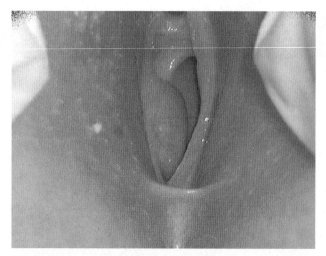

Figure 57-5 Gartner duct cyst. Cystic perihymenal mass in anterolateral wall of vaginal vestibule. Incidental finding in asymptomatic 8-year-old girl evaluated for suspected sexual abuse. (Courtesy of Jayme Coffman, MD.)

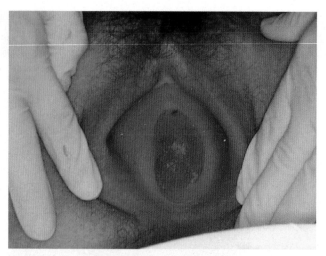

Figure 57-6 Hematocolpos. Bulging midline mass in a 14-year-old girl with imperforate hymen resulting in hematocolpos. This adolescent presented with amenorrhea and lower abdominal mass. (Used with permission from Fleisher GR, Ludwig S, Baskin MN, eds. *Atlas of Pediatric Emergency Medicine*. Philadelphia, PA: Lippincott, Williams & Wilkins; 2004:145.)

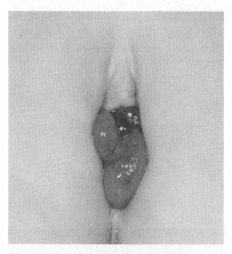

Figure 57-7 Sarcoma botryoides. Grape-like cluster of tissue protruding between the labia of a prepubertal girl. (Used with permission from Emans SJH, Laufer MR, Goldstein DP, eds. *Pediatric and Adolescent Gynecology*. 5th ed. Philadelphia, PA: Lippincott-Raven Publishers; 2005:446–447.)

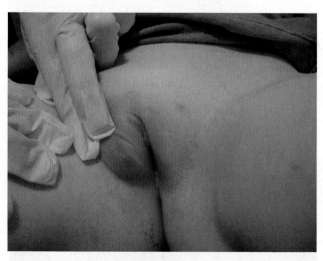

Figure 57-8 Labial abscess. Labial abscess in a 6-year-old girl with a history of poor hygiene. The mass is tender, erythematous, and accompanied by tender inguinal nodes. (Courtesy of Allan R. De Jong, MD.)

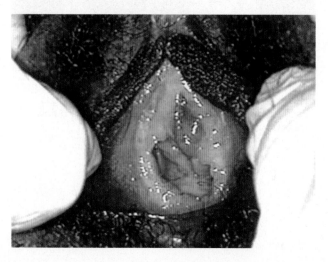

Figure 57-9 Urethral caruncle. Red polypoid mass is seen protruding from a portion of the urethral opening. Incidental finding in an asymptomatic 16-year-old girl who reported being raped 4 months earlier. (Courtesy of Allan R. De Jong, MD.)

DIFFERENTIAL DIAGNOSIS

DIAGNOSIS	ICD-10	DISTINGUISHING CHARACTERISTICS	ASSOCIATED FINDINGS	PREDISPOSING FACTORS	COMPLICATIONS	TREATMENT GUIDELINES
Labial Hypertrophy	N90.6	Painless enlargement of labia minora in adolescents Usually bilateral, about 10% unilateral	Labia minora measures more than 4 cm in span from medial to most lateral point	None known	Genital pruritus and pain	Improved hygiene, but no other recommended treatment Surgical excisions or reductions may be considered in postpubertal girls.
Inguinal Hernia	K40.91 (unilateral) K40.20 (bilateral)	Bulge or lump in mons pubis or labia majora, usually unilateral Often intermittent, increases in size with crying or Valsalva maneuver	May include ovary and/or fallopian tube in hernia Discoloration, pain with incarceration/strangulation	Family history in 10% Male:female prevalence 8:1 Bilateral hernias in girls associated with high risk of testicular feminization	Strangulation Only 2%–3% have testes (testicular feminization) and rarely ovotestes (true hermaphroditism) in sac	Surgical repair
Urethral Prolapse	N36.8	Circular, doughnut-shaped, bright red, purple-to-blue protrusion of the urethral meatus Anterior to hymenal orifice; has urethral meatus in center Usually nontender	Typically presents with painless bleeding or spotting, but may be associated with dysuria or frequency (<25%) May present with urinary retention Predominantly in prepubertal (5- to 8-year-old) black girls (<10% white)	Hereditary predisposition UTIs Increased abdominal pressure Constipation Chronic cough Trauma Lack of estrogen	Strangulated prolapse Urinary obstruction Recurrent/persistent prolapse	Topical therapy with estrogen cream for 2 weeks Surgery recommended for complications
Labial Abscess	N76.4	Acute, painful swelling with overlying redness or discoloration	Enlarged, tender, inguinal lymph nodes common	Trauma, obesity, excessive shaving, poor hygiene, diabetes, folliculitis, or infected cyst	Sepsis	Incision and drainage accompanied by antibiotics
Paraurethral Duct Cyst	N36.8	Glistening, tense, bulging, yellowish white mass Urethral meatus is usually displaced laterally.	May cause dysuria or obstruction May cause deflected urinary stream	Most often noted in neonatal period because of congenital obstruction May be result of acquired obstruction from infection	Secondary infection with abscess of cyst	No treatment for asymptomatic cases Excision, if symptomatic
Gartner Duct Cyst	Q52.4	Visible, palpable, nontender, unilateral perihymenal or perivaginal mass, in anterolateral wall of vaginal vestibule Often translucent with retained, pearly white secretions under surface	Usually asymptomatic Visible, normal vaginal and urethral openings Abnormal ureters or kidneys may be present.	Congenital Vestigial remnants of mesonephric ducts	Secondary infection with abscess of cyst	No treatment for asymptomatic cases Excision, if symptomatic
Bartholin Duct Cyst	N75.0	Visible, palpable, nontender, unilateral mass, medial to labia minora, in posterior part of vaginal vestibule (5 o'clock and 7 o'clock locations) Visible, normal vaginal and urethral openings	Often asymptomatic Infected cysts are accompanied by severe pain and increased swelling.	None with cysts Recurrent infection or abscess of cysts sometimes associated with sexually transmitted infections	Secondary infection with abscess of cyst	Surgical intervention ranging from simple drainage to excision or ablation

(continued)

DIFFERENTIAL DIAGNOSIS *(continued)*

DIAGNOSIS	ICD-10	DISTINGUISHING CHARACTERISTICS	ASSOCIATED FINDINGS	PREDISPOSING FACTORS	COMPLICATIONS	TREATMENT GUIDELINES
Prolapsed Ureterocele	Q62.31	Soft, smooth cystic mass with whitish glistening surface protruding from urethral meatus Commonly present in infancy or early childhood as UTI	No evidence of bleeding Incontinence, voiding dysfunction common May have bladder outlet obstruction	Mostly associated with abnormal insertion of the ureter, duplicating collection system, and obstructed upper pole	Urinary obstruction, UTI, urosepsis 90% of cases have renal pole duplication	Surgical intervention varies depending on severity of clinical situation, size of ureterocele, and associated abnormalities
Hematocolpos	N89.7	Present in neonates as mucocolpos or hydrocolpos with shiny, early grey-to-blue midline mass with hymen stretched over it Present in adolescence as bulging blue-to-red midline mass covered by hymen	Urethra is superior to mass and hymenal opening is absent. Can present as abdominal pain, lower abdominal mass, or amenorrhea	Results from imperforated hymen, transverse hymenal septum, or atretic vagina	Often associated with imperforate hymen, but occasionally associated with more significant genital tract malformations	Surgical incision of imperforate hymen in prepubertal girls or excision of portion of hymen in pubertal girls
Sarcoma Botryoides	C49.5	Lobulated mass protruding or prolapsing through hymenal opening Moist, grape-like clusters	May present as spotting of blood or vaginal discharge A type of rhabdomyosarcoma	Peak incidence <2 years, 90% before 5 years of age	Rare spread of tumor beyond vagina	Surgical excision of mass plus chemotherapy
Urethral Caruncle	N36.2	Thin, reddish polypoid mass or membrane protruding from a portion of urethral opening Usually asymptomatic	Occasionally associated with dysuria, frequency, urgency, or recurrent UTI	Cause unknown	None	Surgical excision or electrocoagulation

Other Diagnoses to Consider

- Labial hematoma

- Lipoma

- Lymphangioma

- Henoch–Schönlein purpura

- Urethral polyps

- Hymenal cysts

- Epithelial inclusion cysts

When to Consider Further Evaluation or Treatment

- Surgical evaluation and intervention are generally not required for labial hypertrophy, urethral prolapse, and asymptomatic cysts.

- Surgical evaluation and intervention are indicated for inguinal hernias, labial abscesses, symptomatic cysts, prolapsed ureteroceles, hematocolpos, sarcoma botryoides, and urethral caruncles.

- Bilateral exploration is recommended up to the age of 5 years for girls with inguinal hernias because bilateral hernias are more common in females than in males.

- Evaluation for commonly associated renal and ureteral malformations is needed for all cases of prolapsed ureterocele.

- Primary therapy for urethral prolapse is sitz baths plus topical therapy with estrogen cream two to three times a day for 2 weeks. Some authors recommend supplementing topical estrogen with topical antibiotics and/or corticosteroids. Surgery is recommended for strangulated prolapse, urinary obstruction, or recurrent/persistent prolapse.

- Labial abscesses and infected cysts require antibiotics and surgical intervention. Antibiotic choice should include coverage for Group B streptococcus, enterococcus, *Escherichia coli*, Proteus species, and *Staphylococcus aureus* including methicillin-resistant *S. aureus*.

SUGGESTED READINGS

Baldwin DD, Landa HM. Common problems in pediatric gynecology. *Urol Clin North Am.* 1995;22:161–176.
Eilber KS, Raz S. Benign cystic lesions of the vagina: a literature review. *J Urol.* 2003;170:717–722.
Emans SJH, Laufer MR, Goldstein DP, eds. *Pediatric and Adolescent Gynecology.* 5th ed. Philadelphia, PA: Lippincott-Raven Publishers; 2005:446–447.
Fleisher GR, Ludwig S, Baskin MN, eds. *Atlas of Pediatric Emergency Medicine.* Philadelphia, PA: Lippincott, Williams & Wilkins; 2004:145.
Kellogg ND, Frasier L. Conditions mistaken for child sexual abuse. In: Reece RM, Christian CW, eds. *Child Abuse: Medical Diagnosis and Management.* 3rd ed. Evanston, IL: American Academy of Pediatrics; 2009:389–425.
Yerkes EB. Urologic issues in the pediatric and adolescent gynecology patient. *Obstet Gynecol Clin N Am.* 2009;36:69–84.

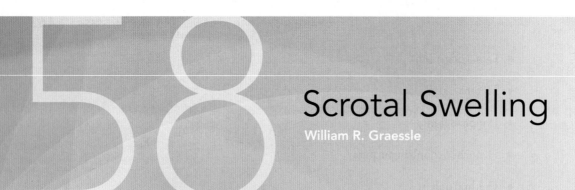

Scrotal Swelling

William R. Graessle

Approach to the Problem

Common causes of scrotal swelling vary by age. Inguinal hernia is a common cause of scrotal swelling at any age. Spermatocele, varicocele, and primary testicular tumors are seen predominantly during adolescence. An acute scrotum may be caused by epididymitis, testicular torsion, or torsion of the testicular appendage (appendix testis torsion). At any age, generalized edema or edema in reaction to local trauma or inflammation may cause scrotal swelling that can be quite significant. To prevent ischemic damage and the need for the removal of the testicle, rapid diagnosis and intervention are essential when testicular torsion is suspected.

Key Points in the History

- A swelling present since birth suggests a hydrocele or hydrocele of the spermatic cord, while the acute onset of scrotal swelling is more suggestive of a reactive hydrocele, testicular torsion, or epididymitis.

- Fluctuation in the swelling size with physical activity or Valsalva maneuvers may be seen with a communicating hydrocele or inguinal hernia.

- A history of sexual activity, urethral discharge, or both may be present in patients with epididymitis.

- Pain, especially acute, raises the concern for testicular torsion.

- A history of nausea, vomiting, or abdominal distension in a patient with a suspected inguinal hernia suggests incarceration.

- Recurrent epididymitis may be seen in patients with dysfunctional voiding.

Key Points in the Physical Examination

- The scrotum of an adolescent male should be examined in the standing position. Varicoceles may be missed when the patient is recumbent.

- Use of a Valsalva maneuver may aid in the detection of hernias, communicating hydroceles and varicoceles.

- Scrotal swelling with fullness at the inguinal ring is consistent with an inguinal hernia or hydrocele of the spermatic cord.

- A smooth mass that transilluminates when a light source is applied directly to the scrotum suggests a hydrocele.

- In testicular torsion, the affected testis may appear to sit higher than the contralateral testes.

- Redness limited to the upper pole of the testis is consistent with torsion of the appendix testis.

- The testicular surface should be smooth; an irregular surface should raise suspicion for a testicular tumor.

- The presence of tenderness, firmness, or discoloration suggests incarceration or strangulation of an inguinal hernia.

- The reduction of an apparent hydrocele is consistent with a communicating hydrocele or an inguinal hernia.

- Edema affecting both sides of the scrotum may occur in patients with generalized edema—for example, in patients with hypoalbuminemia—and in patients with local trauma, including blunt trauma to the perineal area or severe perineal dermatitis.

PHOTOGRAPHS OF SELECTED DIAGNOSES

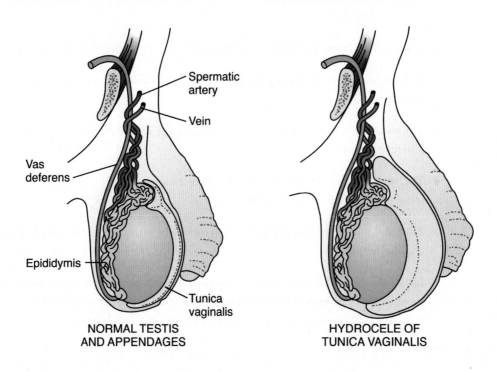

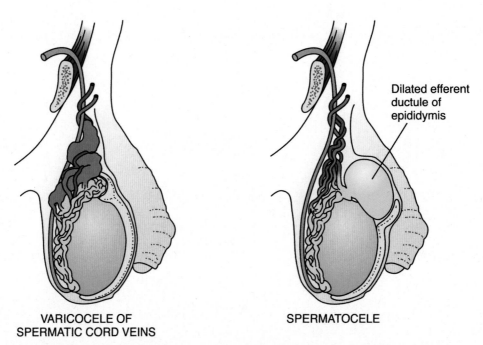

Figure 58-1 **Schematic of a hydrocele, varicocele, and spermatocele.** (Image from Rubin E, Farber JL. *Pathology*. 3rd ed. Philadelphia, PA: Lippincott Williams & Wilkins; 1999.)

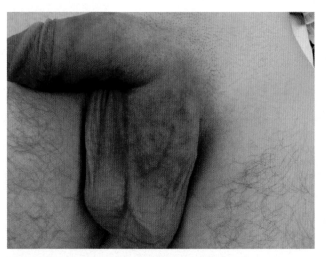

Figure 58-2 Varicocele with "bag of worms" appearance above the testicle. (Courtesy of T. Ernesto Figueroa, MD, FAAP, FACS.)

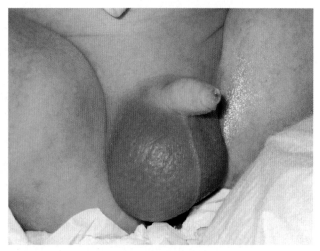

Figure 58-3 Infant with a hydrocele. (Courtesy of T. Ernesto Figueroa, MD, FAAP, FACS.)

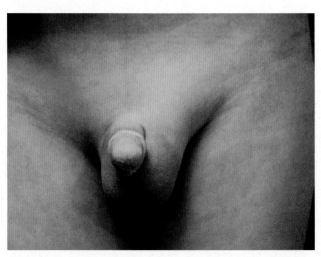

Figure 58-4 Inguinal hernia. Note the fullness near the inguinal ring. (Courtesy of Philip Siu, MD.)

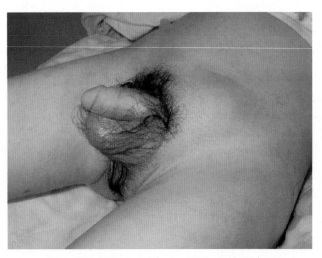

Figure 58-5 Adolescent with testicular torsion. (Courtesy of T. Ernesto Figueroa, MD, FAAP, FACS.)

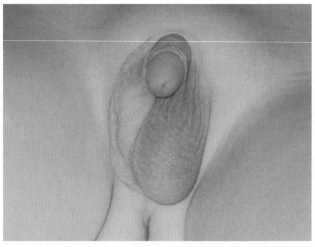

Figure 58-6 Torsion of the appendix testis with reactive hydrocele. (Courtesy of T. Ernesto Figueroa, MD, FAAP, FACS.)

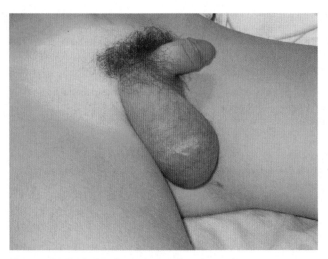

Figure 58-7 Testicular tumor. (Courtesy of T. Ernesto Figueroa, MD, FAAP, FACS.)

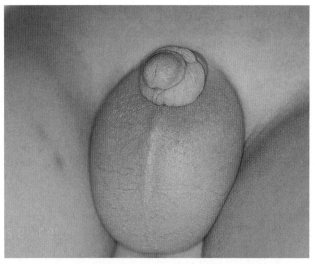

Figure 58-8 Scrotal swelling in a 7-year-old boy with nephrotic syndrome. (Used with permission from Fleisher GR, Ludwig S, Baskin MN. *Atlas of Pediatric Emergency Medicine*. Philadelphia, PA: Lippincott Williams & Wilkins; 2004:304.)

DIFFERENTIAL DIAGNOSIS

DIAGNOSIS		ICD-10	DISTINGUISHING CHARACTERISTICS	AGE
Varicocele		I86.1	Swelling in upper part of scrotum Feels like a "bag of worms" Usually left-sided	10%–15% of postpubertal boys
Hydrocele		P83.5 N43.3	Swelling around testicle Normal cord palpated above the mass Fluctuation of the fluid around the testis is consistent with a communicating hydrocele.	Common in newborns Seen in 5%, two-thirds are bilateral.
Hydrocele of the Spermatic Cord		N43.2	Inguinal fluid mass not in communication with peritoneum or scrotum	Infancy
Hernia Inguinal		K40 Bilateral hernia K40.2	Reducible swelling in inguinal area	Any
Testicular Torsion		N44.0	Enlarged testicle Painful Does not transilluminate	Peak in adolescence with a smaller peak in the neonatal period Can occur at any age
Appendix Testis Torsion		N44.03	Infarcted appendage may be palpated or visible (blue dot sign) at the upper pole of testis	Most commonly at the onset of puberty
Epididymitis		N45.1	Enlargement and tenderness of epididymis. Scrotum may be painful and swollen Testis should be normal.	Adolescents Younger children with urinary tract abnormalities Older children with voiding dysfunction
Spermatocele		N43.40	Nontender cystic swelling separate from the testis	After onset of puberty
Meconium Sequestration		R22.9 (mass, scrotum)	Firm, nodular scrotal mass	Infants and young children
Testicular Cancer		D40.10	Painless mass	More commonly adolescent or young adult

ASSOCIATED FINDINGS	PREDISPOSING FACTORS	TREATMENT GUIDELINES
More pronounced with standing	Acute varicocele may be caused by intra-abdominal venous obstruction.	Treatment is controversial. Referral to urologist to discuss treatment options
Transilluminates If reducible, hernia should be suspected	Congenital May be found in reaction to a torsion of an appendix testis.	Communicating hydroceles and those that fail to resolve spontaneously require surgical intervention.
Often associated with hernia and scrotal hydrocele	Congenital	Referral to urologist for elective surgical repair
Inguinal swelling may be accompanied by scrotal mass. Swelling may be fixed when incarcerated.	Increased intra-abdominal pressure. Ventriculoperitoneal shunt or dialysis catheter: The extra fluid may make an underlying hernia apparent.	Incarcerated hernias require emergent evaluation by a urologist or pediatric surgeon. Reducible hernias should be referred for elective correction.
High-riding testicle Nodular cord swelling superior to testis	Some males predisposed because of a high insertion of tunica vaginalis on cord Lack of posterior anchoring of the testis allows free rotation on the spermatic cord (bell clapper deformity).	Emergent ultrasound imaging and surgical intervention Referral to urology or pediatric surgery
Reactive hydrocele may make differentiation from testicular torsion difficult without imaging.	Cause unknown	Evaluation by urologist or pediatric surgeon if testicular torsion suspected Ultrasound to rule out testicular torsion
Urethral discharge may be present. Pyuria and bacteriuria	Commonly idiopathic Hematogenous spread of viral disease Sexually transmitted diseases	Antibiotics to cover *Chlamydia trachomatis* and *Neisseria gonorrhoeae*
Transilluminates	N/A	Surgical intervention if painful or progressive enlargement Evaluation by urology or pediatric surgery
Usually calcifications on ultrasound	History of meconium peritonitis may be present.	No treatment
Secondary hydrocele may be present. Abdominal mass, prominent inguinal lymph nodes	N/A	Referral to urology and oncology

SECTION 13 • GENITAL AND PERINEAL REGION

Other Diagnoses to Consider

- Henoch–Schönlein purpura

- Leukemic infiltration

- Intraperitoneal hemorrhage

- Inguinal lymphadenopathy

- Generalized edema

When to Consider Further Evaluation or Treatment

- Acute scrotal swelling that suggests the possibility of testicular torsion requires emergent evaluation by a urologist or general surgeon.

- Newborns with a noncommunicating hydrocele can be observed for resolution.

- During the examination of a suspected hydrocele, fluctuation of the volume of fluid suggests a communicating hydrocele or hernia. Communicating hydroceles and hernias should be referred for surgical evaluation and treatment.

- If a hernia is incarcerated or strangulated, the patient should be referred for emergent surgical evaluation.

- Treatment of varicoceles in adolescents is controversial. Patients should be referred to a urologist or pediatric surgeon to discuss treatment options.

- A suspected tumor of the testis requires further evaluation and referral to a urologist. Ultrasound will localize the tumor and may be helpful in differentiating benign tumors from malignant tumors. Tumor markers (e.g., hCG and AFP) may also be helpful.

SUGGESTED READINGS

Fleisher GR, Ludwig S, Baskin MN. *Atlas of Pediatric Emergency Medicine.* Philadelphia, PA: Lippincott Williams & Wilkins; 2004:304.
Leslie JA, Cain MP. Pediatric urologic emergencies and urgencies. *Pediatr Clin North Am.* 2006;53:513–527.
Merrian LS, Herrel L, Kirsch AJ. Inguinal and genital anomalies. *Pediatr Clin North Am.* 2012;59:769–781.
Serefoglu EC, Saitz TR, La Nasa JA, et al. Adolescent varicocele management controversies. *Andrology.* 2013;1:109–115.
Sheldon CA. The pediatric genitourinary examination. *Pediatr Clin North Am.* 2001;48:1339–1380.
Wan J, Bloom DA. Genitourinary problems in adolescent males. *Adolesc Med.* 2003;14:717–731.

PERIANAL AREA AND BUTTOCKS

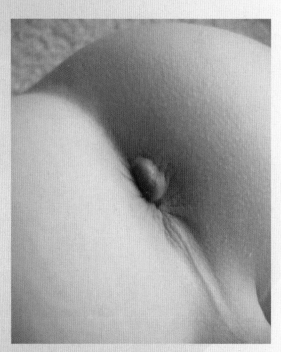

(Courtesy of Michael J. Wilsey, Jr, MD, FAAP.)

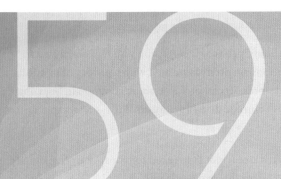

Perianal Swelling

David J. Breland

Approach to the Problem

Clinicians who care for pediatric and adolescent patients know that the complaint of perianal swelling is common, and it encompasses a broad spectrum of pathologic processes. Most perianal conditions are benign and are managed by topical treatments. Sometimes, however, perianal swelling can be associated with systemic illness, such as inflammatory bowel disease. Perianal conditions may present with masses, rectal pain, bleeding, and/or itching, all of which can make the exact diagnosis challenging. Reviewing the patient's history and bowel habits, making note of associated symptoms, and performing a physical examination of the relevant anatomy can often lead to the proper diagnosis and treatment.

Key Points in the History

- Perianal abscesses are one of the most common pediatric disorders of the perineum.

- Abscesses are often classified according to their location in relation to the levator ani and external anal sphincter. The perianal site is the most common.

- Perianal abscesses often arise from the crypts located at the dentate line.

- An early sign of an abscess is an indurated and tender area at the perineum. Oftentimes an infant's constant crying or irritability that is worse with diaper changes is the presenting symptom. Erythema can be present, but is not universal. A digital rectal examination can identify the abscess in most patients.

- A pilonidal abscess is an inflammation in the sacrococcygeal region, is often midline, and is sometimes associated with a draining sinus tract. The abscess may begin at the site of an ingrown hair follicle, located 1 to 2 inches above the anus.

- Rupture of an abscess can lead to the formation of a fistula with persistent drainage. With an abscess or fistula, clinicians should consider associated disease, particularly in older children and adolescents.

- Fifteen percent of patients with Crohn disease will present with perianal abscesses or fistulas. In addition, other systemic conditions such as diabetes, chronic granulomatous disease, neutropenia, leukemia, HIV, as well as immunosuppressive therapy may initially present with a perianal abscess.

- Most cases of rectal prolapse, hemorrhoids, perianal fissures, and skin tags are caused by functional constipation. These conditions are often associated with a history of painful defecation associated with large, hard stools. Rectal prolapse, more common in boys, may also be associated with the diagnoses of chronic diarrhea, intestinal parasites, cystic fibrosis, and malnutrition.

- Patients with a history of blood-streaked stool, blood-streaked toilet paper, or frank blood in the toilet, may have a perianal fissure and/or internal hemorrhoids.

- Hemorrhoids are varices of the perirectal venous plexus. Small asymptomatic hemorrhoids are more common in children. Symptomatic hemorrhoids are not very common in the pediatric age group; however, when present, they can cause bleeding, prolapse, discomfort/pain, fecal soiling, and pruritus.

- External hemorrhoids involve the skin of the anus, and the innervation is associated with the skin. Acute pain and bleeding sometimes occurs when external hemorrhoids are infected.

- Internal hemorrhoids are located under the rectal mucosa and can be associated with hematochezia. When present, internal hemorrhoids may be associated with portal hypertension.

- A thrombosed external hemorrhoid may cause a throbbing, burning pain at the end of defecation, and is often associated with a new bulge or swelling in the anal region.

- Skin tags are often asymptomatic and may be a remnant of a healed fissure (sentinel skin tag), or a previous thrombosed external hemorrhoid. They can also be associated with chronic itching, or problems with hygiene.

- Chronic fissures with large skin tags should raise concern for a possible diagnosis of Crohn disease.

- Human papillomavirus (HPV) causes anogenital warts that are called condyloma acuminata. Most infections are subclinical and the most common manifestations are benign skin lesions. However, the presence of genital warts should raise concern for sexual abuse in children, and HIV infection in adolescent males who have sex with men.

- Anogenital warts can be passed transplacentally, vertically through the birth canal, or via autoinoculation from an HPV lesion on the hands.

Key Points in the Physical Examination

- A perianal abscess is a localized, indurated, tender area visualized at any site around the anal verge. If not visualized, digital examination may reveal an indurated and tender mass.

- Other perianal abscess locations, such as the ischioanal area, may reveal a large, visible fluctuant and tender mass on the buttocks, or a completely normal examination.

- Pilonidal abscess often occurs at the site of an ingrown hair follicle and presents as a boil at the sacral midline 1 to 2 cm above the anus. Often there are accompanying draining sinus tracts or fistulas.

- Patients suspected of having an anal fissure should be placed in a lateral decubitus position for the physical examination. Anal fissures are a superficial split in the skin around the anus, with sharply demarcated edges. More commonly, anal fissures are in the midposterior position, with some occurring in the midanterior position. Fissures located in other positions should raise concerns for inflammatory bowel disease, occult abscesses and infections (e.g., herpes simplex virus or syphilis). Chronic fissures are indurated and are often associated with a sentinel skin tag.

- Rectal prolapse is an abnormal protrusion of one or more mucosal layers of the rectum through the anal opening. Complete rectal prolapse (procidentia) is the most common presentation, and has the appearance of concentric rings of rectal mucosa herniating through the anus.

- External hemorrhoids can be flesh colored, erythematous or bluish (if thrombosed) masses, and are located at the anal opening. Thrombosed hemorrhoids are often firm and painful.

PHOTOGRAPHS OF SELECTED DIAGNOSES

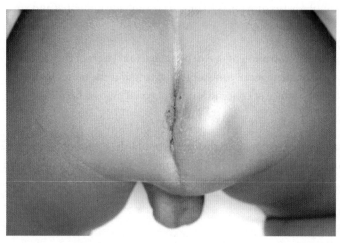

Figure 59-1 Perianal abscess. A 12-month-old male infant presenting with a perirectal mass. (Courtesy of Mark A. Ward, MD.)

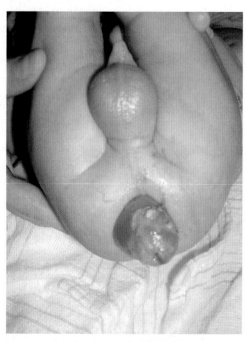

Figure 59-2 Rectal prolapse seen in a male infant. (Courtesy of Mary L. Brandt, MD.)

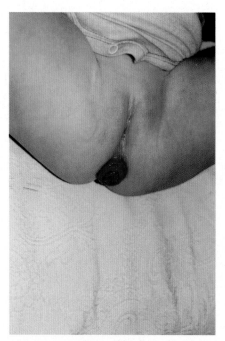

Figure 59-3 Rectal prolapse. Concentric rings of rectal mucosa (all the layers of the rectum) are seen herniating through the anus, indicating a complete prolapse. (Courtesy of Fernando L. Heinen, MD.)

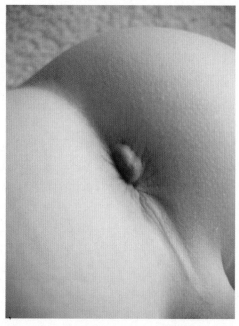

Figure 59-4 External hemorrhoid in a 2-year-old boy with recurrent straining because of chronic constipation. (Courtesy of Michael J. Wilsey, Jr, MD, FAAP.)

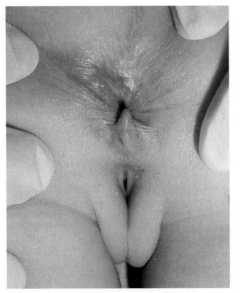

Figure 59-5 **Perianal skin tag.** A "sentinel" perianal skin tag seen in a female infant. (Courtesy of Mary L. Brandt, MD.)

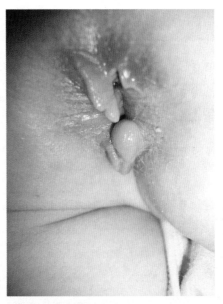

Figure 59-6 **Perianal Crohn disease in a child with multiple large, edematous skin tags and a perianal fissure at the 7 o'clock position.** (Courtesy of Martin Fried, MD.)

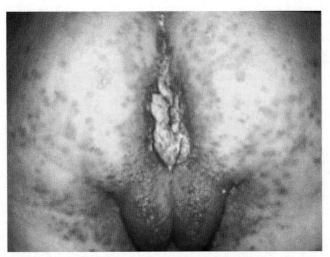

Figure 59-7 **Perianal condylomata seen following sexual abuse.** (Courtesy of Fernando L. Heinen, MD.)

DIFFERENTIAL DIAGNOSIS

DIAGNOSIS		ICD10	DISTINGUISHING CHARACTERISTIC	DISTRIBUTION	DURATION CHRONICITY
Perianal Abscess		K61.0	Tender, fluctuant mass near anus may be palpated on digital examination If abscess ruptures, fistula may develop Pilonidal abscess is midline	Perianal (most common) Ischiorectal Intersphincteric Supralevator	Present until it ruptures spontaneously or is surgically drained
Rectal Prolapse		K62.3	Painless, bright red rectal tissue herniating from anus In mucosal prolapse, radial folds are seen at junction with anal skin In complete prolapse, circular folds are seen at junction with anal skin Occurs most commonly under 4 years old	Anal herniation of rectal mucosa	May become chronic, occurring with most bowel movements (weeks to months)
Hemorrhoid		I84.5	Firm bulge at anal verge May have bluish discoloration Usually asymptomatic External hemorrhoid may be painful when thrombosed	External (below dentate line), most common Internal (above the dentate line), rare in pediatrics	Acute pain that lasts hours to 1–2 weeks (until spontaneously or surgically drained)
Perianal Skin Tag		I84.6	Painless, flesh-colored or hyperpigmented, pedunculated skin or flesh Painful when associated with an anal fissure	Anal verge Sentinel tag forms above Chronic anal fissure	Chronic
Anogenital Warts		A63.0	Types: • Condyloma acuminatum-cauliflower-like lesions • Flat, macular • Papular • Keratotic-thick, crusty, usually multiple	May be found as a discrete lesion or may coalesce to form plaques	N/A

ASSOCIATED FINDINGS	COMPLICATIONS	PREDISPOSING FACTORS	TREATMENT GUIDELINES
Fever (low grade) Perianal pruritus Tenesmus Pain worse with defecation or changing diaper Pelvic pain Mucopurulent discharge	Fistula formation Recurrence Stricture Incontinence	Infancy More common in immunocompromised patients Patients with diabetes	Infants <12 months can do conservative management (local hygiene, Sitz baths, and systemic antibiotics) Pediatric surgery referral for incision, drainage, debridement and systemic antibiotics Sitz baths, stool softeners, and dietary fiber
Usually spontaneously reduced Pruritus Bleeding Tenesmus	Edema and necrosis of prolapsed tissue Fecal incontinence	Constipation (strained defecation) Acute or chronic diarrhea Chronic lung disease Cystic fibrosis Pelvic floor weakness due to myelomeningocele, postanal surgery or Ehlers–Danlos Parasitic infestation, especially trichuriasis (whipworm) Inflammatory polyp Lymphoid hyperplasia Solitary rectal ulcer Hirschsprung disease Malnutrition Congenital hypothyroidism	Conservative management—parents trained to use disposable gloves and lubrication and to gently apply pressure Recurrent/persistent prolapse—examined under anesthesia by pediatric surgeon Emergency center evaluation and surgical consultation for irreducible rectal prolapse
Painless rectal bleeding Occasional discomfort with defecation Anal pruritus	Thrombosis Prolapse Strangulation	Constipation often precedes external hemorrhoids Portal hypertension may precede internal hemorrhoids	Treatment with stool softeners, high-fiber diet, Sitz baths, and topical and systemic analgesics Older patients instructed to manually reduce prolapse hemorrhoid during exacerbations Thrombosed external hemorrhoids may be relieved with cooling packs. Pediatric surgery referral for acutely thrombosed external hemorrhoids within 48–72 hours, symptomatic hemorrhoids
Anal pruritus Rectal bleeding	Hygienic problems—may impair cleaning of perineum when wiping	Constipation Fissure Fistula Injury from rectal surgery Hemorrhoid	Usually no treatment needed Treatment of underlying constipation with stool softeners and high-fiber diet Excised in chronic pruritus or when chronic problems with hygiene
May be friable, pruritic and painful	Cancer (rare)	HPV infection (low-risk types 6, 11) Child sexual abuse Autoinoculation from hand wart HIV/immunocompromised	Evaluate for child sexual abuse Dermatology referral for close observation or ablative therapy with cryotherapy or surgical excision

SECTION 14 ● PERIANAL AREA AND BUTTOCKS

Other Diagnoses to Consider

- Inflammatory bowel disease

- Protruding colonic polyp

- Protruding ileocecal intussusception

- Chronic solitary ulcer

- Hypertrophied anodermal papillae

- Parasitic infection

When to Consider Further Evaluation or Treatment

- Patients with skin tags, anal fissures, perianal abscesses, and fistulas associated with abdominal pain, bloody diarrhea, and weight loss or failure to thrive, with or without delayed puberty should have an evaluation for inflammatory bowel disease, particularly Crohn disease.

- Perianal abscesses are incised and drained in most patients except in patients with known or suspected Crohn disease. Abscesses do not generally need to be cultured unless they persist or recur within days of drainage.

- Thrombosed external hemorrhoids can be excised with the overlying skin under general anesthesia.

- The diagnosis for rectal prolapse is primarily historic, but the clinician should consider stool screening for intestinal parasites or a sweat test for cystic fibrosis.

- Avoid the excision of skin tags associated with a diagnosis of Crohn disease.

- Children who present with anogenital warts should be evaluated for sexual abuse. In addition, an HIV test should be considered in adolescents who are sexually active. Consider vaccination with HPV vaccine that includes types 6 and 11 for boys and girls over the age of 9 years.

SUGGESTED READINGS

Pfefferkorn MD, Fitzgerald JF. Disrders of the anorectum: fissures, fistulas, prolapse, hemorrhoids, tags. In: Wyllie R, Hyams JS, Kay M, eds. *Pediatric Gastrointestinal and Liver Disease.* Philadelphia, PA: Elsevier Saunders; 2011:521–527.

Schubert MC, Sridhar S, Schade RR, et al. What every gastroenterologist needs to know about common anorectal disorders. *World J Gastroenterol.* 2009;15(26):3201–3209.

Sinclair KA, Woods CR, Sinal SH. Venereal warts in children. *Pediatr Rev.* 2011;32(3):115–121.

Stites T, Lund DP. Common anorectal problems. *Semin Pediatr Surg.* 2007;16(1):71–78.

Telega G. Perianal anomalies. In: Liacouras CA, Piccoli DA, eds. *Pediatric Gastroenterology: The Requisites in Pediatrics.* Philadelphia, PA: Mosby Elsevier. 2008:187–191.

Perianal and Buttock Redness

Yolanda N. Evans

Approach to the Problem

Diaper dermatitis is the leading cause of skin irritation and redness in the perianal and buttock regions for infants and younger children. It accounts for more than 1 million clinic visits each year. The term diaper dermatitis is used to describe a large variety of different sources of erythema, and it can often be difficult to distinguish the source of irritation and, therefore, the most effective treatment. Irritant dermatitis is the most common cause of erythema in the perianal region. The cause is multifactorial and includes friction, moisture, and exposure to urine and feces. Exposure to wetness and urine increases the pH of the skin, making it more susceptible to irritants and friction.

Key Points in the History

- Wearing highly absorbent disposable diapers is associated with a decreased incidence of diaper dermatitis.

- Children with diaper dermatitis are more likely to be colonized with yeast than other children. *Candida albicans* may be isolated in up to 80% of infants with perianal irritation that lasts more than 3 days.

- Infection with *Staphylococcus aureus* and Group A beta-hemolytic streptococcus (GABHS) can cause erythema, pruritus, and pain.

- It is important to determine whether the patient has had increased exposure to moisture and irritants from sources such as diarrhea, chemicals, or infrequent diaper changes.

Key Points in the Physical Examination

- Diaper dermatitis can take on a variety of clinical manifestations. Irritant dermatitis begins as erythema on the buttocks and perianal areas, sparing the skin folds.

- An erythematous rash of the groin that affects the skin folds and has perianal papules and pustules is characteristic of a yeast infection.

- Allergic contact dermatitis may begin as mild erythema, later progressing to erythema, and scaling with shiny plaques affecting the buttocks, lower abdomen, and thighs while sparing the skin folds.

- GABHS presents as sharply demarcated areas of painful erythema that involves the vulva and penis.

- *Staphylococcus aureus* infection presents as folliculitis or bullous impetigo with vesicles and denuded areas. Lesions often itch.

- Infestation with *Sarcoptes scabiei* presents with pruritic, erythematous papules in the diaper area, along the wrists, between the fingers and toes, ankles, palms, and soles. Infants may also have lesions along the scalp and face.

PHOTOGRAPHS OF SELECTED DIAGNOSES

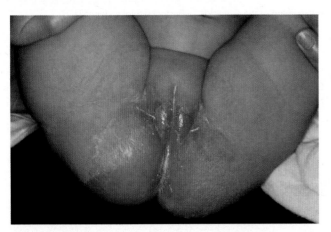

Figure 60-1 Primary irritant diaper dermatitis.
Confluent areas of shiny erythema over labia majora and buttocks. (Courtesy of Jan Edwin Drutz, MD.)

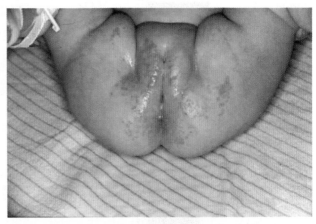

Figure 60-2 Candidal diaper dermatitis. Infant with erythematous rash with satellite lesions in the groin. (Courtesy of Jan Edwin Drutz, MD.)

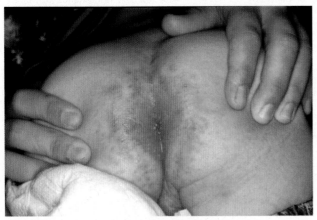

Figure 60-3 Perianal Group A beta-hemolytic streptococcus. Intense erythema is noted in the immediate perianal area of this toddler. (Courtesy of Jan Edwin Drutz, MD.)

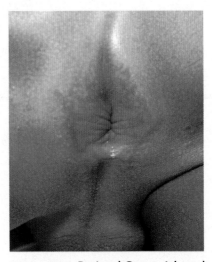

Figure 60-4 Perianal Group A beta-hemolytic streptococcal infection. Perianal streptococcal disease in an African American child. (Courtesy of George A. Datto, III, MD.)

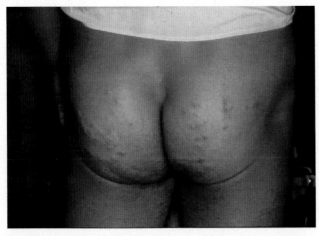

Figure 60-5 Buttock folliculitis. A child with erythematous papules over the posterior buttocks consistent with folliculitis. (Courtesy of Jan Edwin Drutz, MD.)

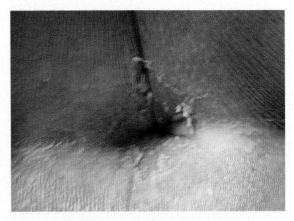

Figure 60-6 Perianal erythema and desquamation in a patient with Kawasaki disease. (Courtesy of Esther K. Chung, MD, MPH.)

DIFFERENTIAL DIAGNOSIS

DIAGNOSIS		ICD 10	DISTINGUISHING CHARACTERISTICS	DISTRIBUTION
Irritant Contact Dermatitis		L22	Papules with sparing of the skin folds	Buttocks, thighs, genitalia
Candidal Diaper Rash		B37.49	Satellite lesions, scaly margins that involve skin folds	Buttocks, perianal, lower abdomen
Perianal Streptococcal Infection		B95.5	Sharp demarcation, perianal erythema with tenderness, pruritus, pain	Perianal and genitalia involvement
Seborrheic Dermatitis		L21.0	Salmon-colored, greasy lesions May be accompanied by erythematous, well-demarcated rash and peripheral satellite lesions, but generally no pustules or erosions Patient generally asymptomatic	Initially may be confined to diaper area After few days, rash extends to involve other body parts with predilection for flexural creases
Allergic Contact Dermatitis		L23.9 Allergic contact dermatitis, unspecified cause	Convex surfaces of diaper area	Convex surfaces of diaper area
Scabies		B86	Pruritic, erythematous papules	Perianal, buttocks, wrists, ankles, in between fingers and toes, axilla

ASSOCIATED FINDINGS	COMPLICATIONS	PREDISPOSING FACTORS	TREATMENT GUIDELINES
Tide water rash (clearly defined borders from diaper elastic bands)	Bacterial or yeast superinfection	Prolonged moisture, diarrhea, chemical exposure	Increase frequency of diaper changes Use highly absorbent diapers Apply water repellent barrier (e.g., zinc oxide)
Oral thrush	Bacterial superinfection	Precedent irritant or other diaper dermatitis; systemic antibiotic treatment	Maintain clean, dry skin Topical antifungal cream or ointment
Strep pharyngitis	Glomerulonephritis	Self-inoculation with oral organisms	Systemic oral antibiotics
Usually begins in the scalp during Infancy Scalp lesions may be somewhat red with yellow, flaky scale	Secondary candidal and/or bacterial infection	Specific etiology unknown Appears to be related to inflammatory reaction of the skin	Clearing of scalp lesions (when present) using antiseborrheic shampoo is generally beneficial Low-potency topical corticosteroid application for short period of time helps clear remaining lesions
Erythematous papules and some skin flaking	Vesicles and eruptions occasionally	Any number of topical substances/agents (e.g., ethylenediamine or rubber) to which patient is highly sensitized	Avoid known sensitizing agents; use mildly potent topical steroids; and consider oral antihistamine
Excoriations and burrows between fingers and toes	N/A	Recent contacts with infected persons	Permethrin application, avoiding eyes and mouth

- Acrodermatitis enteropathica

- Psoriasis

- Folliculitis

- Miliaria rubra

- Granuloma gluteale infantum

- Histiocytosis X

- Syphilis

- Laxative abuse

- Herpes simplex virus infection

- Lichen sclerosis

- Child abuse

- Molluscum contagiosum

When to
Consider
Further
Evaluation
or Treatment

- Diaper dermatitis is the leading cause of redness in the perianal and buttock regions of infants and young children.

- When erythema and rash do not resolve despite appropriate treatment with hygiene, topical steroid, antibiotic, or antifungal treatment, then consider other etiologies.

SUGGESTED READINGS

Nield L, Kamat D. Prevention, diagnosis, and management of diaper dermatitis. *Clin Pediatr.* 2007;46(6):480–486.
Ravanfar P, Wallace JS, Pace NC. Diaper dermatitis: a review and update. *Curr Opin Pediatr.* 2012;24(4):472–479.
Scheinfeld N. Diaper dermatitis: a review and brief and brief survey of eruptions in the diaper area. *Am J Clin Dermatol.* 2005;6(5):273–281.

SKIN

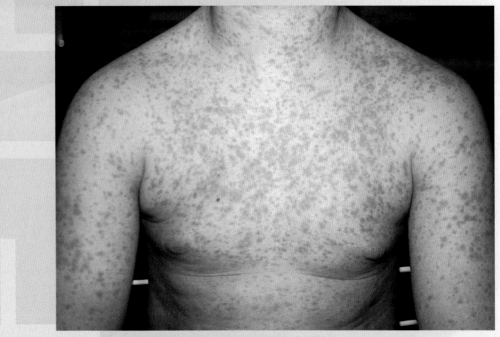

(Courtesy of Kathleen Cronan, MD.)

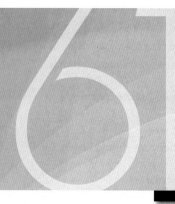

Child Physical Abuse

Christopher C. Stewart

Approach to the Problem

When faced with a concerning cutaneous injury, it is important to consider not only child abuse but also other causes. Age and developmental ability of the patient, as well as the location and type of the lesion(s), help in determining the likelihood of an abusive or nonaccidental cause of cutaneous findings. Common cutaneous injuries seen in child physical abuse include bruises, pattern injuries, and burns. It is important to match the history (or mechanism) of how the findings appeared with the actual observed finding(s). Try to determine whether the mechanism is plausible, based on the child's developmental ability. Photo-documentation can be important for the investigative process, for review by experts, and to document changes. For example, if a suspected bruise does not resolve with time, then it is not a bruise and could be a birthmark.

Key Points in the History

- Obtain a detailed history of the alleged cause of the cutaneous findings, if available.

- Sometimes no history is given, or only potential mechanisms are offered. For example, a caretaker may not have witnessed an actual event, but may believe that something specific happened to explain the findings.

- A vague history such as "fell from chair" is not adequate to match an injury to a mechanism; therefore, it is essential to gather details related to the fall.

- A changing or discrepant history is concerning for abuse.

- Height of the fall, specific details about the fall (i.e., Was it straight down or in an arc? Was there twisting or rotational motion? Were there multiple strikes with the child falling down stairs?), surface onto which the fall occurred, whether there were objects on the floor, and other such information can help evaluate whether the explanation fits the injury.

- Consider detailed questions about the environment, witnesses, and the child's response to the event or injury.

491

- Delay in seeking care is potentially a concerning factor; an explanation for a delay in seeking care should be elicited and can be evaluated as being a reasonable explanation or not.

- For scald injuries, a temperature of the water should be obtained at the scene by investigators.

- Family history of bleeding disorders or other underlying conditions should be obtained.

- Medications, such as recent anticoagulant use, should be assessed.

- Previous accidents resulting in injuries such as fractures, burns, and head trauma can suggest a pattern of abuse and should raise suspicion for child physical abuse.

- Include in the medical record any explanation given by the child or adolescent for the injury, using their exact words, when possible.

Key Points in the Physical Examination

- Corroborate the child's developmental ability.

- Location is a key determinant of suspicion for abuse: buttocks, trunk, neck, ears, genitalia, and upper arms are concerning locations for bruises or other injuries.

- Examine the entire body. Subtle bruising or pattern marks can easily be missed.

- Pattern marks can be suspicious. Linear or other pattern marks should be measured, documented, and photographed.

- Scald burns with sharply demarcated lines, without splash marks, are suspicious for forced immersion.

- Examine behind the ears, as there may be bruises from inflicted trauma.

- Examine the mouth carefully; injuries to the frenulum can result from forced bottle feeding or smothering of a crying baby.

- Perform a genital examination on every child with suspected physical abuse.

- Penile bruises may result from pinching and may reflect physical punishment or an accidental toilet seat injury.

- Photo-documentation can be important for follow-up, expert review, and investigating agencies.

PHOTOGRAPHS OF SELECTED DIAGNOSES

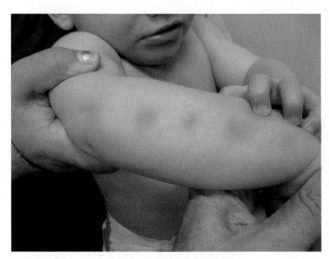

Figure 61-1 Circular bruises. These are typical of fingertip marks from squeezing, shown here on an infant's forearm. (Courtesy of Dr. Jean Labbé.)

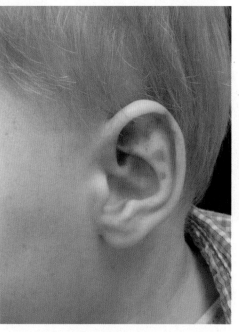

Figure 61-2 Bruise of the external ear. Ear injuries are highly concerning for child physical abuse. (Courtesy of Dr. Jean Labbé.)

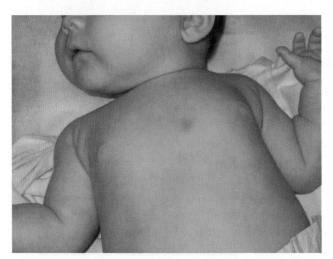

Figure 61-3 Bruise on infant's chest. Both the location of the bruise, and the fact that it is an infant make this less likely to be from an accident. (Courtesy of Dr. Jean Labbé)

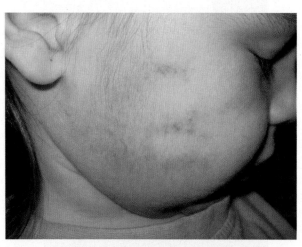

Figure 61-4 Slap mark on child's cheek. Petechial lines or an outline of a hand may be observed in slaps when blood is pushed through the space between the fingers of the slapping hand. (Courtesy of Dr. Jean Labbé.)

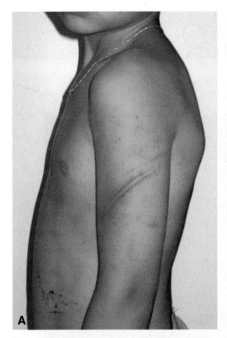
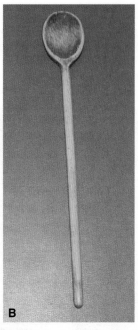

Figure 61-5 Pattern mark on a child's arm (A) from being struck by a wooden spoon. **Wooden spoon (B)** matching the mark on child's arm seen in (A). (Courtesy of Dr. Jean Labbé.)

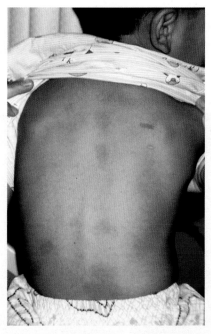

Figure 61-6 Dermal melanocytosis on child's back. These lesions may be mistaken for bruises. Bruises should resolve, however, over days to weeks. (Courtesy of Dr. Jean Labbé.)

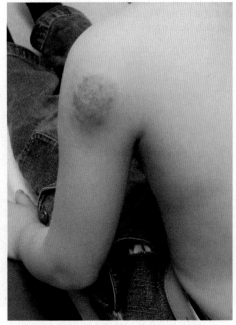

Figure 61-7 Cavernous hemangioma on child's shoulder. This type of lesion is sometimes mistaken for a bruise from an inflicted injury. (Courtesy of Dr. Jean Labbé.)

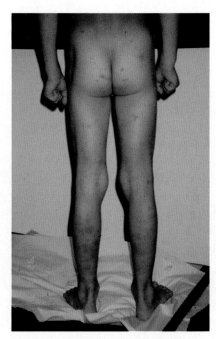

Figure 61-8 Henoch–Schönlein purpura (HSP). The purpuric lesions of HSP may be mistaken for bruises from inflicted injury. (Courtesy of Dr. Jean Labbé.)

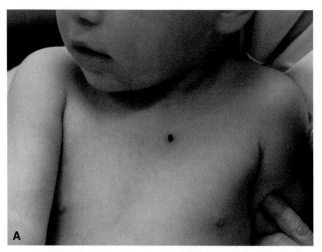

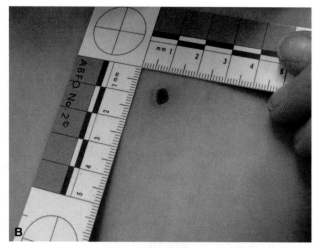

Figure 61-9 **Cigarette burn (A). Close-up of cigarette burn** showing a typical measurement of approximately 8 mm **(B)**. (Courtesy of Dr. Jean Labbé.)

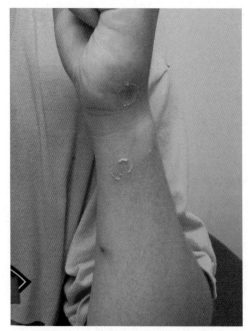

Figure 61-10 **Impetigo.** This entity is sometimes mistaken for a cigarette burn. (Courtesy of Dr. Jean Labbé.)

DIFFERENTIAL DIAGNOSIS

DIAGNOSIS	ICD-10	DISTINGUISHING CHARACTERISTICS	DISTRIBUTION
Accidental Scald Burn Injuries	T30.0 Burn of unspecified body region, unspecified degree	Unusual in children less than 6 months old Nonmobile children less likely to get accidental burns Often have accompanying splash marks	Often on face and chest if child pulls a container of hot liquid onto themselves On parts of body used to explore (palms, fingers rather than the back of the hand)
Accidental Bruises	R58 Ecchymosis	Unusual in children less than 6 months old Children not pulling to a stand are unlikely to get bruises	More likely found on bony prominences: shins, lower arms, elbows, under chin, forehead, hips, ankles
Dermal Melanosis, Slate Grey Nevi, Mongolian Spots	L81.4 Melanosis	Usually present at birth Do not fade over a short period of time Usually on buttocks or back, but may be anywhere Often with irregular borders, indistinct edges More likely blue, bluish-grey	Sacral area, buttocks, back May appear anywhere, but rare on palms, soles, or face
Hemangiomas	D18.0 Hemangioma	May be present at birth or shortly thereafter May grow in size	Often on face scalp or neck, chest or back
Henoch–Schönlein Purpura	D69.0	Starts as erythematous papules or urticarial wheals Develops into groups of petechiae and purpura	Buttocks, lower extremities, belt-line (pressure points), extensor surfaces
Impetigo	L01.0	Painful, red rash with fragile bullae and honey-colored crusting	Nares Can be found anywhere
Erythema Nodosum	L52.0	Reddish painful lumps (nodules) under the skin	Generally on the shins, though may occur in other areas (buttocks, calves, ankles, thighs, and arms)
Contact Dermatitis	L23 Allergic contact dermatitis	Pruritic Eczematous appearance Resolves after exposure removed Poison oak or ivy (urushiol)	Often with pattern associated with bracelet, clothing snaps Periumbilical (belt-line) area

ASSOCIATED FINDINGS	PREDISPOSING FACTORS	TREATMENT GUIDELINES
Lack of other suspicious cutaneous, radiologic, or laboratory findings	Toilet training may be associated with parent frustration leading to abusive immersion scald burns.	Standard burn treatment guidelines For abuse work-up, if less than 2 years old, consider skeletal survey, and possible blood work (liver function tests, lipase) and urinalysis
Lack of other suspicious cutaneous, radiologic, or laboratory findings	Ambulation Underlying coagulopathy	Expect self-resolution If large bruise and concerns for underlying fracture, consider radiographic studies.
N/A	Dark skin pigmentation Individuals of African, Asian, Hispanic, or Mediterranean descent	N/A
May ulcerate	Prematurity Caucasian Female gender	Most superficial hemangiomas resolve without treatment. Cavernous hemangiomas may require treatment with lasers, steroids, and propanolol
Arthritis, abdominal pain, renal disease	Age younger than 10	Supportive treatment NSAIDS for arthritis Steroids for renal disease
Cellulitis, lymphangitis Rarely glomerulonephritis	Breaks in skin from cuts, bites Varicella Humid climates Recent hospitalization	Self-limited Topical antibiotics to cover *Staphylococcus aureus* and Group A beta-hemolytic streptococcus
Fever General ill feeling (malaise) Joint aches	Medications (sulfa-containing) Strep throat Cat-scratch disease Infectious mononucleosis	NSAIDS Steroids may be used. Elevation Hot or cold compresses
Id reaction	Nickel-containing jewelry or clothing snaps Various cosmetic products Leather materials (potassium dichromate) Poison oak or ivy (uroshiol)	Emollients Topical retinoids Antihistamines for itching Topical steroids for itching Alpha-hydroxy acids (including lactic and glycolic acids)

Other
Diagnoses
to Consider

Bruising

- Dermal melanosis, slate grey nevi, mongolian spots

- Hemangiomas

- Henoch–Schönlein purpura

- Cupping, spooning, coining

- Leukemia

- Von Willebrand disease

- Idiopathic thrombocytopenic purpura

- Hemophilia

- Erythema nodosum

Burns

- Epidermolysis bullosa

- Staphylococcal scalded skin syndrome

- (Bullous) impetigo

- Contact dermatitis

- Accidental scald or contact burns

- Phytophotodermatitis

- Chemical burns from home remedies like laxatives

When to
Consider
Further
Evaluation
or Treatment

- In general, whenever there is bruising suspicious for child abuse, a complete blood count and coagulation panel (prothrombin time, partial thromboplastin time, and international normalized ratio) should be obtained to rule out malignancy or bleeding disorder.

- Consider referral to a dermatologist if a medical condition is being considered.

- In children less than 2 years old with concerning cutaneous findings, a skeletal survey should generally be done to look for fractures specific for abuse.

- Consider head imaging and fundoscopic examination in infants or children less than a year of age if suspicious injuries.

- Suspicious injuries should be referred to a child abuse specialist.

- Child protective services or the police should be contacted when appropriate, and may be responsible for scene investigation.

SUGGESTED READINGS

Harris TS. Bruises in children: normal or child abuse? *J Pediatr Health Care*. 2010;24(4):216–221.

Hobbs CJ. ABC of child abuse. Burns and scalds. *BMJ*. 1989;298(6683):1302–1305.

Kos L, Shwayder T. Cutaneous manifestations of child abuse. *Pediatr Dermatol*. 2006;23(4):311–320.

Sugar NF, Taylor JA, Feldman KW. Bruises in infants and toddlers: those who don't cruise rarely bruise. *Arch Pediatr Adolesc Med*. 1999;153(4):399–403.

Swerdlin A, Berkowitz C, Craft N. Cutaneous signs of child abuse. *J Am Acad Dermatol*. 2007;57(3):371–392.

Facial Rashes

Sunitha V. Kaiser and Julie S. O'Brien

Approach to the Problem

Rashes on the face can be an isolated local phenomenon or associated with systemic disease. Clues to the etiology of the rash are found in the anatomic location, distribution, color, type, and the shape of the involved lesions. Many patients and their families are often concerned about the impact of the facial rash on the child's appearance, self-esteem, and interpersonal interactions.

Key Points in the History

- When acne lesions appear in a child under 7, consider an evaluation for endocrinologic abnormalities.

- In a female with acne and oligomenorrhea or hirsutism, consider evaluation for polycystic ovarian syndrome.

- The lesions of impetigo may be distinguished from contact dermatitis in that impetigo lesions are generally painful, whereas contact dermatitis lesions are pruritic.

- Children with eczema frequently have family members with a history of eczema, allergies, or asthma.

- During winter, when the air has lower humidity, facial rashes exacerbated by dry skin such as eczema, pityriasis alba, and lip-licking dermatitis are often worse.

- Autoimmune diseases can present with a chronic erythematous facial rash. Associated fever and arthritis raise the suspicion for these disorders.

Key Points in the Physical Examination

- Focal rashes on the face are seen with impetigo and tinea corporis.

- Symmetric lesions are seen with infectious processes, such as erythema infectiosum or scarlet fever.

- When evaluating acne, it is important to assess the type of lesions (comedone vs inflammatory), the number and distribution of lesions, and the presence of scarring in order to guide therapy.

- In severe cases of eczema, lesions can be found throughout the body; however, lesions in the axilla or groin area should prompt consideration of other diagnoses, such as psoriasis. If pustules are present, consider superinfection with *Staphylococcus aureus*.

- Contact dermatitis presents as a localized skin lesion exposed to an irritant, such as nickel-containing clothing snaps or jewelry.

- Vesicular lesions occur in herpes simplex virus (HSV) and coxsackievirus infections. In herpes infections, the vesicles are grouped or dermatomal.

- Rhus dermatitis and some cases of eczema are associated with vesicular lesions.

- Acne presents with comedones.

- Pearl-like lesions with central umbilication are seen in molluscum contagiosum.

- The facial lesions of tuberous sclerosis are very hard subcutaneous papules. They are often misdiagnosed as acne; look for other dermatologic findings of tuberous sclerosis, including ash leaf spots and shagreen patches.

- Individuals with scaly rashes such as eczema, seborrhea, psoriasis, and pityriasis alba often have skin changes present in other parts of their body.

- Seborrhea classically has a greasy scale, whereas psoriasis has a silvery scale.

- Erythematous plaques sparing the nasolabial folds are characteristic of the malar rash seen in systemic lupus erythematosus.

PHOTOGRAPHS OF SELECTED DIAGNOSES

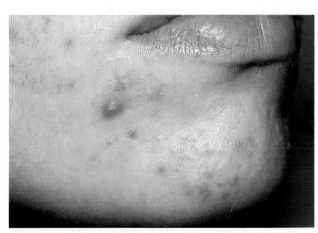

Figure 62-1 Inflammatory acne. Erythematous papules and pustules on chin. (Used with permission from Goodheart HP. *Goodheart's Photoguide to Common Skin Disorders.* 2nd ed. Philadelphia, PA: Lippincott Williams & Wilkins; 2003:14.)

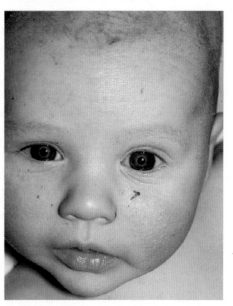

Figure 62-2 Eczema. Symmetric bilateral scaly rash on cheeks. (Used with permission from Goodheart HP. *Goodheart's Photoguide to Common Skin Disorders.* 2nd ed. Philadelphia, PA: Lippincott Williams & Wilkins; 2003:46.)

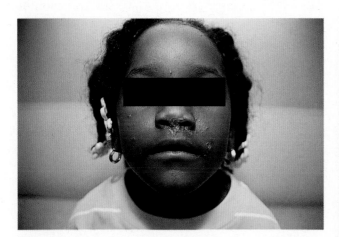

Figure 62-3 Impetigo. Honey-crusted lesions at base of nares that are self-inoculated onto other parts of the face. (Courtesy of George A. Datto, III, MD.)

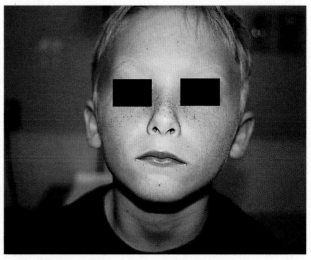

Figure 62-4 Erythema infectiosum. Bilateral erythematous macular rash on cheeks—"slapped cheeks." (Courtesy of George A. Datto, III, MD.)

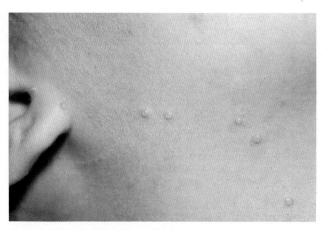

Figure 62-5 **Molluscum contagiosum.** Umbilicated papules on face of child. (Used with permission from Goodheart HP. *Goodheart's Photoguide to Common Skin Disorders.* 2nd ed. Philadelphia, PA: Lippincott Williams & Wilkins; 2003:138.)

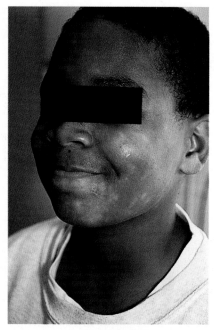

Figure 62-6 **Pityriasis alba.** Hypopigmented scaly macules on cheeks. (Courtesy of George A. Datto, III, MD.)

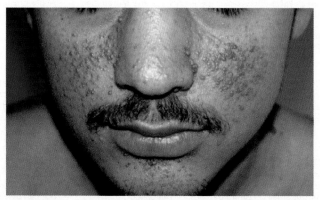

Figure 62-7 **Tuberous sclerosis.** Adenoma sebaceum (angiofibroma). (Used with permission from Goodheart HP. *Goodheart's Photoguide to Common Skin Disorders.* 2nd ed. Philadelphia, PA: Lippincott Williams & Wilkins; 2003:388.)

DIFFERENTIAL DIAGNOSIS

DIAGNOSIS		ICD-10	DISTINGUISHING CHARACTERISTICS	DISTRIBUTION	DURATION/ CHRONICITY
Acne		L700	Obstructive lesions: open comedones—blackheads Closed comedones—whiteheads. Inflammatory lesions: erythematous papules, pustules, or nodules Scars: pits, hypo-/hyperpigmented lesions	Early puberty: blackheads/ whiteheads on midface (midforehead, nose, and chin) Later: inflammatory lesions on the lateral cheeks, lower jaw, back, and chest	Persists throughout adolescent years
Eczema		L20.8	Dry skin, pruritus, scaling, erythematous papules and vesicles ± crusting (acute) Lichenification (chronic)	Infants: extensor surfaces, cheeks, and scalp with sparing of diaper area. Children: flexor surfaces and neck	Chronic waxing and waning course
Impetigo		L01.0	Papules evolve into vesicles then pustules with a golden crust. In bullous impetigo, vesicles enlarge to form flaccid bullae with clear yellow fluid	Face and extremities	Acute presentation
Seborrhea		L21.9	Scaling and poorly defined erythematous patches	In infants: scalp, face, diaper area In adolescents: scalp, face, chest, and intertriginous areas Blepharitis	Chronic—lasting weeks to months in infancy and longer in adolescents
Scarlet Fever		A38.9	Diffuse blanching erythema with numerous small (1–2 mm) papules that give a "sandpaper" quality to the skin	Usually starts on the head/neck, then spreads to trunk, then extremities and ultimately desquamates; palms and soles spared. Rash most marked in skin folds	Acute presentation, but can persist for 1–2 weeks after treatment
Erythema Infectiosum		B08.3	Erythematous "slapped cheek" rash; rash may resolve and then recur with changes in temperature, sun exposure, or stress Less commonly, morbilliform, confluent, and vesicular rashes occur.	Face: confluent red rash on cheeks with circumoral pallor Trunk/Extremities: reticulated, lacelike rash	Acute, brief self-limited
Molluscum Contagiosum		B08.1	Firm, pearly papules (2–5 mm) with a central umbilication	Can occur anywhere on the body, sparing palms, and soles	Chronic, may persist for months to years

ASSOCIATED FINDINGS	COMPLICATIONS	PREDISPOSING FACTORS	TREATMENT GUIDELINES
Signs of pubertal development	Scarring Low self-esteem, depression, anxiety	Pubertal rise in androgens leading to increased sebum production, *Propionibacterium acnes* causing inflammation, abnormal keratinization clogging follicles, genetics	For mild comedonal acne, topical retinoid and/or benzoyl peroxide For mild/moderate inflammatory, topical retinoid and topical antibiotic ± benzoyl peroxide to prevent resistance. For severe inflammatory, topical retinoid and oral antibiotic for 8–12 weeks ± benzoyl peroxide For severe inflammatory or nodular, consider isotretinoin/referral to dermatology For women with premenstrual flares, consider hormonal therapy
Asthma Allergic symptoms	Superinfection with *S. aureus*. Eczema herpeticum	Diminished epidermal barrier function and skin inflammation Genetic factors	Gentle skin care with dye-free, fragrance-free emollients twice daily and avoidance of triggers of symptoms For flares marked by itching, erythema, papules, and lichenification: short courses of topical steroids Calcineurin inhibitors, tacrolimus and pimecrolimus, may be considered in moderate to severe disease in immunocompetent children >2 years For severe disease, consider bleach baths. For those with *S. aureus*, wet wraps and oral antihistamines Oral antibiotics only for superinfection
May occur due to scratching in children with eczema or scabies May evolve to bullous impetigo or be spread through self-inoculation	Cellulitis Poststreptococcal glomerulonephritis	Skin trauma followed by infection with *S. aureus* and/or Group A beta-hemolytic streptococci	If localized and without bullae, use topical mupirocin. If extensive or bullous, use oral antibiotics and consider methicillin-resistant *S. aureus* coverage based on local microbial patterns
Dandruff	Discomfort from itching, bacterial superinfection, social anxiety	Poorly understood, but involves sebum production by sebaceous glands and possible colonization with malassezia	For infants: emollients and soft brush to remove scale; consider topical low-potency corticosteroid or 2% ketoconazole shampoo for scalp or ointment for body For adolescents/adults: scalp—selenium sulfide or ketoconazole shampoo ± topical corticosteroid shampoo; body—topical corticosteroid or ketoconazole
Fever, pharyngitis, perioral pallor, strawberry tongue	Acute otitis media, sinusitis, tonsillopharyngeal abscess, post-strep glomerulonephritis, acute rheumatic fever, streptococcal toxic shock syndrome	Occurs as a result of prior exposure to Group A streptococcus which can cause a delayed-type skin reactivity to pyrogenic exotoxin produced by the organism	Oral penicillin V or amoxicillin If allergic to penicillin, use cephalosporins or macrolides.
25% have classic symptoms: fever and coryza followed by the rash 25% will be asymptomatic during their infection 50% have only nonspecific flu-like symptoms	Arthritis Arthralgias Transient aplastic crisis Chronic anemia in immunocompromised hosts Hydrops fetalis Myocarditis	Caused by parvovirus B19, which replicates in the erythroid progenitor cells Conditions that increase RBC destruction (e.g., sickle cell disease) or decrease RBC production (e.g., iron deficiency anemia) increase the risk of developing transient aplastic crisis.	Rash and prodrome are typically mild and self-limited. In patients with risk factors or concern for symptomatic anemia, follow serial complete blood counts and transfuse as needed.
Pruritus may be present. Molluscum dermatitis occurs when patients develop eczematous plaques surrounding the papules.	Lesions can become irritated, inflamed, or superinfected. Lesions on the eyelid can cause conjunctivitis.	Caused by poxvirus. Possible increased risk with eczema; however, inconclusive evidence	Self-limited Will resolve with time (months to years) No evidence for clinically effective treatment. Cryotherapy with liquid nitrogen can be effective but can result in scaring or hypopigmentation. Surgical removal may be followed by recurrence; cantharidin, potassium hydroxide, or podophyllum may also be used.

(continued)

DIFFERENTIAL DIAGNOSIS *(continued)*

DIAGNOSIS	ICD-10	DISTINGUISHING CHARACTERISTICS	DISTRIBUTION	DURATION/ CHRONICITY
Pityriasis Alba	L30.5	Hypopigmented Oval shaped with poorly defined margins Fine scale	Typically found on cheeks; may also involve neck, upper trunk, and upper arms	Chronic, may last months when appears with a waxing and waning course over years
Angiofibromas—seen with tuberous sclerosis (also called fibroadenomas; previously called adenoma sebaceum)	D10.6— angiofibroma Q85.1— tuberous sclerosis	1–3 mm pink or red subcutaneous papules	Malar distribution: nasolabial folds and cheeks	Chronic
HSV Infection	B00.9	Vesicular lesions	Initial infection often presents as gingivostomatitis with pharyngeal and oral mucosal involvement. Subsequent infections present with perioral lesions, but can be seen around the eye from contact spread	Acute

ASSOCIATED FINDINGS	COMPLICATIONS	PREDISPOSING FACTORS	TREATMENT GUIDELINES
Commonly asymptomatic, but can be pruritic	N/A	Considered mild form of eczema. Typically occurs in darker skinned patients when exposed to more sunlight, highlighting hypopigmentation	Moisturizers alleviate itching and dry skin. Sunscreen can minimize appearance. May consider low-dose topical steroids for more severe cases.
Over 80% of individuals with tuberous sclerosis have dermatologic findings including: • ash leaf spots: hypopigmented macules • shagreen patches: thickened, pebbly skin often on neck or back—resembling an orange peel Patients may also have periungual or subungual fibromas that appear later in adolescence or adulthood.	There is no risk of malignant transformation of the skin lesions associated with tuberous sclerosis. However, complications of the disease include seizure, cardiac rhabdomyomas, and CNS tubers.	Tuberous sclerosis is associated with mutations in chromosome 9q34 and 16q13.3. It is inherited in an autosomal dominant fashion, however 50% of cases are due to new mutations.	Laser therapy has been used but is painful and has a high recurrence rate. Topical rapamycin has been used with some success.
Primary infection often occurs with fever, malaise, myalgias, irritability, and cervical lymphadenopathy. Subsequent perioral lesions are painful.	Herpetic whitlow: infection of the finger Eczema herpeticum in patients with eczema Herpes keratoconjunctivitis: leading cause of corneal blindness in industrialized countries.	Contact with HSV, type 1. Immunocompromised patients are at risk for increased frequency and severity of HSV infections.	Self-limited Treat pain with acetaminophen or ibuprofen. Treatment of gingivostomatitis may require hospitalization for dehydration. Acyclovir is helpful if started within the first 48–72 hours of outbreak. For frequent recurrent outbreaks, consider prophylaxis with acyclovir.

SECTION 15 • SKIN

Other Diagnoses to Consider

- Systemic lupus erythematosus

- Dermatomyositis

- Scarlet fever

- Hemangiomas

- Psoriasis

- Petechiae/Purpura

When to Consider Further Evaluation or Treatment

- Because acne scars may be irreversible, their presence should prompt the clinician to be aggressive in the selection of therapeutic agents and to consider referral to a dermatologist.

- Severe eczema is often infected with *S. aureus,* especially with pustular or eroded lesions.

- For severe seborrheic dermatitis, consider an alternate diagnosis including psoriasis or HIV infection.

- Special precautions should be taken with pregnant women exposed to parvovirus B19. Due to the effect of the virus on red cell production, complications include miscarriage, intrauterine fetal demise, and hydrops fetalis.

SUGGESTED READINGS

Gollnick H, Cunliffe W, Berson D, et al. Management of acne: a report from a global alliance to improve outcomes in acne. *J Am Acad Dermatol.* 2003;49:S1.

Goodheart HP. *Goodheart's Photoguide to Common Skin Disorders.* 3rd ed. Philadelphia, PA: Lippincott Williams & Wilkins; 2008: Chapters 1, 2, 5, 14, and 16.

Krakowski AC, Eichenfield LF, Dohil MA. Management of atopic dermatitis in the pediatric population. *Pediatrics.* 2008;122(4):812.

Krueger DA, Franz DN. Current management of tuberous sclerosis complex. *Paediatr Drugs.* 2008;10(5):299–313.

Naldi L, Rebora A. Clinical practice. Seborrheic dermatitis. *N Engl J Med.* 2009;360(4):387–396.

Paller AS, Mancini AJ, eds. *Hurwitz Clinical Pediatric Dermatology: A Textbook of Skin Disorders of Childhood and Adolescence.* 4th ed. Philadelphia, PA: Elsevier Saunders; 2011:Chapters 3, 4, 14, 15, and 19.

Silverberg N. Pediatric molluscum contagiosum: optimal treatment strategies. *Paediatr Drugs.* 2003;5:505–512.

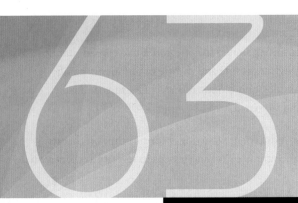

Diffuse Red Rashes

Bethlehem Abebe-Wolpaw

Approach to the Problem

Diffuse red rashes are a common complaint. The differential diagnosis for this type of rash is wide, including minor, self-resolving illnesses that can be managed safely in the outpatient setting to life-threatening conditions that require prompt and aggressive intervention. Diffuse red rashes are most often a result of exposure to sunlight, a number of infections, or medications. In some cases, the combination of exposure to sunlight and medication is the reason for the rash.

Key Points in the History

- The timing of the rash in the setting of medication ingestion is often helpful in determining the etiology.

- Exanthematous drug eruptions usually occur within 5 to 14 days after starting medications. Medications most commonly implicated in drug eruptions include antibiotics (penicillins, sulfonamides), nonsteroidal anti-inflammatory drugs (NSAIDs), and anticonvulsants (carbamazepine, phenytoin). Pruritus is often an associated symptom.

- A severe form of drug eruption known as DRESS (drug rash with eosinophilia and systemic symptoms) usually occurs 2 to 8 weeks after a medication is initiated, most commonly after exposure to anticonvulsants.

- In the majority of cases, the onset of Red Man syndrome is within 60 minutes of initiation of vancomycin infusion.

- The typical prodrome of measles (rubeola) includes fever, malaise, cough, coryza, conjunctivitis, and Koplik spots (small red lesions on mucous membranes with a white central spot) followed on day 3 by the rash that spreads in a cephalocaudal fashion.

- The diffuse painful, sometimes painless, erythema of sunburn occurs 3 to 5 hours after exposure and usually peaks at 12 to 24 hours, after ultraviolet (UV) radiation of as little as 30 minutes duration.

- Drug- and chemical-induced photosensitivity similar in appearance to a typical sunburn results from the combination of UVA light exposure and the use of photosensitizing medications such as NSAIDs, sulfonamides, quinolones, tetracyclines, furosemide, griseofulvin, thiazides, amiodarone, and isoniazid.

- Polymorphous light eruption is a light-induced, nonscarring, pruritic eruption that tends to be most severe at the beginning of the sunny season and lessens in severity as the season progresses.

- Initial symptoms of staphylococcal scalded skin syndrome (SSSS) include fever, malaise, irritability, conjunctivitis, pharyngitis, and impetigo prior to the onset of the rash. SSSS can present at any age but preferentially affects newborns during their first week of life and children under age 5.

- In toxic shock syndrome (TSS), there is typically a focus of infection such as a tampon, soft tissue infection, abscess, or burn.

Key Points in the Physical Examination

- Drug-related rashes usually manifest as generalized morbilliform eruptions, generally starting on the face and trunk, and then spreading distally.

- DRESS is a severe form of a drug reaction that is characterized by fever, erythroderma, lymphadenopathy, facial edema, transaminitis, leukocytosis with eosinophilia, and visceral involvement.

- Erythema, flushing, and pruritus of the face and upper body are typical of Red Man syndrome. Severe reactions include generalized erythema, intense pruritus, and hypotension.

- The typical rash seen in measles is a nonpruritic, blotchy, erythematous, blanching, maculopapular rash that spreads in a cephalocaudal manner. Koplik spots are considered pathognomonic for measles.

- The appearance of erythema on sun-exposed areas that become painful and that spare areas of covered skin aids with diagnosing sunburn as well as drug- and chemical-induced photosensitivity.

- Polymorphous light eruption is limited to sun-exposed areas such as the face, posterior neck, and extremities. Rash occurs within hours and occasionally 1 to 2 days after sun exposure with pruritus as a key finding.

- Parvovirus B19 infection, or erythema infectiosum, causes an intense erythema specifically on the face and a reticulated erythematous rash on the rest of the body.

- Tonsillopharyngitis with fever and sore throat followed by the development of a blanching, confluent erythematous rash with a sandpaper quality is consistent with scarlet fever. Pastia lines are accentuated erythema with petechiae in a linear pattern in skin folds in areas such as the antecubital fossa and axilla.

- The widespread erythroderma of SSSS appears similar to a sunburn, is tender to touch, and is notably prominent in the perioral and flexural areas. The rash then progresses to flaccid bullae that easily rupture. Nikolsky sign (separation of the upper epidermis with gentle pressure or friction) is a classic finding.

- The diffuse blanching erythroderma of TSS, which can also resemble a sunburn, is distinguished by high fevers, abdominal distress, myalgias, headache followed by hypotension, and multisystem organ involvement, as well as subsequent desquamation of the rash.

- The typical petechial rash of Rocky Mountain spotted fever may start as a maculopapular eruption peripherally, which then spreads centrally before becoming petechial.

PHOTOGRAPHS OF SELECTED DIAGNOSES

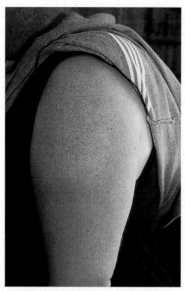

Figure 63-1 Sunburn. Diffuse erythema on lateral aspect of arm. (Courtesy of George A. Datto, III, MD.)

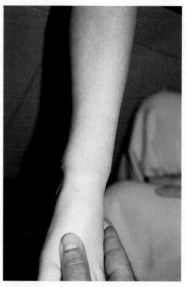

Figure 63-2 Photosensitivity. Edematous and erythematous sharp-bordered lesion that developed on ankle after sun exposure. (Courtesy of George A. Datto, III, MD.)

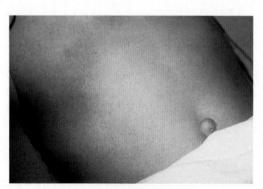

Figure 63-3 Drug rash. Erythroderma with fine morbilliform rash that developed after antibiotic exposure. (Courtesy of George A. Datto, III, MD.)

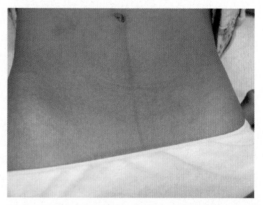

Figure 63-4 Rash seen with scarlet fever. Note the diffuse distribution of this rash that is more intense in the lower abdomen and groin. (Courtesy of Esther K. Chung, MD, MPH.)

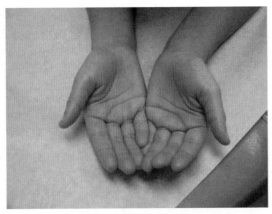

Figure 63-5 **Palmar erythema.** Note the intense palmar redness seen in a child with scarlet fever. (Courtesy of Esther K. Chung, MD, MPH.)

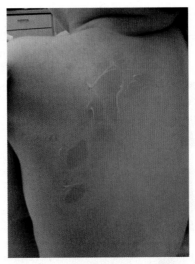

Figure 63-6 **Staphylococcal scalded skin syndrome.** A 4-year-old boy with the characteristic erythema and skin sloughing seen with SSSS. (Courtesy of Bethlehem Abebe-Wolpaw, MD.)

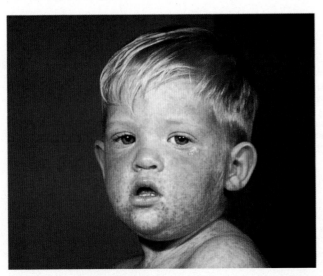

Figure 63-7 **Measles.** Child with measles (rubeola) showing the characteristic conjunctivitis, coryza, and red, blotchy rash that appear around day 3 of illness, first on the face and then becoming more generalized. (Used with permission from Centers for Disease Control and Prevention Public Health Image Library.)

DIFFERENTIAL DIAGNOSIS

DIAGNOSIS		ICD-10	DISTINGUISHING CHARACTERISTICS	DISTRIBUTION	DURATION, CHRONICITY
Sunburn		L55.9	Usually painful erythema to sun-exposed areas	Sun-exposed skin	Peaks at 12–24 hours after sun exposure, resolves 3–7 days later
Photosensitivity		L56.8	Accelerated and/or exaggerated sunburn	Sun-exposed skin	Improves after discontinuation of drug, chemical
Drug Eruption		L27.0	Rapid onset erythema as seen with vancomycin and Red Man syndrome or gradual development of a morbilliform rash	Generalized; may start on face, trunk then spread distally	Resolves over 1–2 weeks following discontinuation of drug
DRESS (Drug rash with eosinophilia and systemic symptoms)		L27.0	A severe form of drug eruption	Widespread, same as above	May see initial improvement then flare 3–4 weeks after the start of the reaction
Scarlet Fever		A38	Blanching, confluent erythematous rash with a sandpaper quality Accentuated erythema with petechiae in a linear pattern found in skin folds such as the antecubital fossa and axilla are known as Pastia lines	Initially the sandpaper-like rash occurs on upper body then becomes more generalized sparing palms and soles. While the sandpaper-like rash spares the palms and soles, there may be erythema notes on the palms, soles, and in the perineal and groin areas.	Rash fades over 5–7 days
Staphyloccocal Scaled Skin Syndrome (SSSS)		L00	Diffuse erythroderma similar to a sunburn, tender to touch Progresses to flaccid bullae that easily rupture Nikolsky sign (separation of the upper epidermis with gentle pressure or friction) is a classic finding	May be patchy or generalized	Resolution of rash in 1–2 weeks
Erythema Infectiosum (Fifth Disease)		B08.3	Intense, nontender facial erythema Reticulated erythematous rash on the rest of the body	Facial erythema that spares nasolabial folds Extremities and trunk with diffusely lacy rash	Resolves 3–7 days after onset

ASSOCIATED FINDINGS	COMPLICATIONS	PREDISPOSING FACTORS	TREATMENT GUIDELINES
Blisters in severe cases Edema followed by desquamation Hyperpigmentation	Systemic symptoms (fever, headache, nausea, vomiting) seen with severe sunburns Secondary infections Increased risk of skin cancer	Inadequate sunscreen application Lack of protective clothing Sun exposure during peak sunlight hours	Avoid sun exposure until symptoms resolve Symptomatic relief with NSAIDs, emollients, cool compresses Consider oral and/or topical steroids for severe cases
Blisters Edema Desquamation	Same as for sunburn above	Drug-induced Plant-induced (furocoumarin is a phototoxic agent found in citrus, parsnips, carrots, and other plants) Baseline sensitivity to sun	Removal and avoidance of causative drug, chemical Symptomatic relief with same agents used for sunburn Liberal use of sunscreen
Pruritus	Secondary infection	Eruption occurs within 5–14 days after initiating medication such as antibiotics, NSAIDs, or anticonvulsants	Discontinuing the drug leads to resolution of the rash Symptomatic treatment with oral antihistamines, topical steroids, oral steroids, emollients Also consider second-generation H_1 blockers
Fever, lymphadenopathy, facial edema, transaminitis, leukocytosis with eosinophilia, and visceral involvement	Secondary infection Systemic involvement (hepatitis, pericarditis/myocarditis, interstitial nephritis, pneumonitis)	Occurs 2–8 weeks after a medication is initiated, most commonly seen with anticonvulsants	Discontinuing the drug is critical in minimizing the associated morbidity and mortality Symptomatic treatment with systemic steroids, topical steroids, antihistamines. Case reports of benefit seen with intravenous immunoglobulin and N-acetylcysteine
Fever, pharyngitis, headache, desquamation, nausea, vomiting, occasionally pruritus	Rheumatic fever, peritonsillar/retropharyngeal abscess, post-streptococcal glomerulonephritis	Group A streptococcal infection, most common focus of infection is tonsillopharyngitis	Penicillin, amoxicillin, macrolides if penicillin-allergic Antihistamines for pruritus
Fever, malaise, irritability, conjunctivitis, pharyngitis, and impetigo prior to the onset of the rash	Fluid losses Bacteremia Sepsis Mortality <5%	Staphylococcal infection	Topical wound care, emollients, gentle handling, analgesics, antibiotics to cover staphylococcus Corticosteroids are contraindicated, can exacerbate dermatitis
Occasionally arthralgias Mild arthritis	Aplastic crisis in patients with hemoglobinopathies Anemia in immunocompromised patients Nonimmune hydrops fetalis in pregnant woman Myocarditis	Parvovirus B19 Rash occurs 2–5 days after nonspecific symptoms of fever, headache, nausea	Usually none needed Symptomatic treatment of arthralgias and pruritus with NSAIDs and antihistamines, respectively

(continued)

SECTION 15 • SKIN

DIFFERENTIAL DIAGNOSIS *(continued)*

DIAGNOSIS	ICD-10	DISTINGUISHING CHARACTERISTICS	DISTRIBUTION	DURATION, CHRONICITY
Toxic Shock Syndrome	A48.3	Diffuse blanching erythroderma similar to a sunburn, followed by subsequent desquamation	Generalized	Diffuse erythroderma along with hypotension present 24–48 hours after initial symptoms, can be fatal
Measles	B05.9	Nonpruritic, blotchy, erythematous, blanching, maculopapular rash Koplik spots are pathognomonic	Rash progresses in a cephalocaudal manner	Lasts 1–2 weeks
Polymorphous Light Eruption	L56.4	Light-induced, nonscarring, pruritic erythematous eruption	Limited to sun-exposed areas such as the face, posterior neck, and extremities	Eruption resolves in 1–2 weeks if light trigger is avoided

ASSOCIATED FINDINGS	COMPLICATIONS	PREDISPOSING FACTORS	TREATMENT GUIDELINES
Fever, abdominal distress, myalgias, headache, hypotension, multisystem organ involvement	Shock, multiorgan dysfunction	Staphylococcus, Group A streptococcus Tampon use, soft tissue infection, abscess, burn	Immediate treatment in an intensive care setting with fluid resuscitation, antibiotics, and vasopressors Removal of focus of infection (tampons, drainage of abscesses)
Fever, malaise, cough, coryza, conjunctivitis, and Koplik spots (small red lesions on mucous membranes with a white central spot)	Pulmonary involvement Encephalitis	Paramyxovirus	Supportive care Vitamin A
Pruritus	N/A	Most severe at the beginning of the sunny season (spring/early summer) and lessens in severity as the season progresses	Sun avoidance Liberal use of sunscreen Sun-protective clothing Symptom relief with topical steroids and sometimes systemic steroids in severe cases

Other Diagnoses to Consider

- Systemic lupus erythematosus

- Dermatomyositis

- Kawasaki disease

- Infectious mononucleosis

- Porphyrias

- Stevens–Johnson syndrome

- Toxic epidermal necrolysis

- Sézary syndrome, a type of cutaneous T-cell lymphoma

- Omenn syndrome, a form of severe combined immunodeficiency with desquamation

When to Consider Further Evaluation or Treatment

- Avoid sun exposure until the resolution of sunburn or photosensitivity rash. Liberal use of sunscreen with minimum of SPF 30 is encouraged. In those with severe or extensive findings, oral and/or topical steroids may be considered.

- Discontinuation of the causative agent in drug-related eruptions is imperative for resolution of symptoms. Antihistamines and topical steroids can alleviate symptoms.

- Diagnosis of streptococcal pharyngitis and/or scarlet fever warrants treatment with penicillin to reduce infectivity, hasten resolution, and prevent rheumatic fever.

- SSSS usually requires hospitalization for young patients, IV antibiotics, as well as close attention to fluid and electrolyte status because of increased fluid losses seen in this syndrome. The rash requires topical wound care similar to that for thermal burns, including analgesics, emollients, and gentle handling.

- Watch for aplastic crisis in patients with hemoglobinopathies who present with parvovirus B19 infection.

- Prompt recognition of TSS is essential to enable immediate treatment in an intensive care setting with fluid resuscitation, antibiotics, and vasopressors as well as removal of focus of infection (tampons, drainage of abscesses).

SUGGESTED READINGS

Aber C, Connelly EA, Schachner LA. Fever and rash in a child: when to worry? *Pediatr Ann.* 2007;36:30–38.
Aronson PL, Florin TA. Pediatric dermatologic emergencies: a case-based approach for the pediatrician. *Pediatr Ann.* 2009;38:109–116.
Berk DR, Bayliss SJ. MRSA, staphylococcal scalded skin syndrome, and other cutaneous bacterial emergencies. *Pediatr Ann.* 2010;39:627–633.
Grossberg AL. Update on pediatric photosensitivity disorders. *Curr Opin Pediatr.* 2013;25:474–479.
Kress DW. Pediatric dermatology emergencies. *Curr Opin Pediatr.* 2011;23:403–406.
Pacha O, Hebert AA. Pediatric photosensitivity disorders. *Dermatol Clin.* 2013;31:317–326.
Segal AR, Doherty KM, Leggott J, et al. Cutaneous reactions to drugs in children. *Pediatrics.* 2007;120:e1082–e1096.
Seth D, Kamat D, Montejo J. DRESS syndrome: a practical approach for primary care practitioners. *Clin Pediatr.* 2008;47:947–952.

Red Patches and Swellings

Eliza Hayes Bakken and Ellen Laves

Approach to the Problem

The key to successful diagnosis of a red rash or swelling is a careful history and physical examination while keeping a broad list of differential diagnoses in mind. Timing, appearance, and progression of the rash; presence of associated signs and symptoms; and recent exposures and activities aid in identifying the etiology and diagnosis. The distribution, appearance, and feel of the skin are also helpful in determining the etiology.

Key Points in the History

- Lesions that change in location, shape, and size over minutes to hours are likely urticarial. They can be caused by an exposure to a new antigen (detergent, perfume, food), but are more commonly caused by viral infections.

- Cellulitis and erysipelas are characterized by erythema and tender swelling surrounding a break in the skin, and may be accompanied by fever.

- Insect bites can be discrete or clustered and are more frequent on exposed surfaces of the skin. Time spent outdoors, near a pet, or with other similarly affected individuals is suggestive.

- A hemangioma may start off as a flat area of telangiectasia with a surrounding ring of pallor. A hemangioma typically increases in size over the child's first months of life prior to involution.

- Hematoma should be suspected with a suggestive history or whenever there is concern for nonaccidental trauma.

- Contact dermatitis is an allergic hypersensitivity response to an irritant or allergen that is usually limited to the area where the exposure occurred and is frequently pruritic.

- Erythema infectiosum is often accompanied by fever, rhinorrhea, and/or arthralgias.

- Pityriasis rosea presents initially as a single patch (the "herald patch") that evolves into a diffuse macular eruption. It is sometimes pruritic. Systemic symptoms are rare.

- Erythema nodosum often occurs in the setting of infection but can also be due to a wide variety of immunologic and oncologic conditions.

Key Points in the Physical Examination

- Noting whether the patient has multiple, clustered, or discrete lesions can help to narrow the differential diagnosis.

- Urticarial lesions have a wheal and flare appearance that can evolve during examination.

- Cellulitis and erysipelas are typically warm and tender. Erysipelas is raised, with well-defined edges, whereas cellulitis lacks defined edges. The presence of fluctuance suggests an underlying abscess.

- Insect bites frequently have a central punctum with surrounding erythema. If multiple bites are present, they are usually grouped rather than randomly scattered.

- A subtle cluster of blanching telangiectasias with a ring of pallor is suggestive of an early hemangioma. They later develop into nonblanching cherry red macules or papules. Bluish discoloration suggests deeper involvement.

- Hematomas may vary in size, shape, and distribution. They are usually tender and not well demarcated. They may change in color from reddish to shades of purple, blue, and green over time.

- Contact dermatitis may present as papular, papulovesicular, or eczematous lesions. Location may implicate the offending stimulus.

- Erythema infectiosum is suggested by a nontender "slapped cheek" erythema, which spares the nasal bridge and periorbital areas, and is typically associated with a lacy or reticular rash that may be seen on the trunk and the extremities.

- Pityriasis rosea initially presents as a pink, scaly, oval patch, followed by the eruption of oval macules with a collarette of scale. Pityriasis rosea often has a "Christmas-tree" distribution, with lesions following skin cleavage lines (Langer lines).

- Erythema nodosum is characterized by tender, raised, reddish blue lesions found on the shins. These lesions may also appear on the buttocks, calves, ankles, thighs, and arms.

PHOTOGRAPHS OF SELECTED DIAGNOSES

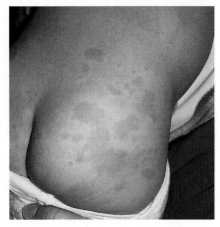

Figure 64-1 Urticaria. Erythematous wheals on buttocks of child. (Courtesy of George A. Datto, III, MD.)

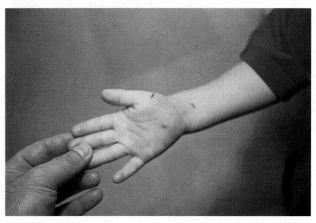

Figure 64-2 Cellulitis. Poorly defined erythematous lesion on hand that developed after skin abrasion. (Courtesy of George A. Datto, III, MD.)

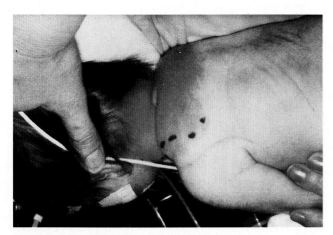

Figure 64-3 Erysipelas. Very erythematous rash on neck with sharply demarcated borders. (Courtesy of George A. Datto, III, MD.)

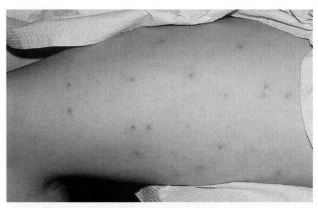

Figure 64-4 Insect bites. These fleabites are grouped in a characteristic nonfollicular, "breakfast, lunch, and dinner" pattern. (Used with permission from Goodheart HP, MD. *Goodheart's Photoguide of Common Skin Disorders.* 2nd ed. Philadelphia, PA: Lippincott Williams & Wilkins; 2003.)

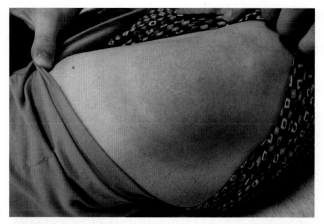

Figure 64-5 Erythema chronicum migrans. Note the central punctum following a tick bite and the ring-like appearance (Courtesy of Paul S. Matz, MD.)

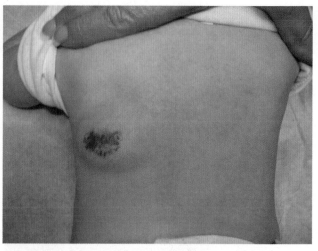

Figure 64-6 Mixed hemangiomas. (Used with permission from Stedman's.)

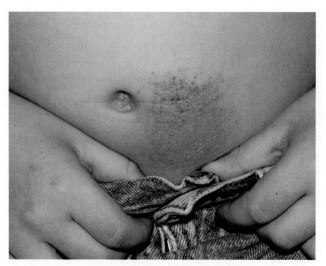

Figure 64-7 Allergic contact dermatitis. This boy developed an eczematous eruption at the site where the nickel snap on his blue jeans contacted his skin. (Used with permission from Goodheart HP, MD. *Goodheart's Photoguide of Common Skin Disorders.* 2nd ed. Philadelphia, PA: Lippincott Williams & Wilkins; 2003.)

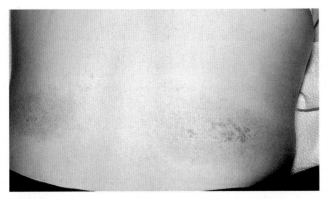

Figure 64-8 Allergic contact dermatitis. This patient reacted to the rubber in the elastic waistband of her underpants. Note sparing at the sites where the garment did not come into constant contact with the skin. (Used with permission from Goodheart HP, MD. *Goodheart's Photoguide of Common Skin Disorders.* 2nd ed. Philadelphia, PA: Lippincott Williams & Wilkins; 2003.)

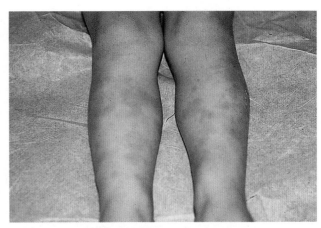

Figure 64-9 Erythema nodosum. Tender erythematous nodules on extensor aspects of lower legs. (Courtesy of George A. Datto, III, MD.)

DIFFERENTIAL DIAGNOSIS

DIAGNOSIS		ICD-10	DISTINGUISHING CHARACTERISTICS	DISTRIBUTION	DURATION/ CHRONICITY
Urticaria		Allergic: L50.0 Idiopathic: L50.1 Unspecified: L50.9	Evanescent, erythematous wheals with surrounding flare	Localized or diffuse	Usually acute in onset and quickly resolving. On occasion can be a chronic condition
Cellulitis		Digit: L03.0 Limb: L03.1 Face: L03.2 Trunk: L03.3 Other sites: L03.8 Unspecified: L03.9	Warm, tender, erythematous lesion without well-demarcated borders	Often occurs at site of trauma/insect bite	Resolving, nonchronic condition, if treated by appropriate antibiotics
Erysipelas		A46	Raised, tender, erythematous lesion with well-demarcated borders	May occur anywhere on the body	Resolving, nonchronic condition if treated by appropriate antibiotics
Insect Bite		T63.4	Pruritic, raised, warm lesion with central punctum	Anywhere, but typically exposed areas	Nonchronic condition
Erythema Chronicum Migrans		A69.20	Bull's eye lesion with central clearing and erythematous borders May see expanding ring lesion	Solitary Multiple lesions with disseminated Lyme disease	Lesion(s) typically resolve(s) following antibiotic therapy
Hemangioma		D18.0	Raised, nontender, erythematous or bluish lesions with surrounding pallor	Head and neck Trunk Extremities Internal organs	50% have involuted by age 5 years, 70% by age 7 years, and 90% by age 9 years
Hematoma		T14.0	Tender, well-demarcated lesions that change color to purple, blue, and green over time	Can occur anywhere on the body	Self-resolving nonchronic lesions

ASSOCIATED FINDINGS	COMPLICATIONS	PREDISPOSING FACTORS	TREATMENT GUIDELINES
Angioedema Pruritus	Respiratory distress, angioedema, hypotension, diarrhea, or vomiting (suggests anaphylaxis)	Food Drugs Infections (often viral) Physical factors	First-line treatment: antihistamines Anaphylaxis: epinephrine
Fever, chills, malaise, pain, warmth	Abscess Lymphangitis Lymphadenitis Sepsis Osteomyelitis Bacteremia	Skin trauma, including lacerations, abrasions, insect bites and other puncture wounds Immunocompromise	Antibiotics covering streptococci and staphylococci. If pustules or abscesses are present, cover for methicillin-resistant *Staphylococcus aureus*
Fever, chills, malaise, pain, warmth	Abscess Bacteremia Streptococcal toxic Shock syndrome Arthritis Lymphadenitis	Diabetes mellitus Immunocompromise Nephrotic syndrome Streptococcal infection	Antibiotics covering group A streptococci. Staphylococci infection is less common
Pruritus	Cellulitis Consider exposure to venomous spider if patient has other systemic signs/symptoms	Time spent outdoors at dusk or dawn, and/or near water Exposure to flea-infested animals	Oral antihistamines Topical corticosteroids
Fever Myalgias Arthralgias Arthritis Pain Pruritus	Arrhythmia Meningitis Cranial neuropathies Carditis	Ixodes (deer) tick bite and infection with the spirochete, *Borrelia burgdorferi*	Antibiotic therapy Appropriate antibiotic therapy should be initiated
Multiple superficial lesions may be associated with internal hemangiomas	Visual problems Airway compromise Ulceration Disfigurement Kasabach–Merritt syndrome	Generally nonhereditary but 10% of patients have a positive family history of such lesions	Generally conservative Dermatology referral if on face, if multiple lesions present Consider abdominal ultrasound if multiple lesions present
Fracture can be present	N/A	Trauma	Supportive care X-ray if concern for fracture

Other Diagnoses to Consider

- Erythema multiforme

- Stevens–Johnsons syndrome

- Dermatographia

- Tinea cruris

- Tinea corporis

- Rubeola

- Langerhans cell histiocytosis

When to Consider Further Evaluation or Treatment

- Urticaria with another sign of anaphylaxis (angioedema, wheezing, hypotension, or vomiting) warrants emergent epinephrine administration. Urticaria after exposure to a new food or medication may represent an allergy. Recommend future avoidance of the offending agent.

- Cellulitis that does not improve within 72 hours of starting systemic antibiotics should be reevaluated. Consider broader spectrum antibiotics or admission for intravenous antibiotics and observation. Abscesses often require incision and drainage.

- Insect bites that are associated with other systemic symptoms should prompt additional workup and treatment for superinfection or anaphylaxis. If concern for venomous spider bite, prompt hospitalization and possible antivenom administration are indicated.

- Hemangiomas on the face should prompt a referral to a pediatric dermatologist as treatment may be indicated to prevent disfigurement. Hemangiomas near the eye can obstruct vision and lead to amblyopia. The presence of a very large hemangioma or multiple hemangiomas should raise suspicion for a genetic syndrome and/or internal lesions as seen with hemangiomatosis.

- Large hematomas may overlie boney fractures. Multiple hematomas, especially in unusual sites should prompt consideration of child physical abuse.

SUGGESTED READINGS

Bisno A. Current concepts: streptococcal infections of the skin and soft tissues. *N Engl J Med.* 1996;334(4):240–245.

Hartzell LD, Buckmiller LM. Current management of infantile hemangiomas and their common associated conditions. *Otolaryngol Clin N Am.* 2012;45(3):545–556.

Kakourou T, Drosatou P, Psychou F, et al. Erythema nodosum in children: a prospective study. *J Am Acad Dermatol.* 2001;44(1):17–21.

Kelly BP. Superficial fungal infections. *Pediatr Rev.* 2012;33(4):e22–e37.

Khangura S, Wallace J, Kissoon N, et al. Management of cellulitis in a pediatric emergency department. *Pediatr Emerg Care.* 2007;23:805–811.

Scott LA, Stone MS. Viral exanthems. *Dermatol Online J.* 2003;9(3):4.

Sicherer S, Leung D. Advances in allergic skin disease, anaphylaxis, and hypersensitivity reactions to foods, drugs and insects in 2007. *J Allergy Clin Immunol.* 2008;121:1351–1358.

Linear Red Rashes

Liana K. McCabe

Approach to the Problem

The pattern of a rash can be quite helpful in identifying its etiology. Linear patterns of rashes may be seen in many conditions. In particular, linear red rashes are commonly seen in infectious and inflammatory conditions. They may also be the result of other systemic processes.

Key Points in the History

- A linear red rash that develops after outdoor activity should raise the suspicion of rhus dermatitis due to the exposure to poison ivy, oak, or sumac.

- Rhus dermatitis, scabies, and cutaneous larva migrans are intensely pruritic lesions.

- Children with scabies may have a close contact, who also has an itchy rash. It is helpful to inquire if the parent or another household contact also has a rash, particularly if they share a sleeping surface or bed with the child.

- Lichen striatus may start as a small area of papules that then spreads into a linear distribution.

- Lichen striatus is twice as common in girls than in boys.

- Outdoor exposure to soil or sand that is shared with dogs or cats (e.g., sandboxes) is often a predisposing factor in patients affected with cutaneous larva migrans.

- Linear epidermal nevus, which is not typically pruritic, appears at birth or shortly thereafter.

- Lymphangitis is the secondary manifestation of infection at a distal site. Systemic symptoms of fever, chills, and malaise are often present.

Key Points in the Physical Examination

- Rhus dermatitis is seen on exposed skin, particularly the areas that were exposed while outdoors.

- Excoriation surrounding a linear rash suggests pruritus and scratching, which may lead to bacterial superinfection.

- Red rashes may not be as apparent in individuals with darker skin; therefore, it is important to assess patients in adequate lighting.

- Lichen striatus may appear to be mildly hypopigmented or flesh-colored.

- Infants with scabies often have a generalized rash that includes the soles of their feet. In young children, the rash of scabies is typically seen in the axilla and groin. Older children will often have lesions in the web spaces of their fingers and toes.

- An advancing serpiginous eruption in the skin that is intensely pruritic is virtually pathognomonic for cutaneous larva migrans.

- The Koebner phenomenon is commonly seen in linear rashes such as rhus dermatitis, linear psoriasis, and lichen planus.

PHOTOGRAPHS OF SELECTED DIAGNOSES

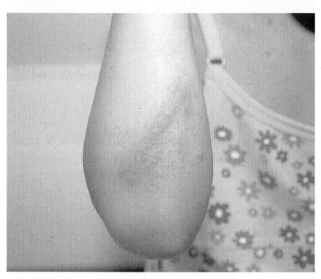

Figure 65-1 Rhus dermatitis. Linear papules and vesicles following exposure to poison ivy. (Courtesy of George A. Datto, III, MD.)

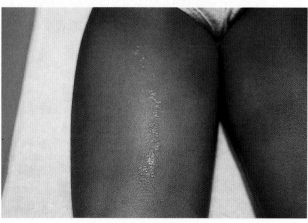

Figure 65-2 Lichen striatus. Small, shiny, hypopigmented papules in a linear distribution on the posterior thigh. (Courtesy of George A. Datto, III, MD.)

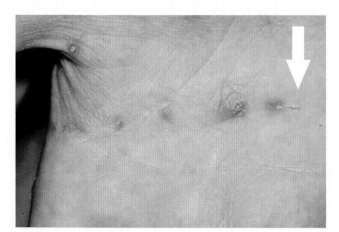

Figure 65-3 Scabies. This close-up view shows a burrow (*arrow*) on the palm. (From Goodheart HP, MD. *Goodheart's Photoguide of Common Skin Disorders.* 2nd ed. Philadelphia, PA: Lippincott Williams & Wilkins; 2003.)

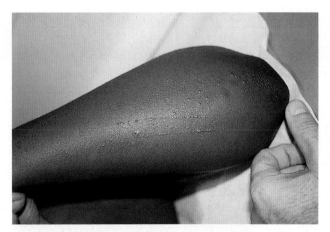

Figure 65-4 Koebner phenomenon. Papulovesicular eruption in a linear distribution on the forearm of a child with an Id reaction (autosensitization dermatitis) associated with tinea capitis. (Courtesy of George A. Datto, III, MD.)

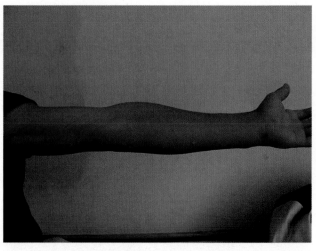

Figure 65-5 Lymphangitis. Linear red streak proximal to skin infection. (Courtesy of Paul S. Matz, MD.)

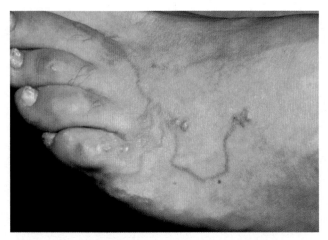

Figure 65-6 Cutaneous larva migrans. Serpiginous red streaks on sole of foot. (Used with permission from Goodheart HP. *Goodheart's Photoguide of Common Skin Disorders.* 2nd ed. Philadelphia, PA: Lippincott Williams & Wilkins; 2003:315.)

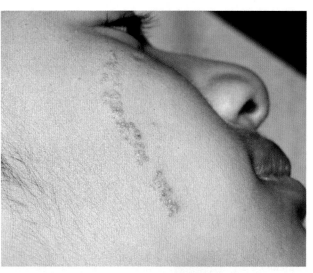

Figure 65-7 Linear epidermal nevus. Warty, linear lesions on face. (Used with permission from Goodheart HP. *Goodheart's Photoguide of Common Skin Disorders.* 2nd ed. Philadelphia, PA: Lippincott Williams & Wilkins; 2003:9.)

DIFFERENTIAL DIAGNOSIS

DIAGNOSIS		ICD-10	DISTINGUISHING CHARACTERISTICS	DISTRIBUTION	DURATION/ CHRONICITY
Rhus Dermatitis		L24.7	Multiple types of lesions, including papules, vesicles, or bullae with straw-colored fluid inside that are pruritic	Often on arms and legs or other exposed surfaces of the skin May be transmitted to other sites by scratching	Acute but may persist for weeks
Scabies		B86	Linear burrows with adjacent papules Often seen are areas of excoriation due to the intense pruritus	Infant—lesions are often generalized to the entire body. Toddler—lesions may be pronounced in the axilla and groin. Children—lesions often seen specifically within the webs of fingers and toes.	Acute, but itching and rash may persist for 1–2 weeks after treatment
Lichen Striatus		L44.2	Flat-topped papules in unilateral streaks and swirls Overlying dusky scale with mild erythema	Along lines of Blaschko Usually on extremities, upper back, or neck	Chronic
Koebner Phenomenon		L30.9 Dermatitis, unspecified	Raised papulovesicular lesion at sites of trauma or irritation	Tend to be linear due to scratching or brushing against offending agent	Chronic waxing and waning presentation
Lymphangitis		I89.1	Warm, painful, erythematous streak(s) that extends proximal to an injury or infection	Usually proximal to site of infection along the lymphatic drainage lines	Acute
Cutaneous Larva Migrans		B76.9	Erythematous, tortuous or serpent-like lesions that may progress Larvae migrate at about 1–2 cm per day Occasional bullae	Often found on the lower extremities or hands	Chronic, lasting weeks to months
Linear Epidermal Nevus		D23.9	Linear papules that appear smooth and then may become wart-like or scaly	May occur on any part of the body, but commonly found on the face, trunk, or extremities	Chronic

ASSOCIATED FINDINGS	COMPLICATIONS	PREDISPOSING FACTORS	TREATMENT GUIDELINES
Pruritus Koebner phenomen on (new lesions develop after trauma) Edema	Bacterial superinfection	Contact with poison oak, ivy, or sumac Indirect contact with clothing, pets that brushed against plant, or smoke from burning plant	Antihistamine for itch Topical or systemic corticosteroids
Intense pruritus Other family members with similar symptoms	Bacterial superinfection	*Sarcoptes scabiei*	5% permethrin cream for patients >2 months Oral antihistamines and topical steroids may be used to treat symptoms.
Hypopigmentation may be associated Asymptomatic	None	Unclear cause May be triggered by viral infection	Fades without treatment in 1–2 years Lubricants and topical steroids may decrease scale and inflammation.
Seen in rhus dermatitis, psoriasis, pityriasis rubra pilaris, lichen nitidus	None	Variety of underlying conditions	Treat the underlying diagnosis
Local lymphadenopathy Fever	Bacteremia Sepsis	Infection due to: *Staphylococcus aureus* Group A streptococcus	Culture Antibiotic active against gram-positive organisms Some cases of nodular lymphangitis may require surgical debridement.
Local lymph nodes are enlarged and tender. Pruritus	N/A	Most commonly caused by dog/cat hookworm, *Ancyclostoma braziliense*	If untreated, larvae will die in a few months. Topical antifungals will hasten treatment
Most lesions appear at birth, and 95% present by 7 years of age	Cosmetic concern	N/A	Topical retinoids or keratolytics May be excised or ablated with laser therapy.

Other Diagnoses to Consider

- Striae

- Contact dermatitis

- Linear psoriasis

- Linear morphea (localized scleroderma)

When to Consider Further Evaluation or Treatment

- Rhus dermatitis may be treated with systemic corticosteroids when severe or extensive in distribution. If systemic steroids are used, start with a 48-hour course of steroids, followed by a 2- to 3-week taper.

- Scabies should be treated with 5% permethrin if the patient is older than 2 months. The lotion should be applied from head to toe, and then washed off 8 to 14 hours later. Treatment may need to be repeated 1 week later if symptoms worsen. Treatment is recommended for all household contacts, when possible.

- Resistant scabies is increasing in prevalence; therefore, if there is no improvement after two treatments with permethrin, another treatment such as ivermectin, precipitated sulphur, or benzyl benzoate should be considered.

- For scabies, all bedding, clothing, towels and stuffed animals that the person has touched during the 3 days prior to treatment should be laundered in a washer with hot water. Mites do not survive more than 3 days in the absence of skin contact, so items that cannot be washed can be placed in a plastic bag for at least 3 days.

- Itching associated with scabies may last for several weeks after mites are eliminated. Steroid creams or oral steroids may be necessary if itching is severe.

- If desired by the patient for cosmetic reasons, linear epidermal nevus may be treated with topical retinoids or keratolytics. If these agents are unsuccessful, the lesion can be excised or ablated by laser therapy.

- If lymphangitis is suspected, appropriate antibiotic coverage should be initiated and the source of infection should be investigated.

SUGGESTED READINGS

American Academy of Pediatrics. *Red Book: 2012 Report of the Committee on Infectious Diseases.* In: Pickering LK, ed. 29th ed. Elk Grove Village, IL: American Academy of Pediatrics; 2012:298–299, 641–643.

Cohen BA. *Pediatric Dermatology.* 3rd ed. Baltimore, MD: Elsevier Mosby; 2005.

Goodheart HP. *Goodheart's Photoguide to Common Skin Disorders.* 3rd ed. Philadelphia, PA: Lippincott Williams & Wilkins; 2008:11, 361–362.

Paller AS, Mancini AJ, eds. *Hurwitz Clinical Pediatric Dermatology: A Textbook of Skin Disorders of Childhood and Adolescence.* 4th ed. Philadelphia, PA: Elsevier Saunders; 2011.

Weston WL, Lane AT, Morelli JG. eds. *Color Textbook of Pediatric Dermatology.* 4th ed. St. Louis, MO: Mosby; 2007.

Zitelli BJ, McIntire SC, Nowalk AJ. eds. *Zitelli and Davis's Atlas of Pediatric Physical Diagnosis.* 6th ed. Philadelphia, PA: Mosby; 2012.

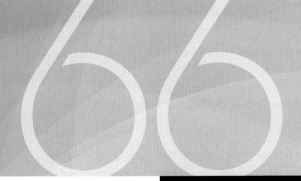

Focal Red Bumps

Ilse A. Larson

Approach to the Problem

Focal red bumps are common in pediatric patients. Etiologies include self-limited, benign diagnoses such as insect bites and erythema toxicum neonatorum; more serious infectious causes like furuncles, carbuncles, abscesses, and cat-scratch disease; and tumors including hemangiomas, pyogenic granulomas, and Spitz nevi.

Key Points in the History

- Erythema toxicum neonatorum is a common, self-resolving rash seen in newborns with onset in the first 24 to 48 hours of life.

- Insect bites may not have a known exposure. Household members may be affected differently, with younger patients experiencing more pronounced local reactions.

- Furuncles, carbuncles, and abscesses are more common in patients and families with a history of recurrent skin infections and/or methicillin-resistant *Staphylococcus aureus* (MRSA) colonization.

- Hemangiomas typically arise between 2 and 4 weeks of age, but may have a precursor lesion that is sometimes detected at birth.

- Hemangiomas have a phase of rapid growth beginning at 4 to 8 weeks of age and continued expansion through 6 to 9 months of age. This is followed by slowed growth and eventual involution beginning in the second year of life. Hemangiomas typically completely involute by age 7 to 9.

- Pyogenic granulomas tend to grow rapidly and bleed easily. They typically arise later in childhood than hemangiomas.

Key Points in the Physical Examination

- Erythema toxicum neonatorum may appear as isolated lesions that resemble flea bites or as coalescent lesions.

- Insect bites, particularly mosquito bites, tend to have induration that is particularly apparent the day after the insect bite. A central punctum can help to distinguish an insect bite from other swelling.

SECTION 15 • SKIN

535

- A furuncle is a deep bacterial folliculitis. Confluence of several adjacent furuncles can create a carbuncle, which can become further organized into a walled-off abscess. These lesions are all typically tender and warm.

- Although pyogenic granulomas can resemble hemangiomas, only the former exhibit a hypopigmented collarette.

- Stroking a mastocytoma can result in formation of a wheal with swelling and itchiness that occurs within minutes, Darier sign. Patients with mastocytomas may also have dermatographism of unaffected skin.

- The papules associated with cat-scratch disease are oftentimes less pronounced than the accompanying regional lymphadenopathy, which is typically tender and erythematous.

PHOTOGRAPHS OF SELECTED DIAGNOSES

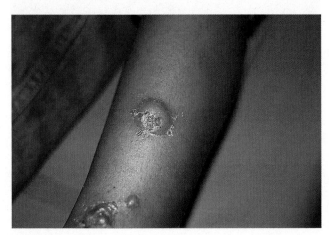

Figure 66-1 **Insect bite.** This insect bite occurred during summer. Note the vesicular reaction. (Courtesy of George A. Datto, III, MD.)

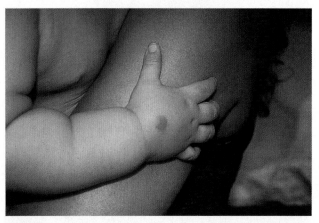

Figure 66-2 **Insect bite.** Erythematous wheal on dorsum of hand. (Courtesy of George A. Datto, III, MD.)

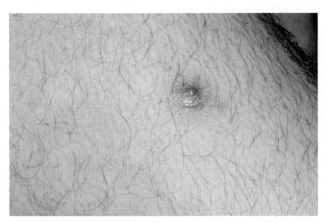

Figure 66-3 **Furuncle.** Painful, red nodule with central pustule. (Used with permission from Goodheart HP. *Goodheart's Photoguide of Common Skin Disorders.* 2nd ed. Philadelphia, PA: Lippincott Williams & Wilkins; 2003:126.)

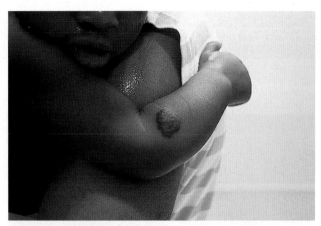

Figure 66-4 Hemangioma on the forearm of an infant with darkly pigmented skin. The lesion appears more purple in color than red.
(Courtesy of George A. Datto, III, MD.)

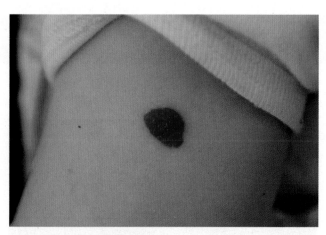

Figure 66-5 Hemangioma. Note the distinct borders and deep red color.
(Courtesy of Susan A. Fisher-Owens, MD, MPH.)

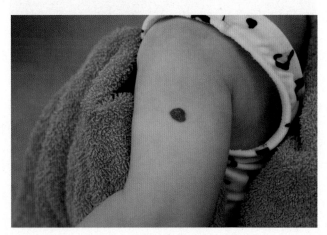

Figure 66-6 Involuting hemangioma. Note the central gray discoloration as the hemangioma begins to involute.
(Courtesy of Susan A. Fisher-Owens, MD, MPH.)

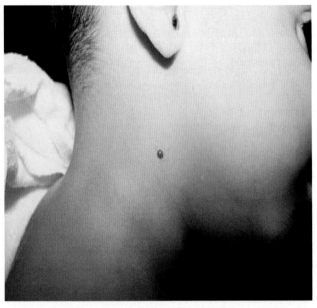

Figure 66-7 **Pyogenic granuloma.** Vascular lesion with surrounding collarette. (Courtesy of Kathleen Cronan, MD.)

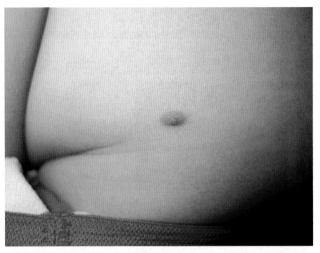

Figure 66-8 **Spitz Nevus.** (Used with permission from Stedman's.)

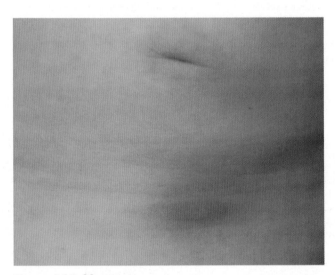

Figure 66-9 **Mastocytoma.** (Used with permission from Stedman's.)

DIFFERENTIAL DIAGNOSIS

DIAGNOSIS		ICD-10	DISTINGUISHING CHARACTERISTICS	DISTRIBUTION
Erythema Toxicum Neonatorum		P83.1	Most common in term infants (up to 50% of term infants) Erythematous lesions with central papule	Anywhere, but usually spares palms and soles
Insect Bites		T63.4	Oftentimes pruritic, erythematous, and warm Usually nontender May have central punctum Flea and bedbug bites tend to be in clusters—"breakfast, lunch, and dinner"	Most commonly found on exposed areas
Furuncle/Carbuncle		L02.9	Warm, swollen, tender nodule with central ulceration, may have purulent discharge	Hair-bearing areas, follicular distribution
Abscess		L02.9	Warm, swollen, tender	Frequently on buttocks or trunk
Hemangioma		D18.0	Superficial hemangiomas are erythematous with well-defined borders Deep hemangiomas have a blue hue and ill-defined borders Arise between 2 and 4 weeks of age	Anywhere, but commonly on head, neck, or trunk
Pyogenic Granuloma		L98.0	Benign vascular tumor, bright red, can be pedunculated, often has collarette of hypopigmentation Grows rapidly Bleeds easily	Most common on hands, fingers, or face
Spitz Nevus		D22.9	Solitary pink-red nodule, sharply circumscribed and dome-shaped	Usually on face
Mastocytoma		D47.9	Red or red-brown macular lesion, which can become tense and raised with stroking, Darier sign May occur as an isolated lesion or as multiple lesions as with mastocytosis	Typically on trunk
Cat-Scratch Disease		078.3	Raised erythematous papule(s) at the site of the scratch, develops 3–10 days after inoculation	Exposed skin

DURATION/ CHRONICITY	ASSOCIATED FINDINGS	PREDISPOSING FACTORS	TREATMENT GUIDELINES
Starts at 24 to 48 hours of life and can last 1 to 2 weeks	Eosinophils are present in the fluid from an unroofed lesion and on biopsy.	None	None, lesions self-resolve within first 2 weeks of life
Acute presentation	Can be associated with papular urticaria—a delayed hypersensitivity reaction involving pruritic erythematous papules arranged in clusters May be associated with transmission of insect-borne illnesses	Exposure, especially outdoors	Cool compresses, topical antihistamines, topical corticosteroids, or systemic antihistamines for pruritus Avoidance of causative insect
Acute presentation; occasionally recurrent lesions occur in hair-bearing areas	None	Skin trauma MRSA colonization	Incision and drainage ± antibiotics
Acute onset Occasionally recurrent	Can be associated with fever	Skin trauma MRSA colonization	Incision and drainage ± antibiotics
Chronic, appears shortly after birth, slowly grows in first 6–12 months and slowly involutes, with resolution in most cases by 2–4 years of age	Complications include ulceration and subsequent superinfection	Male: female ratio 1:2 More common in preterm or very-low-birth weight infants	Observation Refer for treatment if location is periorbital, in the "beard distribution," midline over the lumbosacral spine or scalp, in the diaper area or in other areas prone to friction. Treatment options include topical or systemic beta-blockers, oral corticosteroids, or pulsed dye laser.
Acute to chronic in presentation Lasts weeks to months	Bleeding may be a complication.	Can be triggered by trauma or medications Most common in school-aged children	Refer to dermatology. Excision by cauterization or laser therapy
Grows over 3–6 months; then stabilizes	May have overlying telangiectasia	None	Refer to dermatology for definitive diagnosis if resembles a melanoma Otherwise, conservative management
May present at birth or develop by 1–2 months of age Oftentimes, persists	Often associated with dermatographism of uninvolved skin Manipulation of the lesion or drug exposure (to opiates, polymyxin B or acetylsalicylic acid) can cause massive histamine release, leading to flushing, tachycardia, hypotension, wheezing, syncope, diarrhea, or vomiting	None	For solitary lesions, typically no treatment is necessary. For children with systemic symptoms, can treat with hydroxyzine or UV phototherapy. Refer to dermatology if concerns for mastocytosis.
Develops 3–10 days after inoculation	Painful, erythematous regional lymphadenopathy May be associated with fever, fatigue, headache, and other systemic symptoms	Exposure to cats, although inoculation can also come from splinters, thorns, or dog scratches	Most cases spontaneously resolve. Antibiotics can be used in severe cases.

Other Diagnoses to Consider

- PHACES syndrome (posterior fossa malformations, hemangiomas, arterial anomalies, cardiac defects, eye anomalies, and sternal clefting)

- Kasabach–Merritt syndrome

- Traumatic hematoma

- Nonaccidental trauma

- Erythema nodosum

- Panniculitis

- Impetigo

- Allergic/contact dermatitis

- Acne

When to Consider Further Evaluation and Treatment

- Patients with recurrent furuncles, carbuncles, or abscesses may benefit from pharmacologic MRSA eradication. These patients may also warrant evaluation for an underlying immunodeficiency.

- Hemangiomas that are near the eye, in the beard distribution, in the diaper area, midline on the scalp, or over the spine should be evaluated by a dermatologist.

- Spitz nevi can resemble melanoma; consider referral to a dermatologist for definitive diagnosis, given the need for prompt treatment of the latter condition.

- Patients with multiple mastocytomas, mastocytosis, or systemic symptoms resulting from manipulation of their lesions should be referred to a dermatologist for further evaluation.

SUGGESTED READINGS

Briley LD, Phillips CM. Cutaneous mastocytoma: a review focusing on the pediatric population. *Clin Pediatr.* 2008;47:757–761.
Chen TS, Eichenfield LF, Friedlander ST. *Infantile hemangiomas: an update on pathogenesis and therapy. Pediatrics.* 2013;131:99–108.
Eichenfield LF, Friedan IL, Esterly NB, eds. *Neonatal Dermatology.* 2nd ed. Philadelphia, PA: Elsevier; 2008:91.
Weston WL, Lane AT, Morelli JG. *Color Textbook of Pediatric Dermatology.* 4th ed. Philadelphia, PA: Mosby; 2007:73–74, 227, 237–255.

Raised Red Rashes

Kathleen Cronan
and Lee R. Atkinson-McEvoy

Approach to the Problem

Raised red rashes are common in pediatrics and can be concerning to parents and practitioners. The majority of raised red rashes, however, are not indicative of serious illness. Many red rashes have associated symptoms that may be helpful in making a final diagnosis. For example, symptoms of fatigue, fever, and lymphadenopathy suggest infectious mononucleosis. Complications can occur in some individuals with certain red rashes. For example, exposure of a pregnant woman to parvovirus may place her fetus at risk. At times, typical eruptions may not follow a predicted pattern—the distribution may be atypical, the season may not fit, or the age may be unusual. These diagnostic challenges emphasize the importance of a detailed history and astute observation.

Key Points in the History

- High fever for 3 to 5 days followed by acute defervescence that precedes the rash eruption is characteristic of roseola.

- Classic characteristics in the history aid in the diagnosis. For example, a history of "slapped cheeks" indicates Fifth disease; the presence of Koplik spots (clustered white papules in the buccal mucosa opposite the second molars) denotes measles.

- Individuals acutely affected by infectious mononucleosis are at risk for rash development following exposure to penicillins; however, those with infectious mononucleosis may also develop a rash in the absence of penicillin exposure.

- Antibiotic exposure is associated with a drug rash and erythema multiforme.

- Pruritus is typical in erythema multiforme, varicella, hot tub folliculitis, and scabies.

- Seasonal occurrence can provide clues to the diagnosis: late summer and fall would be the season for coxsackievirus, for example; spring and fall is when erythema multiforme, for example, may be seen.

- Family members with a similar rash may suggest scabies.

- The location of rash origin is important. For example, a red rash that begins on the scalp and travels downward is characteristic of measles.

- Erythema may be more apparent in light-skinned children.

- The size and types of papules may support specific diagnoses: fine micropapules indicate scarlet fever; target lesions denote erythema multiforme.

- Papules and vesicles in combination may indicate scabies or impetigo.

- The color of the lesions aids in the diagnosis of the rash: rose-pink lesions are seen in roseola; red maculopapular lesions, in measles; and brownish lesions on the palms and soles, in syphilis.

- Red lesions on the palms and soles are present in syphilis, measles, erythema multiforme, scabies, and Gianotti–Crosti syndrome.

- Symmetric lesions may be noted in erythema multiforme, syphilis, and Gianotti–Crosti syndrome.

- Diffuse mucosal inflammation (i.e., urethritis, conjunctivitis, pharyngitis) is seen in Kawasaki disease.

- There are often oral mucous membrane findings in infectious mononucleosis, erythema multiforme, roseola, Kawasaki disease, and measles.

- Conjunctivitis is seen in Kawasaki disease and measles.

- In syphilis, the rash follows lines of cleavage.

- Periorbital edema is associated with roseola and infectious mononucleosis.

- Measles presents with Koplik spots (gray-white papules) on the buccal mucosa and dark red macules and papules that start on the head and spread caudally.

PHOTOGRAPHS OF SELECTED DIAGNOSES

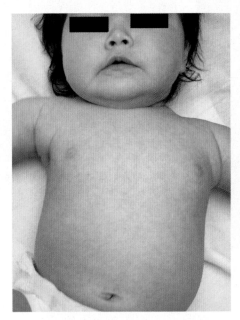

Figure 67-1 Roseola. Rose pink-colored rash on the trunk of an infant. (Courtesy of John Loiselle, MD.)

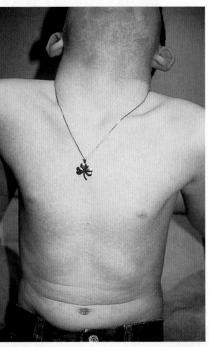

Figure 67-2 Scarlet fever. Fine, sandpapery rash on the trunk and neck. (Courtesy of George A. Datto, III, MD.)

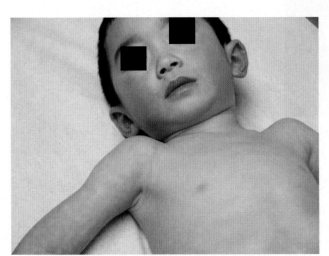

Figure 67-3 Erythema infectiosum. Erythematous "slapped" cheeks along with erythematous rash on extensor surfaces of arms. (Courtesy of Philip Siu, MD.)

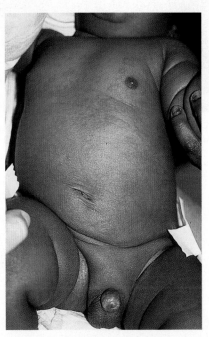

Figure 67-4 Kawasaki disease. Erythematous maculopapular rash that started in the groin and spread onto the trunk. (Courtesy of George A. Datto, III, MD.)

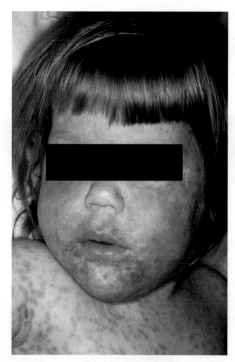

Figure 67-5 Infectious mononucleosis. (Courtesy of Kathleen Cronan, MD.)

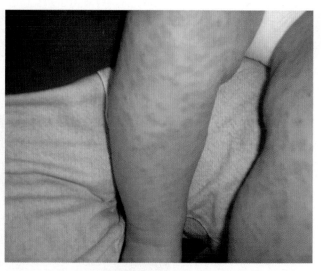

Figure 67-6 **Gianotti–Crosti syndrome.** Note the reddish-brown papular lesions on the extremities. (Courtesy of John Loiselle, MD.)

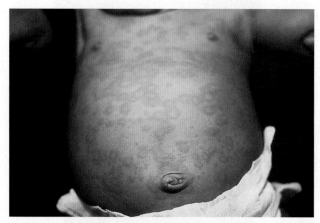

Figure 67-7 **Erythema multiforme.** Target-shaped lesions in an infant. (Courtesy of George A. Datto, III, MD.)

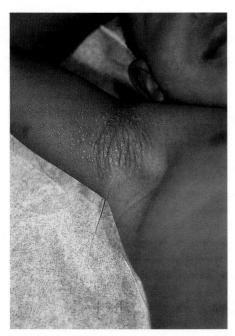

Figure 67-8 **Scabies.** Note the lesions in the axilla of a child. (Courtesy of George A. Datto, III, MD.)

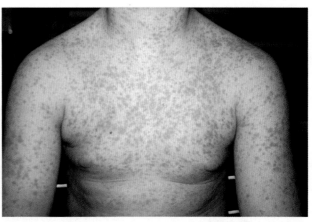

Figure 67-9 **Measles.** Lesions typically start on the head and travel downward. (Courtesy of Kathleen Cronan, MD.)

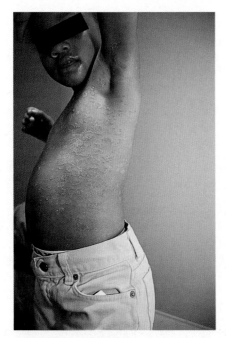

Figure 67-10 **Unilateral laterothoracic exanthem.** Pink, scaly rash involving the axilla and trunk on the right side of this child. (Courtesy of George A. Datto, III, MD.)

DIFFERENTIAL DIAGNOSIS

DIAGNOSIS		ICD-10	DISTINGUISHING CHARACTERISTICS	DISTRIBUTION	DURATION/ CHRONICITY
Roseola		B08.20	Rose-pink lesions that blanch with pressure Rarely coalesce <2 years of age	Trunk Extremities Neck Face	Brief Self-limited
Scarlet Fever		A38.9	Erythematous rash that blanches with pressure Generalized sandpaper rash that may or may not be pruritic Desquamation on hands and feet School age	Begins in axillae and groin, then generalizes Often seen on the face and neck areas	Brief Self-limited
Erythema Infectiosum (Fifth Disease)		B08.3	Three stages: • Erythematous blush "Slapped cheeks" appearance • Lacy reticulated pattern eruption on the trunk and extensor surfaces of the extremities • Waxing and waning of rash over 1–3 weeks	Face Extremities Trunk Proximal extremities	Brief Self-limited
Kawasaki Disease		M30.3	Maculopapular to morbilliform rash Generally less than age 6 but cases of children older than 9 years described	Often starts in groin	Can last from days to weeks
Infectious Mononucleosis		B27.80	Macular or maculopapular, morbilliform eruption Exanthem occurs in 5%–10% of patients Older children and adolescents	Trunk Upper arms Face Forearms Thighs	Brief Self-limited
Gianotti–Crosti Syndrome		L44.4	Monomorphous red to red-brown papules 1–6 years of age	Begins on extensor surfaces of legs and arms Buttocks Cheeks Symmetric distribution	Lasts 8–12 weeks
Erythema Multiforme		L51.9	Papules that develop into erythematous rings with papules or vesicles that evolve into a dusky clearing in the center (target lesion)	Trunk, face, neck, palms, soles, dorsal hands, and feet; extensor surfaces of arms and legs Symmetric distribution Oral lesions—buccal mucosa	Usually lasts 2–3 weeks
Scabies		B86	Papules, pustules, vesicles, and even nodules in some cases Linear burrows	Infants—trunk, palms, soles, neck, face Older children—flexural areas, interdigital spaces, wrists, axillae	Can last several weeks

ASSOCIATED FINDINGS	COMPLICATIONS	PREDISPOSING FACTORS	TREATMENT GUIDELINES
Rash preceded by high fever Periorbital edema Leukopenia Bulging fontanelle	Febrile seizures	Human herpes virus 6 or 7	None needed
Fever, malaise, sore throat, palatal petechiae, abdominal pain, tonsillopharyngitis, strawberry tongue Perioral pallor Pastia lines Tender anterior cervical adenopathy	Glomerulonephritis Rheumatic fever	Group A beta-hemolytic streptococcus (GABHS)	Treat with penicillin for 10 days (consider clindamycin or erythromycin in penicillin allergic patient)
Low-grade fever Aches and pains Mild arthritis Arthralgia	Red-cell aplasia Nonimmune fetal hydrops	Parvovirus B19	None needed
High fever for 5 days Lymphadenopathy Swelling of hands and feet Mucositis Irritability	Coronary artery aneurysms Infants and children older than 9 with greatest risk of complications	Unknown	IVIG and aspirin
Fever Headache Malaise Pharyngitis Lymphadenopathy Periorbital swelling (Hoagland sign) Splenomegaly Hepatomegaly	Splenic rupture Upper airway obstruction Neurological symptoms Hemolytic anemia	Epstein–Barr virus	Treat symptoms (fever, pharyngitis) as needed
Fever Cough Lymphadenopathy Hepatomegaly in hepatitis B virus—associated cases	None	Viral infections Hepatitis B virus infection (rare in United States)	None needed
Low-grade fever Arthralgias Malaise	None	Viral infections (usually HSV-1) Drugs	Removal of inciting antigen, if possible Oral antihistamines If recurrent HSV infection, consider acyclovir prophylaxis
Intense pruritus especially at night	Secondary infection Id reaction Eczematous changes	*Sarcoptes scabiei*	Permethrin 5% cream is the treatment of choice, may need to be repeated in 1 week

(continued)

SECTION 15 • SKIN

DIFFERENTIAL DIAGNOSIS (*continued*)

DIAGNOSIS	ICD-10	DISTINGUISHING CHARACTERISTICS	DISTRIBUTION	DURATION/ CHRONICITY
Measles	B05.9	Erythematous maculopapular lesions followed by brawny desquamation Enanthem—Koplik spots	Progresses from scalp to hairline to face to neck to trunk to upper and lower extremities to feet	Lasts 1–2 weeks
Asymmetric Lateral Exanthem of Childhood (Asymmetric Periflexural Exanthem OR Unilateral Laterothoracic Exanthem)	R21 (rash or other nonspecific eruption)	Lesions start on the trunk and extend to the axilla Pink-red, scaly papules Age 1–5 years	Also involves arms and thighs Often becomes bilateral within 2 weeks	Lasts 3–6 weeks (occasionally up to 4 months)
Hot Tub Folliculitis	R21 (rash or other nonspecific eruption)	Pruritic papules may change to pustules or nodules Occurs 1–2 days after exposure	Torso, buttocks, legs Hot tub exposed areas	Brief Self-limited

ASSOCIATED FINDINGS	COMPLICATIONS	PREDISPOSING FACTORS	TREATMENT GUIDELINES
Cough Coryza Fever Conjunctivitis Ill appearance	Pneumonia Encephalitis	Paramyxovirus	No specific treatment Single oral dose of 200,000 IU of vitamin A recommended in children with poor nutrition or vitamin A deficiency
Pruritus Localized lymphadenopathy Usually follows low-grade fever, sore throat, rhinorrhea, or diarrhea	None	Unknown	None
Occasional fever Malaise Headache	Cellulitis	*Pseudomonas aeruginosa*	Topical antipruritic agents can help relieve symptoms. When severe, consider antibiotics with coverage against Pseudomonas

Other Diagnoses to Consider

- Drug eruptions

- Urticaria

- Contact dermatitis

- Henoch–Schönlein purpura

- Meningococcal disease

- Varicella (particularly in children who have received varicella vaccine for whom the rash may be atypical)

- Other viral exanthem

When to Consider Further Evaluation or Treatment

- A second course of permethrin 5% cream is often necessary 1 week following the initial dose in the treatment of scabies. Family members should also be treated, and bedding and clothing should be washed in the hottest water possible or dry-cleaned.

- In patients with diagnosed measles and poor nutrition or vitamin A deficiency, vitamin A supplementation is recommended. Measles is associated with significant complications, including pneumonia, encephalitis, myocarditis, and the late-occurring subacute sclerosing panencephalitis. If these are suspected, appropriate referrals and inpatient management should be sought.

- Fever and petechiae or purpura should always be considered as high risk for meningococcemia, and appropriate testing and treatment should be instituted promptly.

- Patients with suspected Kawasaki disease should be evaluated for coronary artery aneurysm formation.

- Acute abdominal pain in a child with infectious mononucleosis warrants an evaluation of the spleen for possible rupture.

- Patients with roseola erythema infectiosum should be instructed to avoid contact with pregnant women until the infection subsides due to the risk of nonimmune hydrops in the fetus.

SUGGESTED READINGS

Cherry JD. Roseola infantum (exanthem subitum). In: Feigin RD, Cherry JD, Demmler-Harrison GJ, Kaplan SL. eds. *Feigin and Cherry's Textbook of Pediatric Infectious Diseases*. 6th ed. Philadelphia, PA: Saunders; 2009:780.

Currie BJ, McCarthy JS. Permethrin and ivermectin for scabies. *N Engl J Med*. 2010;362:717–725.

Dyer JA. Childhood viral exanthems. *Pediatr Ann*. 2007;36(1):21–29.

Kwon NH, Kim JE, Cho BK, et al. Gianotti-Crosti syndrome following novel Influenza A (H1N1) vaccination. *Ann Dermatol*. 2011;23(4):554–555.

Luzuriaga K, Sullivan JL. Infectious mononucleosis. *N Engl J Med*. 2010;362:1993–2000.

Paller AS, Mancini AJ, eds. *Hurwitz Clinical Pediatric Dermatology: A Textbook of Skin Disorders of Childhood and Adolescence*. 4th ed. Philadelphia, PA: Elsevier Saunders; 2011.

Vesicular Rashes

Darren M. Fiore

Approach to the Problem

A vesicle is a raised skin lesion filled with clear fluid that is less than 1 cm in diameter. A raised, clear fluid-filled lesion larger than 1 cm is referred to as a bulla. In childhood, there are many diseases that manifest as vesicular rashes, the most familiar of which is the rash seen with herpes simplex virus (HSV) infection. Other viral and bacterial infections also may present with vesiculobullous lesions as may many noninfectious processes, including allergic and immune-mediated diseases, mechanical disorders of the skin, burns, and insect bites.

Vesicular eruptions may be benign and self-limited or may be progressive and life threatening. Early identification of potentially serious disease and prompt attention to complications are critical, particularly in infants and immunocompromised hosts.

Key Points in the History

- Recurrent herpetic skin outbreaks in the same location almost always represent the reactivation of a latent infection rather than a new primary infection.

- Immunocompromised hosts may have disseminated disease due to HSV, varicella zoster virus (VZV), and coxsackievirus infections.

- Primary HSV lesions are often associated with fever and systemic symptoms, whereas secondary lesions or reactivation of HSV lesions are usually not.

- The reactivation of HSV or VZV, known as "shingles," is typically preceded by a prodrome of pain, tingling, itching, or burning at the site.

- In assessing vesicular rashes in the neonate, a detailed maternal history is necessary to elicit possible HSV exposure.

- Lethargy, poor feeding, temperature instability, jaundice, irritability, or seizures in an infant with vesicular lesions should raise suspicion for neonatal HSV infection.

- Frequently accompanying genital HSV is painful inguinal adenopathy, dysuria, urinary retention, and vaginal discharge. However, most primary genital HSV infections are asymptomatic.

- Primary VZV infection or chickenpox is very contagious; therefore, a history of household or school exposure in a child with characteristic lesions is highly suggestive.

- Children vaccinated against VZV may still develop chickenpox, though the disease course is milder.

- When contact dermatitis is suspected, a detailed environmental exposure history is warranted.

- Symptoms of allergic contact dermatitis may not manifest for 6 to 24 hours after the exposure. Symptoms are often worse with second or subsequent exposures.

- A history of outdoor exposure can indicate rhus dermatitis—poison oak, poison ivy, or poison sumac.

Key Points in the Physical Examination

- Grouped vesicles on an erythematous base are the hallmark of HSV infection; however, in immunocompromised patients, the erythematous base is not always apparent.

- HSV lesions on skin or mucous membranes may appear vesicular or, if they have ruptured, the lesions may appear eroded or ulcerated.

- Lesions of neonatal herpes often appear at 5 to 14 days of life; lesions appearing in the first 2 days of life suggest intrauterine exposure. Intrauterine-acquired HSV may not present with vesicles but rather scarring.

- The oral vesicles and ulcers of HSV tend to form more anteriorly on the gingivae, tongue, and hard palate; whereas, the lesions of hand-foot-and-mouth disease are typically more posterior on the soft palate, tonsillar pillars, and posterior oropharynx.

- Primary HSV infection of the eye may appear as blepharitis or keratoconjunctivitis. Signs include corneal or conjunctival erythema, watery discharge, lid swelling, and preauricular adenopathy.

- Lesions of primary VZV infection or chickenpox progress from papules to vesicles to erosions with crust. They occur in successive crops over 2 to 5 days and are predominant on the trunk, face, and scalp and progress in a centripetal distribution.

- Smallpox lesions spread centrifugally, with lesions concentrated on the extremities and spreading inward. A distinguishing feature of smallpox is the central umbilication of the lesions. Children with this disease are typically very ill.

- The presence of a dermatomal vesicular eruption is consistent with the diagnosis of shingles or reactivation of VZV infection.

- Extensive herpes zoster skin lesions may indicate an underlying immunodeficiency and an increased risk of visceral involvement.

- Lesions of contact dermatitis are typically limited to the area of exposure. The skin is often erythematous and edematous with vesiculation and weeping.

- Papular urticaria is characterized by recurrent crops of pruritic papulovesicles on skin areas exposed to insect bites.

PHOTOGRAPHS OF SELECTED DIAGNOSES

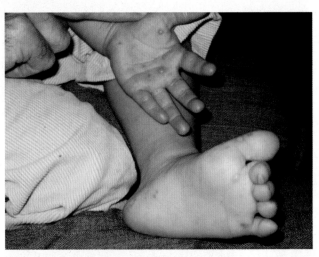

Figure 68-1 **Hand-foot-and-mouth disease.** Vesicles on palms and soles. (Courtesy of Philip Siu, MD.)

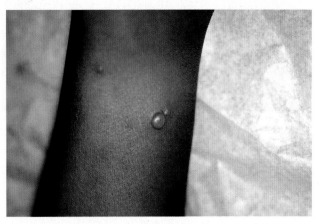

Figure 68-2 **Papular urticaria.** Vesicular lesion following an insect bite on the lower leg of a child. (Courtesy of Shirley P. Klein, MD, FAAP.)

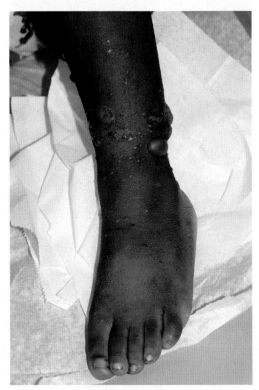

Figure 68-3 **Papular urticaria.** Vesiculobullous eruption secondary to insect bites on exposed area. (Courtesy of Ilona J. Frieden, MD.)

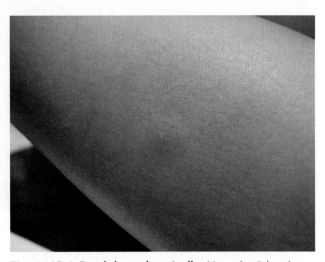

Figure 68-4 **Breakthrough varicella.** Note the "dewdrop-on-a-rose-petal" appearance of this lesion in a child previously immunized against varicella. (Courtesy of Esther K. Chung, MD, MPH.)

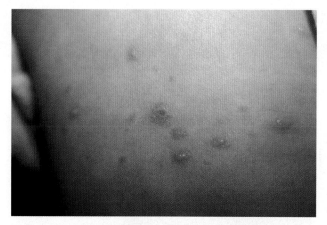

Figure 68-5 **Varicella.** Note the various stages of the lesions: papular, vesicular, and crusted. (Courtesy of Shirley P. Klein, MD, FAAP.)

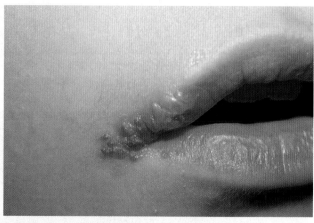

Figure 68-6 **Herpes labialis.** Grouped vesicles predominantly on one portion of the lip. (Courtesy of Ilona J. Frieden, MD.)

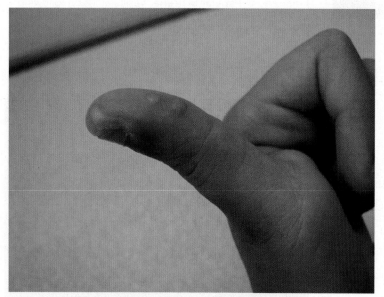

Figure 68-7 **Herpetic whitlow.** A group of vesicular lesions on the distal phalanx. (Courtesy of Paul S. Matz, MD.)

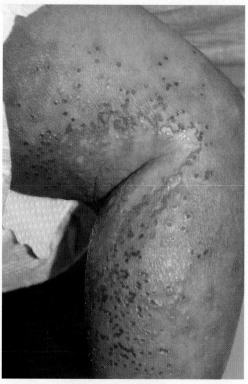

Figure 68-8 **Eczema herpeticum.** Multiple eroded vesicles with umbilication and crusting overlying a patch of eczematous skin. (Courtesy of Ilona J. Frieden, MD.)

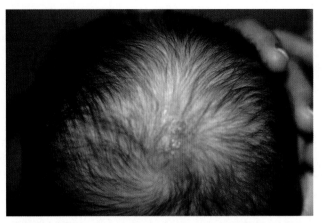

Figure 68-9 **Neonatal herpes.** Scalp erythema and vesicle at site of scalp electrode. (Courtesy of Shirley P. Klein, MD, FAAP.)

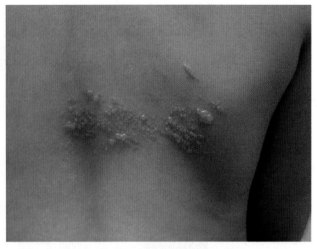

Figure 68-10 **Herpes zoster.** Grouped vesicles on an erythematous base in a dermatomal distribution. (Courtesy of Hans B. Kersten, MD.)

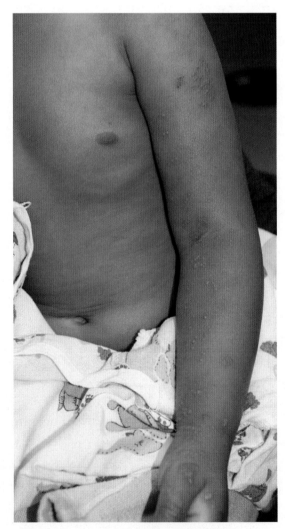

Figure 68-11 **Herpes zoster.** Grouped vesicles and erosions on an erythematous base in a C6 dermatomal distribution. (Courtesy of Ilona J. Frieden, MD.)

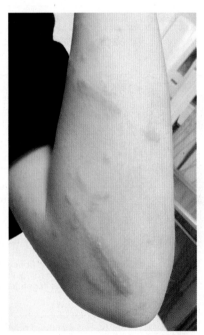

Figure 68-12 **Contact dermatitis.** Erythema and vesicle formation in a linear pattern characteristic of poison ivy. (Courtesy of Darren Fiore, MD.)

DIFFERENTIAL DIAGNOSIS

DIAGNOSIS	ICD-10	DISTINGUISHING CHARACTERISTICS	DISTRIBUTION	DURATION/ CHRONICITY
Hand-Foot-and-Mouth-Disease	B08.4	Elongated, thin-walled vesicles that may ulcerate	Palms, soles, palate, and posterior pharynx Characteristic lack of truncal involvement	5–7 days
Papular Urticaria	L50.8	Erythematous papules with urticarial flare in clusters, may progress to vesicles or bullae	Clustered lesions on shoulders, arms, legs, and buttocks	Recurrent crops last 2–10 days The illness may persist for months.
Varicella (Chickenpox)	B01.9	Crops of lesions in different stages (papules, vesicles on erythematous base, crusted erosions)	Entire body and oral mucous membranes	10 days
Primary HSV Infections (see below)				
• Gingivostomatitis	B00.2	Perioral and intraoral vesicles and crusting	Perioral skin, gingivae, buccal mucosa, palate, tongue	7–10 days
• Herpes Labialis	B00.1	Grouped vesicles on one portion of the lip; often recurrent	Most common location is lower lip	7–10 days
• Keratoconjunctivitis	H19.1	Red, irritated eye with concomitant periocular vesicles	Vesicles on eyelid or face Conjunctivitis (often bilateral) Corneal ulcerations	14–21 days
• Herpetic Whitlow	B00.8	Grouped vesicles on fingers	One or more fingers; often on terminal phalanx (thumb is most common)	7–10 days
• Genital Herpes	B00.1	May range from asymptomatic infection to painful, grouped vesicles in genital area	External genitalia, labia, vaginal mucosa, cervix, penis, scrotum, thighs	5–15 days
• Eczema Herpeticum	B00.0	Generalized HSV infection in patients with atopic dermatitis, characterized by widespread vesicles and crusting associated with fever and malaise	Seen in skin areas affected by atopic dermatitis, with predilection for upper body and head	2–6 weeks
Neonatal HSV	P35.2	Three disease patterns: mucocutaneous, CNS, and disseminated—all may have vesicular and/or eroded lesions Onset in first 4 weeks of life	Lesions can appear anywhere on skin (or at site of fetal scalp electrode) and commonly on oral mucosa	14–21 days
Secondary (Recurrent) HSV	B00.9	Grouped vesicles at or near site of primary eruption	At or near site of initial lesion, often less severe	5–7 days

ASSOCIATED FINDINGS	COMPLICATIONS	PREDISPOSING FACTORS	TREATMENT GUIDELINES
Fever Sore throat Painful oral lesions Anorexia	Mouth pain Dehydration	Exposure to coxsackievirus, most commonly A16, and other enteroviruses	Supportive care Analgesia Hydration
Pruritus	Bacterial superinfection Recurrent lesions if exposure continues	Delayed hypersensitivity reaction to fleas, mosquitoes, lice, scabies, or other mites	Remove offending insect or minimize child's exposure. N,N-Diethyl-meta-toluamide (DEET)-containing insect repellants may help. Treat urticaria and pruritus with antihistamines.
Prodrome of fever, malaise, sore throat, anorexia Lesions are pruritic.	Secondary bacterial infection of skin lesions Scarring Reye syndrome and encephalitis are rare.	Exposure to VZV, particularly day care or household exposure	Self-limited disease (in immunocompetent patients) requiring no systemic treatment Pruritus can be managed with cool compresses, calamine lotion, and antihistamines. Vaccination universally recommended for children ≥12 months of age Varicella zoster immune globulin (VZIG) postexposure prophylaxis exists for certain high-risk populations.
Fever, cervical adenopathy, irritability, mouth pain	Pain Dehydration	HSV-1 (or less commonly HSV-2) exposure via infected saliva	Analgesics, antipyretics, and hydration consider systemic antiviral therapy
Usually after febrile illness or upper respiratory tract infection (URI) (hence, colloquial term "cold sore")	Pain	HSV-1 (or less commonly HSV-2) exposure via infected saliva	OTC topical anesthetics may temporarily reduce pain associated with eroded lesions
Eye pain, photophobia, blurred vision	Corneal scarring Visual impairment	Typically HSV-1 exposure (HSV-2 conjunctivitis more often seen in neonates)	Topical or systemic antiviral therapy is required. Referral to an ophthalmologist is typically recommended.
Often a concomitant oral HSV infection (fingers are auto-inoculated via saliva) Pain and tingling of finger	Pain Recurrences are common.	Skin breakdown (e.g., torn cuticle or thumb-sucking)	Analgesics Topical antiviral therapy may shorten duration of symptoms and viral shedding. Systemic therapy generally not recommended
Fever, lymphadenopathy, malaise, dysuria	Vesicle rupture leading to painful ulcers Cervicitis Urethritis	Predominantly caused by HSV-2 transmitted via sexual contact	Analgesia and systemic antiviral therapy are required for primary genital herpes. Chronic suppressive therapy is required for recurrent disease.
Atopic dermatitis, fever, fatigue, keratoconjunctivitis	Pain Secondary bacterial infection Systemic viremia	Atopic dermatitis and HSV exposure	Parenteral acyclovir therapy
Temperature instability, poor feeding, lethargy, jaundice	Sepsis, DIC, shock, meningitis, seizures, death	Maternal HSV at time of delivery (increased with primary infection)	Parenteral acyclovir therapy
Prodrome of pain, burning, or tingling Lymphadenopathy Usually no fever or systemic symptoms (as in primary infection)	Pain Recurrence	Physical or emotional stress (e.g., bacterial infection, URI, surgery, sunburn) or immunocompromise	Analgesics Treatment of recurrent HSV with systemic antiviral therapy early during prodromal phase may abort or shorten the duration of the eruption. Chronic suppressive therapy may benefit children with frequent recurrences.

SECTION 15 • SKIN

(continued)

DIFFERENTIAL DIAGNOSIS *(continued)*

DIAGNOSIS	ICD-10	DISTINGUISHING CHARACTERISTICS	DISTRIBUTION	DURATION/ CHRONICITY
Other Non-HSV Rashes				
Herpes Zoster (Shingles)	B02.9	Clustered vesicles on erythematous base	Dermatomal distribution Unilateral thoracic dermatomal eruption is most common, but head, neck, buttocks eruptions do occur.	10 days
Variola (Smallpox)	B03	Papular and vesicular rash; often papules have central umbilication	Face, arms, and legs > trunk Lesions may be seen in mouth and throat.	10–14 days
Contact Dermatitis	L23.9	Erythema, vesiculation, and oozing	Limited to area of contact with offending substance Often linear pattern in rhus dermatitis	2–3 weeks

ASSOCIATED FINDINGS	COMPLICATIONS	PREDISPOSING FACTORS	TREATMENT GUIDELINES
Outbreak is often preceded by dermatomal pain. Lesions can be pruritic.	Pain Recurrent outbreaks	Represents reactivation of a prior varicella infection	Supportive care and analgesics
Prodrome of fever, malaise, myalgia	Disseminated infection (sepsis, osteomyelitis, pneumonia, encephalitis)	Exposure to variola virus Considered a possible agent of bioterrorism	Supportive care Vaccine exists for exposed individuals. Confirmed or suspected cases should be isolated.
Pruritus Pain	Repeated exposure may cause more widespread eruption of an Id reaction	Delayed hypersensitivity reaction Common sources of contact allergens include poison ivy and oak (which cause a Rhus dermatitis), nickel, shoes, perfumes, soaps, cosmetics, topical medications, and alcohol	Topical corticosteroids for localized lesions Systemic corticosteroids for more widespread (>10% skin surface) involvement Avoidance of offending contact allergen is critical.

Other Diagnoses to Consider

- Incontinentia pigmenti

- Photosensitivity reactions

- Bullous impetigo

- Eczema herpeticum

- Staphylococcal scalded skin syndrome

- Langerhans cell histiocytosis

- Pemphigus

When to Consider Further Evaluation or Treatment

- HSV infections are often diagnosed clinically; however, diagnostic testing should be performed in uncertain or complex cases. A Tzank smear is a rapid, but not sensitive and not specific test. For more definitive results, consider viral culture, DNA detection, or direct fluorescent antibody testing.

- The use of systemic antiviral therapy in uncomplicated cutaneous HSV infections is not always warranted; treatment *may* shorten the duration of illness if initiated early in the first 72 hours of symptoms or in cases of severe disease.

- HSV and VZV infections in immunocompromised hosts or neonates may disseminate rapidly, and consultation with an infectious disease specialist and/or a neonatologist is recommended.

- The presence of HSV-2 in young children should raise concerns for child sexual abuse.

- Vesicular lesions may become bacterially superinfected, typically by staphylococci, and may require systemic antibiotics.

- HSV or VZV keratoconjunctivitis should be referred to an ophthalmologist for evaluation and treatment. Similarly, in young patients with periorbital HSV lesions, evaluation by pediatric ophthalmology may be helpful to rule out ocular involvement.

- Recurrent episodes of genital herpes may be treated with episodic or chronic suppressive antiviral medication.

- The last documented case of smallpox in the United States was in 1949, and the last case in the world was in 1977. Any confirmed or suspected case of smallpox must be reported to public health officials.

- Immunocompromised patients exposed to VZV are candidates for VZIG and should be referred to an infectious disease specialist.

- Atypical, recurrent or poorly healing, contact dermatitis should be referred to a dermatologist for further evaluation.

SUGGESTED READINGS

Chayavichitslip P, Buckwalter JV, Krakowski AC, et al. Herpes simplex. *Pediatr Rev.* 2009;30:119–130.

Cohen B. *Pediatric Dermatology.* 3rd ed. London: Mosby; 2005:101–120.

Eichenfield LF, Frieden IJ, Esterly NB, eds. *Neonatal Dermatology.* 2nd ed. Philadelphia, PA: Elsevier; 2008:131–158.

Gnann JW Jr, Whitley RJ. Clinical practice: herpes zoster. *N Engl J Med.* 2002;347:340–346.

Weston WL, Lane AT, Morelli JG. *Color Textbook of Pediatric Dermatology.* 4th ed. Philadelphia, PA: Mosby; 2007:127–138, 195–212.

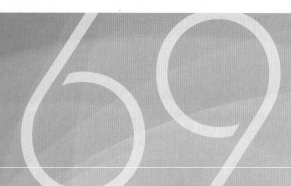

Nonblanching Rashes

William R. Graessle

Approach to the Problem

The child who presents with a nonblanching rash requires careful evaluation. Purpuric lesions, including petechiae and ecchymoses, usually result from vascular injury or disorders of hemostasis. The underlying etiology may be trauma, a simple viral infection, or a more serious condition such as leukemia or a bleeding disorder. When a nonblanching rash is seen in association with fever, serious bacterial infection, including meningococcemia, must be considered.

Key Points in the History

- A history of fever makes an infectious etiology more likely.

- Acute presentation of a nonblanching rash is more concerning than a rash that has been present for more than a couple of weeks.

- The location and pattern of spread may give a clue to the diagnosis: Rocky Mountain spotted fever (RMSF) tends to begin peripherally; Henoch–Schönlein purpura tends to primarily involve the lower extremities and buttocks.

- The presence of photophobia, headache, or both, in association with a nonblanching rash, raises the suspicion for meningococcal or other bacterial meningitis.

- A history of trauma may be the cause of the nonblanching lesions: localized bruising may follow blunt trauma, and petechiae may be seen in areas of friction or scratching.

- Significant ecchymotic lesions in the absence of a history of trauma should raise suspicion for child physical abuse or a bleeding disorder.

- Forceful coughing or vomiting may cause petechiae, particularly on the face and upper chest.

- Accompanying fatigue may be caused by anemia because of bone marrow suppression or infiltration as seen with leukemia.

- A history of tick bites or travel or activities associated with tick exposure should raise suspicion for RMSF or ehrlichiosis.

- Mongolian spots are present at birth and, though they may fade, they generally do not undergo color changes over time. In contrast, ecchymoses change color over time and eventually resolve.

- A history of easy bruising or excessive bleeding in the patient, or a family history of a bleeding disorder, should raise suspicion for hemophilia or von Willebrand disease.

- Familiarity with home remedies found in certain Asian cultures, such as coining and cupping, is essential.

Key Points in the Physical Examination

- Petechiae are nonblanching macules up to 2 mm in diameter caused by the extravasation of blood from capillaries. Mucosal bleeding sometimes is referred to as "wet purpura."

- Forceful coughing or vomiting may cause petechiae on the face and chest, above the nipple line.

- Purpura, seen with inflammatory injury to the smaller blood vessels, are elevated, firm, hemorrhagic plaques located predominantly on dependent surfaces.

- Ecchymoses are larger areas of bleeding into the skin. There is a characteristic change in color as they age, changing from red to purple to green to yellow-brown as the heme is degraded.

- Deep bleeding and hemarthroses are seen with clotting factor deficiencies, whereas petechiae are more commonly seen with thrombocytopenia.

- Ecchymoses that are not explained easily by accidental trauma should raise the suspicion of child physical abuse. Ecchymoses, uncommonly caused by infection, usually are indicative of trauma—accidental and nonaccidental—or a bleeding disorder. Bruising in normally active children is predominantly found on the pretibial surfaces.

- Cupping and coining are practices used by some Asian cultures to treat acute illnesses. Each has a characteristic appearance, and petechiae and ecchymoses may be seen in both.

SECTION 15 • SKIN

PHOTOGRAPHS OF SELECTED DIAGNOSES

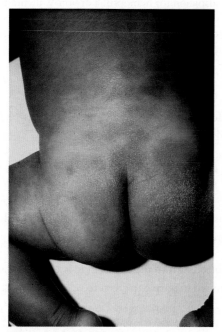

Figure 69-1 Mongolian spots. Blue nevi in the typical sacral area. (Courtesy of Sidney Sussman, MD.)

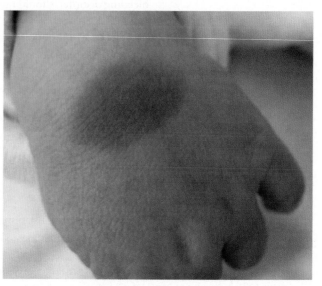

Figure 69-2 Mongolian spot on the hand. (Courtesy of Esther K. Chung, MD, MPH.)

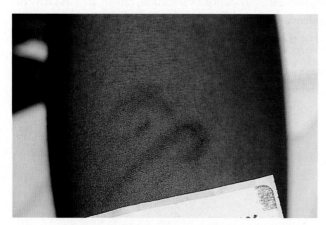

Figure 69-3 Child physical abuse. Curvilinear bruising from a looped cord. (Used with permission from Fleisher GR, Ludwig S, Baskin MN. *Atlas of Pediatric Emergency Medicine*. Philadelphia, PA: Lippincott Williams & Wilkins; 2004:425.)

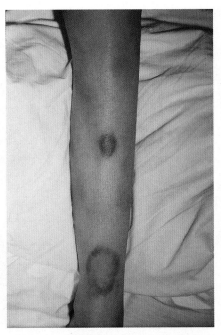

Figure 69-4 Ecchymoses in a patient with hemophilia.
(Courtesy of Sidney Sussman, MD.)

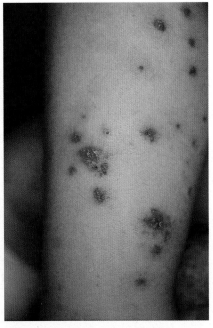

Figure 69-5 Henoch–Schönlein purpura. Note the palpable purpura on the posterior aspects of this child's leg. (Courtesy of Steven Manders, MD.)

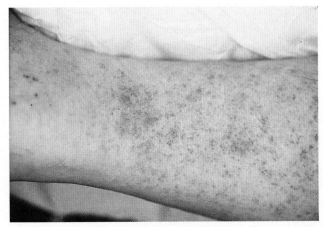

Figure 69-6 Rocky Mountain spotted fever. Note the multiple petechial lesions on the forearm. (Courtesy of Steven Manders, MD.)

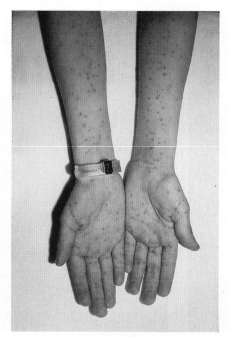

Figure 69-7 **Rocky Mountain spotted fever.** (Courtesy of Sidney Sussman, MD.)

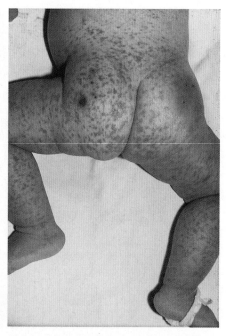

Figure 69-8 **Petechiae and ecchymoses in a patient with idiopathic thrombocytopenic purpura.** (Courtesy of Sidney Sussman, MD.)

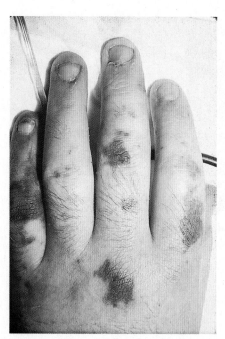

Figure 69-9 **Purpura fulminans in a patient with meningococcemia.** (Courtesy of Steven Manders, MD.)

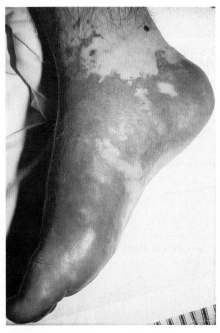

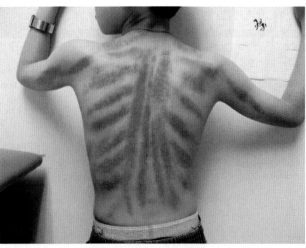

Figure 69-11 Coining. Note the linear petechiae and ecchymoses over the back that are characteristic for this healing practice used by some Asian cultures. (Courtesy of Philip Siu, MD.)

Figure 69-10 Purpura fulminans. Purpura on the foot of the same patient in Figure 69.9. (Courtesy of Steven Manders, MD.)

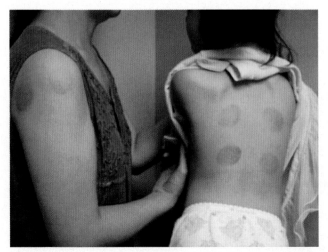

Figure 69-12 Cupping. Note the circular bruises on the mother's arm and the child's back that are the result of cupping, a healing practice used by some Asian cultures. (Courtesy of Philip Siu, MD.)

DIFFERENTIAL DIAGNOSIS

DIAGNOSIS		ICD-10	DISTINGUISHING CHARACTERISTICS	DISTRIBUTION
Mongolian Spots		Q82.8 Other specified congenital malformations of skin	Blue-gray lesions present at birth No color or size changes with time as one would see with ecchymoses	Most commonly in lumbosacral area, but upper back, shoulders, and extremities also commonly affected
Child Physical Abuse		T74.12XA	Ecchymoses in unusual locations or patterns	Anywhere on the body
Henoch–Schönlein Purpura		D69 Purpura and other hemorrhagic conditions	Initially urticarial, progresses to palpable purpura	Typically, buttocks and extensor surfaces of extremities, but any area of body may be involved
Rocky Mountain Spotted Fever		A77.0	Initially macular, gradually develops petechial, purpuric, and ecchymotic features	Begins around ankles and wrists; progresses to involve the entire body, including palms and soles
Idiopathic Thrombocytopenic Purpura		D69.3	Petechiae, ecchymoses, and mucosal bleeding	Generalized petechiae
Purpura Fulminans		D69 Purpura and other hemorrhagic conditions	Palpable purpura, undergoes necrosis	Symmetrical distribution Often begins on dependent surfaces
Coining		R23.3 Petechiae	Linear ecchymotic lesions	Usually back or chest
Cupping		R23.3 Petechiae	Petechiae, ecchymoses, and occasionally first-degree and second-degree burns	Cups placed in area of discomfort—back, abdomen

ASSOCIATED FINDINGS	PREDISPOSING FACTORS	COMPLICATIONS	TREATMENT GUIDELINES
No reddened appearance	Congenital Ethnicities with darker skin, including Asians, Hispanics, and those of African descent	N/A	No treatment required
Retinal hemorrhages, swelling of extremities, unusual skin marks, bucket-handle fractures, spiral fractures, multiple rib fractures, subdural hematomas	Teens and single parents, poverty, substance abuse, domestic violence, and parents who were physically abused as children Young and mentally retarded children are at greater risk.	Head injury Internal injury (liver and spleen laceration, intestinal rupture)	Remove from situation where injury occurred. Refer to child protective services. Consult ophthalmology in young children to rule out retinal hemorrhages.
Abdominal pain, vomiting, periarticular and joint swelling, scrotal edema Elevated ESR (erythrocyte sedimentation rate) and thrombocytosis	Preceding upper respiratory tract infection or other viral syndrome	Gastrointestinal (GI) bleeding Intussusception Renal disease	Consider steroid treatment
Fever, chills, severe headache, myalgias, and GI symptoms (i.e., nausea, vomiting, and diarrhea)	Tick bite Most commonly eastern and southern United States 90% occur between April and September	Hyponatremia DIC Shock	Doxycycline
Child otherwise well-appearing	Preceding viral illness in 50%–65% of cases Most commonly 1–4 years of age	Intracranial hemorrhage	Steroids and intravenous immunoglobulin are used. Treatment is controversial.
Ill-appearing child with features of septic shock—hypotension and poor perfusion	Commonly caused by meningococcemia, but may be seen with other bacterial causes of sepsis	Septic shock	Fluids Broad-spectrum antibiotics
Usually performed on an individual with an acute illness	Vigorous rubbing with coin or spoon sometimes after application of a medicated ointment	N/A	Lesions self-resolve
Usually performed on an individual with an acute illness	Cup applied to skin after igniting alcohol to create a vacuum	N/A	Lesions self-resolve

Other Diagnoses to Consider

- Leukemia

- Aplastic anemia

- Hemolytic uremic syndrome

- Systemic lupus erythematosus

- Liver disease

- Coagulation disorders

- Drug-induced thrombocytopenia

- Wiskott–Aldrich syndrome

When to Consider Further Evaluation or Treatment

- Patients with generalized petechiae or petechiae that are not easily explained by trauma should have a complete blood count. If the diagnosis of thrombocytopenia is established, further evaluation for a specific etiology should occur.

- An ill-appearing child with petechiae or purpura requires urgent evaluation and may need empiric treatment for an infectious etiology, such as bacterial sepsis or RMSF.

- Patients with ecchymoses suspicious for nonaccidental trauma should be evaluated further with coagulation studies and radiographic studies. Referral to child protective services should also be made.

- Patients with significant thrombocytopenia or involvement of other cell lines (anemia and/or white cell abnormalities) should be evaluated by a hematologist.

SUGGESTED READINGS

D'Orazio JA, Neely J, Farhoudi N. ITP in children: pathophysiology and current treatment approaches. *J Pediatr Hematol Oncol.* 2013;35(1):1–13.

Fleisher GR, Ludwig S, Baskin MN. *Atlas of Pediatric Emergency Medicine.* Philadelphia, PA: Lippincott Williams & Wilkins; 2004:425.

Leung AKC, Chan KW. Evaluating the child with purpura. *Am Fam Physician.* 2001;64(3):419–428.

Mudd SS, Findlay JS. The cutaneous manifestations and common mimickers of physical child abuse. *J Pediatr Health Care.* 2004;18(3):123–129.

Reyes MA, Eichenfield LF. Purpura. In: Long SS. ed. *Principles and Practice of Pediatric Infectious Diseases.* 4th ed. New York, NY: Elsevier; 2012:441–444.

Singh-Behl D, LaRosa SP, Tomecki KJ. Tick-borne infections. *Dermatol Clin.* 2003;21(2):237–244.

Weiss PF. Pediatric vasculitis. *Pediatr Clin North Am.* 2012;59(2):407–423.

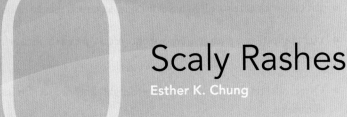

Scaly Rashes

Esther K. Chung

Approach to the Problem

The most common scaly rash in pediatrics is atopic dermatitis (eczema), which affects 15% to 20% of the pediatric population. While eczema tends to be chronic in nature, some patients have symptoms primarily during cold and dry weather. Other common causes of scaly rash include pityriasis rosea, tinea corporis, and seborrhea. Psoriasis and ichthyosis are less common. Initial lesions of pityriasis may at times be mistaken for tinea corporis, and ichthyosis may at times be mislabeled as severely dry skin. In general, most dry and scaly rashes tend to be pruritic in nature.

Key Points in the History

- The duration of symptoms will help to distinguish acute and subacute rashes, such as tinea corporis, from more chronic conditions, such as eczema.

- A family history of atopy should raise suspicion for eczema.

- Eczema generally spares the groin and diaper areas, whereas seborrhea does not.

- A solitary lesion may suggest tinea corporis or may be the herald patch seen in pityriasis rosea.

- Tinea corporis worsens with topical steroids, whereas eczema generally improves.

- Eczema on the face of young infants may have a circular area of erythema and may be misdiagnosed as tinea corporis.

- Cold weather generally exacerbates eczema, but some patients report worsening in the summer and winter months.

- In pityriasis rosea, the rash often starts as a single isolated lesion, a herald patch, followed by a more generalized rash occurring 5 to 10 days later.

- In the event a child shares a bed with another individual who denies pruritus or rash, a diagnosis of scabies is unlikely.

- Psoriasis affects 1% to 3% of the population, but it is uncommon in African Americans.

- Patients with eczema often have dry skin, keratosis pilaris, or both.

- Lichenification is pathognomic of chronic atopic dermatitis when it appears in the expected distribution.

- Often, allergic shiners and Dennie–Morgan lines are seen in individuals with atopic dermatitis.

- Seborrhea generally stays within the hairline, whereas psoriasis extends beyond the hairline.

- In ectopic allergic contact dermatitis, the rash may not be in the expected location as can be seen with nail polish (tosylamide/formaldehyde) allergy.

- Lesions associated with tinea corporis tend to be round, whereas the herald patch in pityriasis rosea is oval.

- The generalized rash of pityriasis rosea classically runs parallel to the lines of skin cleavage, in a "Christmas-tree" distribution.

- In some individuals, the scaly lesions of pityriasis may be found in the pubic, inguinal, and axillary areas, and this is referred to as "inverse pityriasis rosea."

- Postinflammatory hypopigmentation commonly occurs following eczema, pityriasis, and tinea. Hypopigmentation can be distressing to families; therefore, discussing this early in the course of the disease may be helpful.

PHOTOGRAPHS OF SELECTED DIAGNOSES

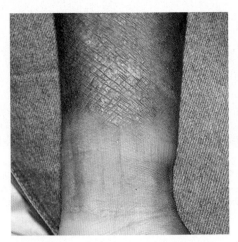

Figure 70-1 Atopic dermatitis. This lesion shows no evidence of active inflammation. Lichenification and postinflammatory hyperpigmentation are apparent. (Used with permission from Goodheart HP. *Goodheart's Photoguide to Common Skin Disorders.* 2nd ed. Philadelphia, PA: Lippincott Williams & Wilkins; 2003:44.)

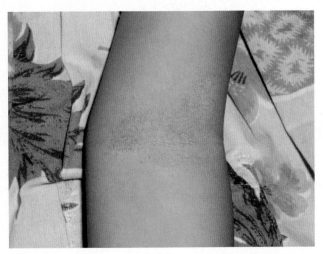

Figure 70-2 Atopic dermatitis. Note the areas of dryness, hypo- and hyperpigmentation and lichenification in the antecubital fossa of this 5-year-old. (Courtesy of Esther K. Chung, MD.)

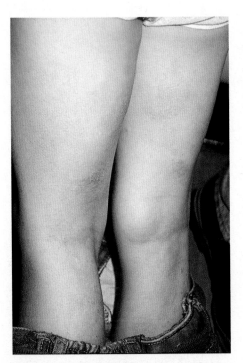

Figure 70-3 Nummular eczema. "Coin-shaped" patches and plaques are located on the legs. (Used with permission from Goodheart HP. *Goodheart's Photoguide to Common Skin Disorders.* 2nd ed. Philadelphia, PA: Lippincott Williams & Wilkins; 2003:87.)

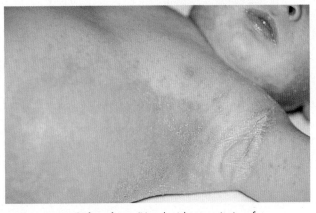

Figure 70-4 Seborrhea. (Used with permission from Fleisher GR, Ludwig S, Baskin MN. *Atlas of Pediatric Emergency Medicine.* Philadelphia, PA: Lippincott Williams & Wilkins; 2004:85.)

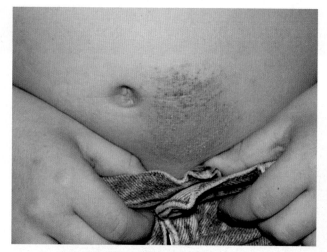

Figure 70-5 **Allergic contact dermatitis.** This boy developed an eczematous eruption at the site where the nickel snap on his blue jeans contacted his skin. (Used with permission from Goodheart HP. *Goodheart's Photoguide to Common Skin Disorders.* 2nd ed. Philadelphia, PA: Lippincott Williams & Wilkins; 2003:67.)

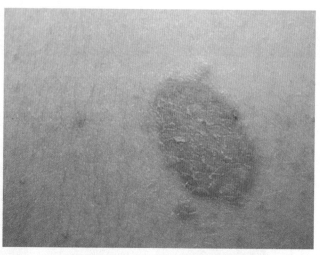

Figure 70-6 **Variation in pityriasis rosea.** In light skin, a "classic" oval erythematous, scaly herald plaque. (Used with permission from Burkhart C, Morrell D, Goldsmith LA, et al. *VisualDx: Essential Pediatric Dermatology.* Philadelphia, PA: Lippincott Williams & Wilkins; 2009.)

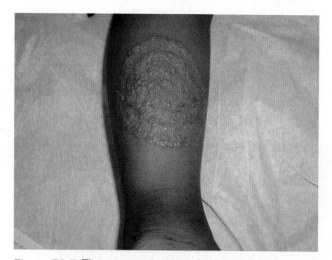

Figure 70-7 **Tinea corporis.** Note the large size of this lesion that was made worse by the use of topical steroids. (Courtesy of Esther K. Chung, MD.)

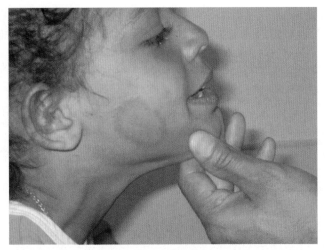

Figure 70-8 Tinea corporis on the face. (Courtesy of George A. Datto, III, MD.)

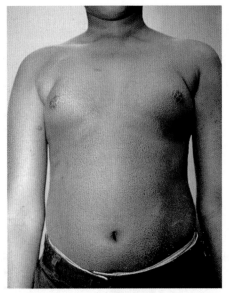

Figure 70-9 Ichthyosis vulgaris. (Courtesy of George A. Datto, III, MD.)

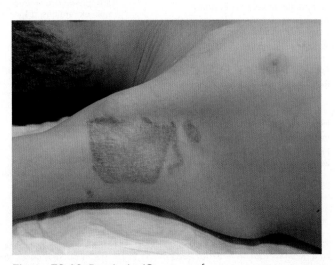

Figure 70-10 Psoriasis. (Courtesy of George A. Datto, III, MD.)

DIFFERENTIAL DIAGNOSIS

DIAGNOSIS	ICD-10	DISTINGUISHING CHARACTERISTICS	DISTRIBUTION
Atopic Dermatitis	L20.9 Atopic dermatitis, unspecified	• Erythema, papules, vesicles in early infancy • Dry, pruritic, scaly patches in young children • May present after the newborn period • Many individuals only have the condition as young children; some adults are affected	• Often begins on the face in young infants • Often begins on extensor surfaces and trunk in older infants • Antecubital and popliteal fossae, face, and neck in older children and adults • Frequently spares the groin
Nummular Eczema	L30.0 Nummular dermatitis	• Starts as vesicles, papules • Erythematous, coin-shaped lesions • May or may not see pruritus • May occur only during the winter months	Extensor surfaces of the extremities
Seborrhea	L21.1 (infantile) L21 (dermatitis)	• Greasy, yellow or salmon-colored • Nonpruritic or very mildly pruritic • Appears at 1 month of age and disappears at between 8 and 12 months of age • Reappears in adolescence	Scalp (as cradle cap), nasolabial folds, postauricular areas, cheeks, trunk, extremities, diaper area, and intertriginous areas
Irritant Contact Dermatitis	L24.9 Irritant contact dermatitis, unspecified	• Focal, mild erythema • Resolves shortly after the irritant is removed	Chin, cheeks, extensor surfaces, diaper area
Allergic Contact Dermatitis	L23.9 Allergic contact dermatitis, unspecified	• May occur in children as young as 6 months • Increased risk in females • Pruritic, eczematous dermatitis appears 24–48 hours after exposure	• Geometric or linear configuration • "Jean snap dermatitis"—periumbilical area • Midline chest with nickel snaps on infant clothing
Pityriasis Rosea	L42	• 70%–80% begin with a single patch followed by a general eruption 5–10 days later of smaller, more ovoid lesions • Oval shape with flat, pink, brown center with an elevated border that is erythematous with a collarette of fine scales • The rash may be more common in young children and in African Americans • Peak incidence in adolescence	• Trunk, upper arms, neck, and thighs but may occur anywhere on the body • When in the pubic, inguinal, and axillary areas; some use the term "inverse" pityriasis rosea
Tinea Corporis	B35.4	• Round, scaly patches with a papular, vesicular, or pustular border with clear center • Most commonly in children, but may be seen at any age	• Predilection for nonhairy areas of the face, trunk, and extremities • Asymmetric distribution
Ichthyosis Vulgaris	Q80.0	• Scales on the tibia may be thick and plate-like • Hyperkeratosis • Rarely occurs before 3 months of life • Scaling on the face is generally limited to childhood and decreases with age	• Extensor surfaces • Flexural surfaces generally spared • May see chapping and accentuation of palmar markings
Psoriasis	L40.9 Psoriasis unspecified L40.4 Guttate psoriasis	• Round, sharply demarcated, deep-red lesion with a silvery scale attached at the center of the lesion • Drop-like lesions are seen in guttate psoriasis • Unpredictable exacerbations and remissions • Prolonged course	• Extensor surfaces, scalp, genital regions, and lumbosacral areas • Typically, a bilateral, symmetric pattern of lesions

ASSOCIATED FINDINGS	PREDISPOSING FACTORS	TREATMENT GUIDELINES
• Keratosis pilaris • Ichthyosis vulgaris • 4%–12% of patients develop cataracts • Cutaneous infection resulting from *S. aureus*, strep • Eczema herpeticum (herpes simplex) • Eczema vaccinatum (vaccinia) • Id reaction • Irritability • Daytime tiredness	• Worse during the winter months • Worsened by frequent bathing • Allergenic foods • Inhalant allergens • Dust mites	• Topical steroids • Calcineurin inhibitors (second line) • Antibiotics for skin infections (e.g., staph infections) • Oral antihistamines to reduce itching and to possibly improve overall sleeping • Moisturizers • Humidified air • Avoidance of irritant and allergic triggers • Avoid simultaneous use of oral and topical antihistamines as this may result in toxicity • Excess use of camphor containing, topical, anti-itch lotions may result in toxicity.
N/A	• Worse during winter months • Manifestation of dry skin (xerosis), ichthyosis (but not necessarily atopy)	• Lukewarm, cool baths • Emollients • Topical steroids • Tar preparations • Oral antihistamines
N/A	Puberty	• Antiseborrheic shampoos containing selenium sulfide, salicylic acid, or zinc pyrithione • Topical steroids in some instances • Ketoconazole foam, gel, or shampoo
N/A	• Soaps, detergents • Salivary secretions • Urine and feces	Irritant avoidance/removal
Id reaction	• Nickel-containing snaps, piercings, belts • Cosmetic products • Fragrant and deodorant products • Leather materials (potassium dichromate) • Rubber materials (carba mix; thiuram) • Poison ivy (uroshiol) • Para-phenylenediamine found in hair dye, henna tattoos	• Allergen avoidance. Epicutaneous patch testing can help in some instances to identify allergens. • Short courses of topical or oral steroids
• Prodrome of headache, malaise, and pharyngitis may be reported • The rash, seen in secondary syphilis, may be similar and should not be overlooked	Associated with preceding viral illness	• Self-limited • Topical antipruritics, sparingly • Oral antihistamines • Exposure to UV light hastens resolution • Oral erythromycin (one study)
N/A	• Warm, humid climates • Contact with an infected individual • Systemic disease such as diabetes mellitus and immunodeficiency	Topical antifungal creams
Keratosis pilaris	• Worse in cold and dry weather • Atopy	• Emollients • Topical retinoids • Antihistamines for itching • Topical steroids for itching • Alpha-hydroxy acids (including lactic and glycolic acids)
• 25%–50% with nail pits • Geographic tongue • Psoriatic arthritis • Psoriatic uveitis	Stress, trauma, strep infection (such as guttate psoriasis), climate, and certain medications may be precipitating factors in fewer than half of patients	• Emollients • Topical steroids • Avoid irritants • Tar preparations

Other
Diagnoses
to Consider

- Scabies

- Letterer–Siwe disease (a form of histiocytosis consisting of lymphadenopathy, hepatosplenomegaly, and a seborrhea-like rash)

- Leiner disease (seborrhea-like dermatitis, diarrhea, wasting and dystrophy, and recurrent gram-negative infection)

- Netherton syndrome ("bamboo hair," congenital ichthyosiform erythroderma, and atopic diathesis)

- Acrodermatitis enteropathica (autosomal recessive disorder; listlessness, diarrhea, failure to thrive, low-serum zinc)

- Zinc deficiency

- Wiskott–Aldrich syndrome (diarrhea, purpura, and susceptibility to infection)

- Phenylketonuria (mental retardation, seizures, blond hair, and eczema)

- Hyper IgE syndrome (recurrent sinopulmonary and cutaneous infections, markedly elevated IgE levels, and chronic dermatitis)

- Lichen striatus

- Systemic lupus erythematosus

When to
Consider
Further
Evaluation
or Treatment

- Further evaluation and treatment should be considered for dry scaly rashes that fail to improve in spite of frequent moisturizing.

- Most dry, scaly rashes are due to atopic dermatitis and will respond to emollients and the use of mild topical steroids.

- Severe and complicated cases of eczema warrant consultation with a dermatologist.

- Because tinea corporis worsens with use of topical steroids, use only these agents when there is a low suspicion for tinea corporis.

- Pityriasis rosea is generally self-limited and resolves by 6 weeks generally; however, it may last as long as 5 months.

- With pityriasis rosea, exposure to UV light hastens resolution.

- Keep in mind that allergic contact dermatitis may last for weeks to months after removal of the allergen, even with the use of topical steroids.

- An asymptomatic focal scaly lesion followed by fever and leucopenia should raise suspicion for systemic lupus erythematosus.

SUGGESTED READINGS

Chuh AA, Dofitas BL, Comisel GG, et al. Interventions for pityriasis rosea. *Cochrane Database Syst Rev.* 2007;18:CD005068.

Huang CF, Wang WM, Chiang CP. Scaly ear rash as the herald of a young girl with juvenile systemic lupus erythematosus. *Ann Dermatol.* 2011;23:S333–S337.

Kress D. What's your diagnosis? Scaly pubic plaques in a 2-year-old girl—or an "inverse" rash. In: Traeger TKD (Section Ed.) Pedi Gyn-Derm. *J Pediatr Adolesc Gynecol.* 2007;20:109–111.

Krol A, Krafchik B. The differential diagnosis of atopic dermatitis in childhood. *Dermatol Ther.* 2006(19);73–82.

Larsen S, Hanifin JM. Epidemiology of atopic dermatitis. *Immunol Clin North Am.* 2002;22:1–24.

Militello G, Jacob SE, Crawford GH. Allergic contact dermatitis in children. *Curr Opin Pediatr.* 2006;18:385–390.

Schon MP, Boehncke WH. Psoriasis. *N Engl J Med.* 2005;352:1899–1912.

Sheu J, Huang JT. Erythematous scaly plaques and papules in a 9-month-old infant. *J Pediatr.* 2013;163:1222.

Fine, Bumpy Rashes

Shonul A. Jain

Approach to the Problem

Fine, bumpy rashes are a common complaint seen in the pediatric outpatient setting. They may be acute or chronic, and may be so subtle and asymptomatic that they are not noted for a period of time. The most classic example of a fine, bumpy rash is the sandpaper rash of scarlet fever, but this category of rashes also includes nonspecific rashes such as viral exanthems, heat rashes, drug reactions, and rarer lichenoid eruptions. Most of these conditions are benign and self-limited, and at times it may not be possible to make the exact diagnosis. It is important to note, however, that there are serious conditions such as toxic shock syndrome (TSS) that may initially present as a mild rash. It is important to have a high clinical suspicion for these serious disorders, particularly when systemic symptoms accompany the rash.

Key Points in the History

- Scarlet fever is generally seen with the accompanying symptoms of fever, headache, sore throat, and abdominal pain; the rash usually appears 24 to 48 hours after the onset of symptoms.

- Folliculitis, which occurs in all skin types, is not always infectious but also may be caused by chemical irritation or physical injury from shaving.

- Keratosis pilaris is often prominent in patients with underlying atopic dermatitis or obesity. Many patients with keratosis pilaris have a family member with this condition.

- Lichen nitidus is usually a chronic, nonpruritic, asymptomatic condition.

- Though usually precipitated by heat, miliaria can occur in the winter in association with fever, overbundling, or the use of certain ointments.

- Fine papular eruptions are the most frequent of all cutaneous drug reactions, classically due to ampicillin or amoxicillin, and are often identical in appearance to viral exanthems.

- Penicillin therapy in patients with Epstein–Barr virus infection may result in a morbilliform (measles-like) exanthem, which is considered to be a drug reaction.

- Scarlet fever often produces Pastia lines, linear rows of petechiae, in the skin folds, particularly in the antecubital and popliteal fossae and the inguinal area.

- Scarlet fever is most often associated with pharyngitis, but may also be seen with other group A streptococcal skin infections such as cellulitis.

- In patients with more skin pigmentation, the rash of scarlet fever may not readily appear erythematous; therefore, it is important to examine patients in bright lighting.

- The Koebner phenomenon, linear papules along the lines of skin trauma, is a hallmark of lichen nitidus and presents in almost all cases.

- Keratosis pilaris, which is rough in texture, occurs along the extensor surfaces of extremities.

- Folliculitis, which may consist of pustules of varying size, is usually confined to hair-bearing areas such as the scalp, forearms, groin, and legs. Often the hair follicle cannot be seen in folliculitis.

- Miliaria is often found on the face and upper trunk and back.

PHOTOGRAPHS OF SELECTED DIAGNOSES

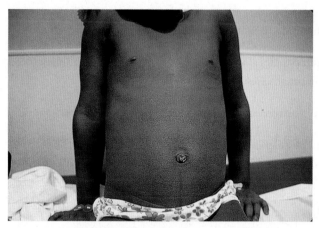

Figure 71-1 Scarlet fever. Fine papules, "sandpaperlike" rash on trunk of child with scarlet fever. (Courtesy of George A. Datto, III, MD.)

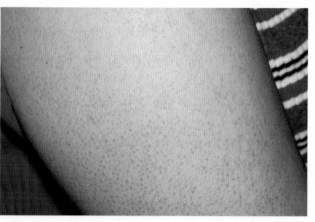

Figure 71-2 Keratosis pilaris. Tiny, rough-textured, follicular papules on lateral upper arms. (Used with permission from Goodheart HP. *Goodheart's Photoguide to Common Skin Disorders.* 2nd ed. Philadelphia, PA: Lippincott Williams & Wilkins; 2003:49.)

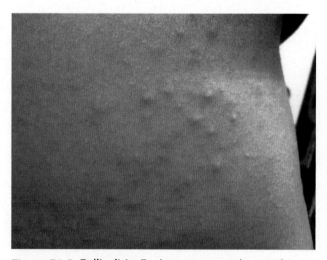

Figure 71-3 Folliculitis. Erythematous papulovesicular lesions on abdomen after exposure in a hot tub. (Courtesy of Lee R. Atkinson-McEvoy, MD.)

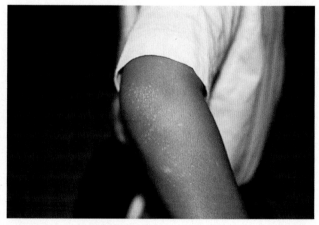

Figure 71-4 Lichen nitidus. Shiny small papules on elbow. (Courtesy of George A. Datto, III, MD.)

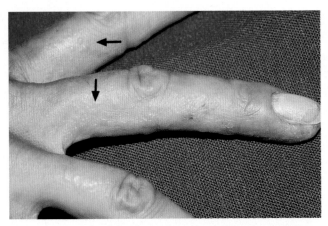

Figure 71-5 Dyshidrotic eczema. Note the fine, fluid-filled bumps on the fingers as depicted by the *arrows*. (Used with permission from Goodheart HP. *Goodheart's Photoguide to Common Skin Disorders*. 2nd ed. Philadelphia, PA: Lippincott Williams & Wilkins; 2003:60.)

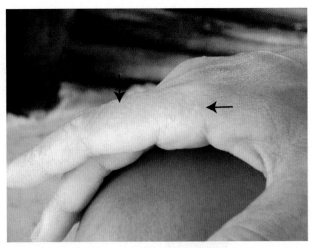

Figure 71-6 Dyshidrotic eczema. Note the fine, fluid-filled bumps on the finger (as depicted by the *arrows*) and the distal area of peeling. (Courtesy of Esther K. Chung, MD, MPH.)

DIFFERENTIAL DIAGNOSIS

DIAGNOSIS		ICD-10	DISTINGUISHING CHARACTERISTICS	DISTRIBUTION	DURATION/ CHRONICITY
Scarlet Fever		A38	Erythematous "sandpaperlike" pinpoint papules Desquamation of tips of fingers and toes	Generalized Concentrates on trunk and skin folds Palms and soles are often erythematous	Rash appears 2–4 days after onset of other symptoms
Keratosis Pilaris		L85.8	Perifollicular Rough 1–2 mm papules	Posterolateral upper arms Anterior thighs	Chronic
Folliculitis		L73.9	Perifollicular inflammation May be painless or tender	Any hair-bearing area—most commonly affecting the face, arms, legs, and axillae	Acute onset
Lichen Nitidus		L44.1	Flesh-colored, monomorphous papules Sharply demarcated	Cluster in groups Trunk Upper extremities Glans penis	Slowly progressive May remain for years Spontaneously resolves
Miliaria Rubra (Heat Rash)		L74.0	Erythematous, fine papules	Face Neck Upper trunk	Spontaneous resolution in 2–3 days
Drug Allergy		T88.7	Erythematous maculopapular rash May be confluent	Generalized Mucous membranes Often spares palms and soles	Begins 7–10 days after starting drug Resolves 1–2 weeks after discontinuation

ASSOCIATED FINDINGS	COMPLICATIONS	PREDISPOSING FACTORS	TREATMENT GUIDELINES
Fever Exudative pharyngitis Strawberry tongue Pastia lines	Suppurative complications Rheumatic fever Glomerulonephritis	Group A streptococcus	Antimicrobial therapy—penicillin, macrolides, cephalosporins
Dry skin	Folliculitis superinfection	Obesity Family history of keratosis pilaris Atopic dermatitis Insulin resistance	Keratolytics Retinoids Mild topical corticosteroids
Hair shaft Pustules present when infected	Cellulitis	Shaving Curly hair Chemical irritants Staphylococcal infection	Modified shaving techniques Laser hair removal Antibiotics, only if infected
Not pruritic Koebner phenomenon	None	Unknown	If persistent, trial of topical corticosteroids
"Prickly" or itchy sensation	None	Heat Tight-fitting clothes Emollients	Cool baths Loose-fitting clothes Avoid oil-based lubricants
Itching Fever Exfoliation	Generally does not progress to anaphylaxis if not urticarial	Ampicillin Amoxicillin Sulfonamides Any medication	Stop offending drug Cool compresses Topical corticosteroids for symptom relief

SECTION 15 • SKIN

Other Diagnoses to Consider

- Nonspecific viral exanthem

- TSS (early phase)

- Kawasaki disease

- Contact dermatitis (early phase)

- "Id" reaction (autoeczematization to various stimuli, particularly fungi, that results in a symmetrical eczematous, maculopapular, or papulovesicular rash)

- Lichen spinulosus (papular rash with a spine or horn at each hair follicle)

- Keratosis follicularis or Darier disease (hereditary skin disorder where keratotic papules coalesce to form crusty, warty plaques)

- Dyshidrotic eczema

When to Consider Further Evaluation or Treatment

- Most fine, bumpy rashes are benign and self-limited. Any persistent rash or a rash associated with systemic symptoms, such as fever or altered mental status, warrants further evaluation.

- If a rash is bothersome and does not respond to initial therapy, further management should be determined after consultation with a pediatric dermatologist.

- The initial rash of TSS may mimic scarlet fever. The presence of high fever, mental status changes, headache, or early shock-like symptoms should raise suspicion for TSS and warrants immediate evaluation and management.

SUGGESTED READINGS

Goodheart HP. *Goodheart's Photoguide to Common Skin Disorders*. 3rd ed. Philadelphia, PA: Lippincott Williams & Wilkins; 2008:60.
Habif T. *Clinical Dermatology*. 5th ed. St. Louis, MO: Mosby; 2009:263, 351–355, 464–466, 486–488.
Hwang S. Keratosis pilaris: a common follicular hyperkeratosis. *Cutis* 2008;82:177–180.
Paller AS. *Hurwitz Clinical Pediatric Dermatology*. 4th ed. Philadelphia, PA: WB Saunders; 2011:106–107.
Shulman ST. Clinical practice guidelines for the diagnosis and management of Group A streptococcal pharyngitis: 2012 update by the Infectious Disease Society of America. *Clin Infect Dis*. 2012;55:1279–1282.
Tilly JT, Drolet BA. Lichenoid eruptions in children. *J Am Acad Dermatol*. 2004;51:606–624.

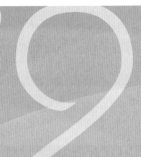

Hypopigmented Rashes

Andrew Saunders
and Lee R. Atkinson-McEvoy

Approach to the Problem

Disorders of pigment are often a significant concern to parents. Even for benign conditions, the cosmetic impact is of importance to patients and families. Hypopigmented lesions may be congenital or acquired, with the latter often occurring in association with inflammation or infection. Congenital lesions appear within the first year of life; as the skin is exposed to sunlight, the normal skin acquires more color and the lesions remain light relative to the normal skin.

Key Points in the History

- A history of rash or other lesion prior to the development of a hypopigmented area suggests postinflammatory hypopigmentation. This condition resolves with time.

- In patients with vitiligo, there is a positive family history in 30% of cases.

- Half of the cases of vitiligo are present in childhood, usually in adolescence.

- Pityriasis alba is common in children with atopy.

- Ash leaf spots may occur in isolation or in association with tuberous sclerosis.

- Piebaldism is an autosomal dominant condition.

- A hyperpigmented nevus is initially present before the development of a halo nevus.

Key Points in the Physical Examination

- Nevoid hypopigmentation, formerly known as Hypomelanosis of Ito, follows the lines of Blaschko in a linear pattern on the extremities and in whorls on the trunk.

- Vitiligo, which may be irregularly shaped, displays hypopigmented and depigmented macules of varying sizes. Vitiligo may involve mucous membranes and hair.

- Patients with piebaldism have a white forelock with hypopigmentation of the adjacent scalp and forehead. The pattern is triangular and enhances with a Wood lamp.

- Ash leaf macules enhance under a Wood lamp.

- Scale frequently accompanies tinea versicolor and may be seen with pityriasis alba. Tinea versicolor infections by *Microsporum* sp. and *Malassezia furfur* tend to fluoresce with Wood lamp examination.

PHOTOGRAPHS OF SELECTED DIAGNOSES

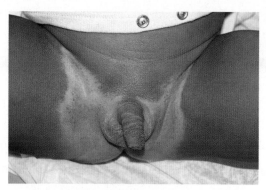

Figure 72-1 Postinflammatory hypopigmentation following a diaper dermatitis. (Courtesy of Ilona J. Frieden, MD.)

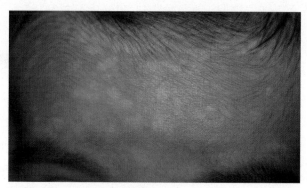

Figure 72-2 Tinea versicolor. Hypopigmented scaly lesions on the forehead of a 22-month-old boy. (Courtesy of Ilona J. Frieden, MD.)

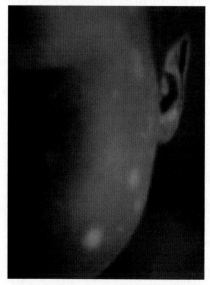

Figure 72-3 Tinea versicolor under Wood lamp. Note the blue-whitish fluorescence. (Courtesy of Paul S. Matz, MD.)

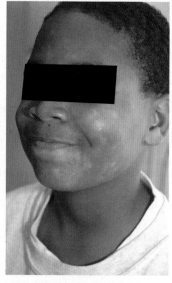

Figure 72-4 Pityriasis alba. (Courtesy of George A. Datto, III, MD.)

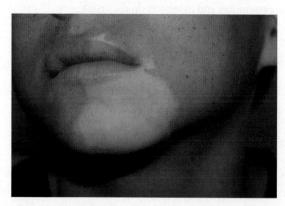

Figure 72-5 Vitiligo. Segmental vitiligo in an 11-year-old child. (Courtesy of Ilona J. Frieden, MD.)

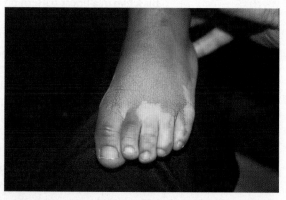

Figure 72-6 Segmental vitiligo on the foot of a child. (Courtesy of George A. Datto, III, MD.)

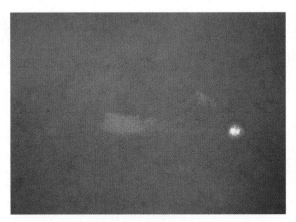

Figure 72-7 Ash leaf macule. Hypopigmented macules on the torso of a child with tuberous sclerosis. (Courtesy of Ilona J. Frieden, MD.)

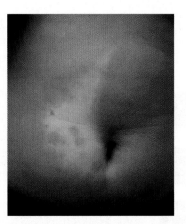

Figure 72-8 Piebaldism. Hypopigmented lesion on a child associated with a white forelock. (Courtesy of Amy Gilliam, MD.)

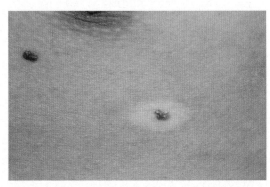

Figure 72-9 Halo nevus. Hypopigmented lesion surrounding an inflamed compound nevus. (From Goodheart HP. *Goodheart's Photoguide of Common Skin Disorders.* 2nd ed. Philadelphia, PA: Lippincott Williams & Wilkins; 2003.)

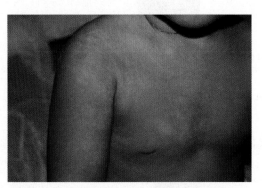

Figure 72-10 Nevoid hypopigmentation (formerly referred to as hypomelanosis of Ito). Linear swirl pattern of hypopigmentation on shoulder. (Courtesy of Ilona J. Frieden, MD.)

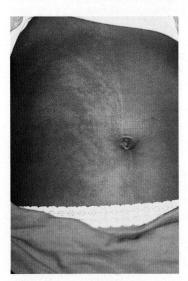

Figure 72-11 Nevoid hypopigmentation (formerly referred to as hypomelanosis of Ito). Linear swirl pattern clearly following the lines of Blaschko. (Courtesy of George A. Datto, III, MD.)

SECTION 15 • SKIN

DIFFERENTIAL DIAGNOSIS

DIAGNOSIS		ICD-10	DISTINGUISHING CHARACTERISTICS	DISTRIBUTION	DURATION/ CHRONICITY
Postinflammatory Hypopigmentation		L81.9	Area of hypopigmentation	Diffuse	Subacute to chronic
Tinea Versicolor		B36.0	Scaly annular confluent hypopigmented lesions on the chest, shoulder, and/or back	Upper chest, shoulder, and/ or back	Subacute to chronic
Pityriasis Alba		L30.5	Hypopigmented macules on the face, moving from place to place	Usually in sun-exposed areas Most often on the face	Chronic, waxing, and waning
Vitiligo		L80	Hypopigmented macules involving mucous membranes	Extensor surfaces of the extremities, face, and neck, but can be diffuse	Chronic
Ash Leaf Macule		Q85.1 (tuberous sclerosis) L81.9 (isolated ash leaf macule)	Discrete hypopigmented macule that enhances with Wood's lamp	Diffuse	Chronic
Piebaldism		E70.3	Rare condition Segmented white patch of scalp involving hair and skin Enhances with a Wood's lamp	Often on scalp, usually frontal	Chronic
Nevus Depigmentosus (Nevus Achromicus)		L81.9	Hypopigmented macule present at or shortly after birth	May occur anywhere	Chronic
Halo Nevus		L81.9	Hypopigmented ring surrounding nevus	May occur anywhere; most commonly on the back	Subacute to chronic
Nevoid Hypopigmentation (Hypomelanosis of Ito)		L81.9	Linear or whorled hypopigmented macule	Follows Blaschko lines on trunk or extremities	Chronic

ASSOCIATED FINDINGS	COMPLICATIONS	PREDISPOSING FACTORS	TREATMENT GUIDELINES
Areas of inflammation	None	Previous area of inflammation or infection	Sunscreen to protect the area from UV rays Treat inflammation or infection appropriately to minimize development
Rare complaints of pruritus	May be difficult to treat	Fungal infection with *M. furfur* or *Microsporum* sp. Thrives in hot, humid climates	Ketoconazole shampoo or selenium sulfide 2.5% applied daily for 1 week, then monthly for 3 months
Other signs of atopy such as atopic dermatitis, allergic rhinitis, or asthma	None	Sun exposure Dry skin	Sunscreen to prevent inflammation from sun exposure Emollients/moisturizers to face
None	Cosmetic concerns	Often genetic/familial	Sunscreen to protect the area from UV rays Cosmetic cover up if considered disfiguring Psoralen with UVA radiation in children over 12 years has been successful Refer to dermatologist for treatment
When associated with tuberous sclerosis: angiofibromas on face and nose, seizures, renal tumors, periungual fibromas, Shagreen patch (connective tissue nevus)	Lesions themselves do not cause complications, but many with associated findings in tuberous sclerosis	Autosomal dominant 100% penetrance 60% spontaneous mutation rate	None for macules If associated with tuberous sclerosis, should see appropriate specialists for associated symptoms
None	None	Autosomal dominant inheritance	Sunscreen to protect the area from UV rays
None	None	None	Sunscreen to protect the area from UV rays
Usually none, more common if family or patient history of vitiligo	None	Inflammation of preexisting nevus	None
None	None	None	Sunscreen to protect the area from UV rays

Other Diagnoses to Consider

- Idiopathic guttate hypomelanosis

- Chemical-induced hypopigmentation

- Albinism, partial

- Nevus anemicus (congenital macules that do not redden in response to vigorous rubbing)

- Waardenburg syndrome (autosomal dominant condition with white forelock, white patches on skin, heterochromia of irises, sensorineural deafness, and other defects)

When to Consider Further Evaluation or Treatment

- When tuberous sclerosis is suspected in a child with an ash leaf macule, referrals for the management of associated conditions should be made to genetics, pediatric neurology, and pediatric dermatology. Imaging should be done to identify tubers, which can occur in any organ and lead to sequelae.

- Patients with vitiligo should be seen by pediatric dermatologists for potential treatment to minimize cosmetic disfigurement.

- The central nevus in a halo nevus must be examined for atypical features.

SUGGESTED READINGS

Chan Y, Tay Y. Hypopigmentation disorders. In: Eichenfield, LF, Frieden IJ, Esterly NB. eds. *Neonatal Dermatology*. 2nd ed. Philadelphia, PA: Saunders Elsevier; 2008:375–396.

Lio PA. Little white spots: an approach to hypopigmented macules. *Arch Dis Child Educ Pract Ed.* 2008;93:98–102.

Taïeb A, Picardo M. Vitiligo. *N Eng J Med.* 2009;360:160–169.

Weinberg S, Prose NS, Kristal L, eds. *Color Atlas of Pediatric Dermatology*. 4th ed. New York, NY: McGraw Hill; 2007:267–284.

73

Hyperpigmented Rashes

Lee R. Atkinson-McEvoy

Approach to the Problem

Hyperpigmented lesions are caused by localized melanin deposition in the skin. Congenital lesions may occur over time as sun exposure increases the amount of melanin contained within these lesions. Patients and their families frequently have concerns about the cosmetic effects of these lesions and the malignant potential of certain lesions. A careful history and examination, following the lesions closely over time, and referring to appropriate specialists when needed, can reassure patients and families and often result in the correct diagnosis and management.

Key Points in the History

- A history of pustules present at birth that evolve into hyperpigmented macules is characteristic of neonatal pustular melanosis.

- Café au lait spots grow proportionally to overall body growth in the first few years of life and then stabilize.

- Café au lait spots may be a benign familial trait. A family history of neurofibromatosis and the presence of more than six café au lait spots should raise suspicion for neurofibromatosis.

- Only 1% of pigmented lesions at birth are congenital melanocytic nevi.

- Freckles are common in light-skinned, red-haired individuals, and are an autosomal-dominant, inherited trait.

- Freckles are induced by sunlight and are more prominent in the summer and fade in the winter.

- Acanthosis nigricans is associated with overweight/obesity, polycystic ovary syndrome, and the metabolic syndrome—particularly in association with diabetes mellitus with insulin resistance.

- Dermal melanocytosis (previously called Mongolian spots) fades after the first 5 to 10 years of life.

- A combination of small 1 to 3 mm hyperpigmented macules and pustules is seen in neonatal pustular melanosis.

- A complaint of a "dirty neck" is frequently associated with the physical finding of acanthosis nigricans, which is commonly seen in association with an elevated body mass index.

- Acanthosis nigricans has a velvety quality and may have papillomatous growths within the area of hyperpigmentation.

- Weight loss can result in improvement or resolution of acanthosis nigricans.

- Dermal melanocytosis is often seen in the sacral or gluteal areas, but may also be present elsewhere on the body, including the dorsum of the hand, the upper back, and the shoulders.

- Congenital melanocytic nevi vary in size and may be associated with hair often darker and longer than in surrounding areas.

- Tinea versicolor may be hyperpigmented or hypopigmented and often has scale.

- Blue nevi get their bluish color from the location of the melanocytes deep in the dermis.

- Nevoid hypermelanosis follows Blaschko lines on the extremities and appears linear; on the trunk, it can have a whorled pattern.

- In neurofibromatosis type 1, there are more than six café au lait macules at least 0.5 cm in size in prepubertal children, and there are associated findings of axillary or inguinal freckling, Lisch nodules (iris hamartomas), and neurofibromas.

PHOTOGRAPHS OF SELECTED DIAGNOSES

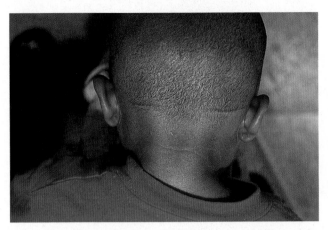

Figure 73-1 Postinflammatory hyperpigmentation.
Hyperpigmented linear lesions following skin trauma from a razor. (Courtesy of George A. Datto, III, MD.)

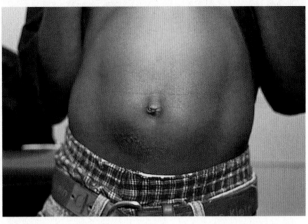

Figure 73-2 Hyperpigmentation resulting from nickel dermatitis. (Courtesy of George A. Datto, III, MD.)

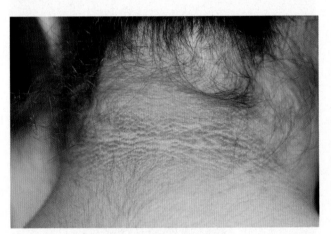

Figure 73-3 Acanthosis nigricans. Thickened velvety, hyperpigmented epidermis in the neck of obese child. (Courtesy of Ilona J. Frieden, MD.)

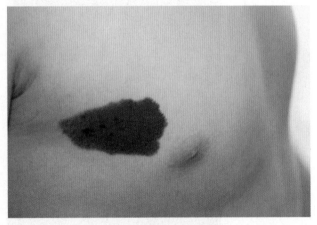

Figure 73-4 Congenital melanocytic nevus. A medium-sized, congenital, pigmented nevus on the trunk of an infant. (Courtesy of Ilona J. Frieden, MD.)

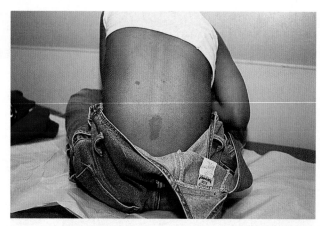

Figure 73-5 Café au lait spots. Multiple café au lait spots on the back of a child. (Courtesy of George A. Datto, III, MD.)

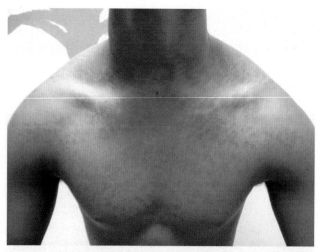

Figure 73-6 Tinea versicolor. While often hypopigmented, this rash may be hyperpigmented as in this individual. (Courtesy of Paul S. Matz, MD.)

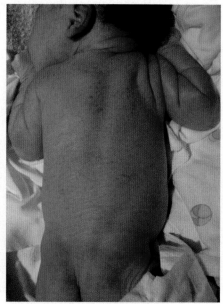

Figure 73-7 Neonatal pustular melanosis. Small hyperpigmented macules seen in a newborn. Often associated with pustules. (Courtesy of Amy Gilliam, MD.)

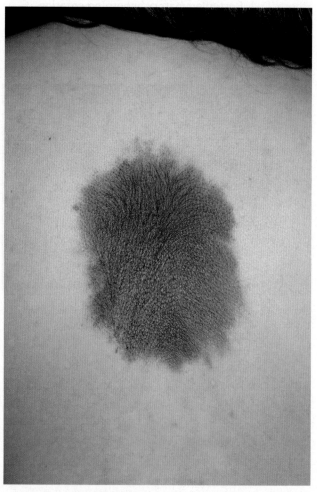

Figure 73-8 Congenital blue nevus. Bluish-discolored nevus that persists. (Courtesy of Ilona J. Frieden, MD.)

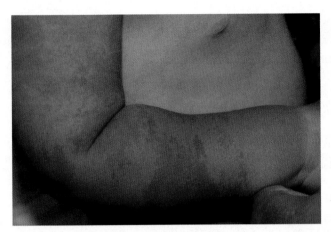

Figure 73-9 Nevoid hyperpigmentation. Previously called hypermelanosis of Ito, an irregular patterned area of hyperpigmentation. (Courtesy of Ilona J. Frieden, MD.)

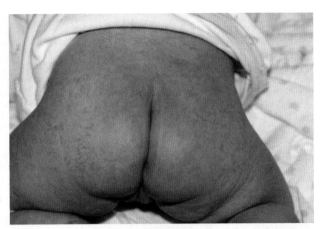

Figure 73-10 Dermal melanocytosis. Slate gray-colored macule on back of infant. (Courtesy of Ilona J. Frieden, MD.)

DIFFERENTIAL DIAGNOSIS

DIAGNOSIS		ICD-10	DISTINGUISHING CHARACTERISTICS	DISTRIBUTION	DURATION/ CHRONICITY
Postinflammatory Hyperpigmentation		L81.0	Increased pigment in area of previous injury or inflammation	Anywhere	Acute to chronic
Acanthosis Nigricans		L83	Velvety, hyperpigmented thickened skin in the skin folds	Frequently on neck, but can be seen in axilla, flexural surfaces	Chronic
Congenital Melanocytic Nevus (CMN)		D22.x Lip, x = 0 Eyelid, x = 1 Ear, x = 2 Face, x = 3 Scalp or neck, x = 4 Trunk, x = 5 Upper limb, x = 6 Lower limb, x = 7 Skin NOS, x = 9	Giant CMN >20 cm Large CMN 1.5–20 cm Small CMN <1.5 cm	Anywhere	Chronic
Café au Lait Spots		L81.3	Hyperpigmented macules	Anywhere	Chronic
Tinea Versicolor		B36.0	Scaly hyperpigmented or hypopigmented oval lesions that may be confluent	Usually on the chest, upper back, or shoulder	Chronic
Neonatal Pustular Melanosis		R21	1–3 mm hyperpigmented macules with accompanying pustules	Diffuse	Acute
Blue Nevus		D22.x Lip, x = 0 Eyelid, x = 1 Ear, x = 2 Face, x = 3 Scalp or neck, x = 4 Trunk, x = 5 Upper limb, x = 6 Lower limb, x = 7 Skin NOS, x = 9	Collection of melanocytes in deep dermis Small dome-shaped nodules	Anywhere	Chronic

ASSOCIATED FINDINGS	COMPLICATIONS	PREDISPOSING FACTORS	TREATMENT GUIDELINES
Healing site of injury or inflammation	Permanent hyperpigmentation	Inflammatory lesion	Treat inflammation/injury when present
Obesity	Associated with metabolic syndrome (diabetes mellitus, fatty liver, elevated cholesterol)	Obesity/overweight	Weight loss can result in improvement of appearance
None	Cosmetic concerns Giant CMN in the head and neck region is associated with leptomeningeal melanocytosis and associated with neurological disorders such as epilepsy. Lesions over the spine can be associated with underlying spinal defects.	None	Refer to dermatology due to risk of malignant change
Can be familial with numerous café au lait spots without other associated features Consider neurofibromatosis type I when there are more than six cafe au lait spots greater than or equal to 0.5 cm in size, axillary freckling, neurofibromas, or Lisch nodules. Consider McCune Albright syndrome when there are a small number of large, dark, cafe au lait spots with jagged edges.	Specific to associated conditions	Hereditary	If isolated, no further management If associated with neurofibromatosis type 1 or other genetic syndrome, appropriate management of underlying condition
Rare complaints of pruritus	May be difficult to treat	Infection with fungus, *Malassezia furfur* or *Microsporum* sp. Thrives in hot, humid climates	Ketoconazole shampoo or selenium sulfide 2.5% applied daily for 1 week then monthly for 3 months
None	None	None	None
None	Cosmetic concerns	None	Low risk of malignant change

(continued)

SECTION 15 • SKIN

DIFFERENTIAL DIAGNOSIS *(continued)*

DIAGNOSIS	ICD-10	DISTINGUISHING CHARACTERISTICS	DISTRIBUTION	DURATION/ CHRONICITY
Nevoid Hyperpigmentation	L81.9	Linear or whorled areas of hyperpigmentation	Usually on trunk	Chronic Present at birth or develops shortly afterwards May be more apparent in the first 2 years of life
Dermal Melanocytosis (Previously Called Mongolian Spot)	D22.5	Blue-gray area of hyperpigmentation Caused by melanocytes in deep dermis	75% are in the sacro-gluteal area but can occur elsewhere	Chronic, fades in the first 5–10 years of life
Freckles (Ephelis)	L81.2	Red-tan macules 2–3 mm in size	Usually on face, arms, chest, and back Can occur in any sun-exposed area	Chronic, first appear at age 3–5 years

ASSOCIATED FINDINGS	COMPLICATIONS	PREDISPOSING FACTORS	TREATMENT GUIDELINES
None	None	None	None
None	None	Common among infants of African, Hispanic and Asian descent	None needed
Most common in children with fair skin, blue eyes, and light hair Autosomal-dominant inheritance	None	Sun exposure	None for freckles but, because these patients often have fairer skin, they should use sunscreen to prevent sunburn

Other Diagnoses to Consider

- Hormone-induced hyperpigmentation of the genitalia in normal newborns

- Xeroderma pigmentosa

- McCune–Albright syndrome

- Lentigines (such as Peutz–Jeghers syndrome)

- Other syndromes with associated café au lait spots, including Noonan syndrome, LEOPARD, Costello syndrome, and Cardio-Facio-Cutaneous syndrome

- Malignant melanoma

When to Consider Further Evaluation or Treatment

- Congenital melanocytic nevi have potential for malignant transformation, so they should be referred to a dermatologist for potential excision.

- Multiple café au lait spots with any associated abnormalities of the eye, seizures, developmental abnormalities, endocrine dyscrasias, or any other abnormalities should be investigated for neurofibromatosis type 1, McCune–Albright syndrome, and other associated syndromes.

- If tinea versicolor does not respond to topical treatments, consider further management with alternative topical or oral antifungal treatment.

- Children with acanthosis nigricans who are significantly overweight should be evaluated for diabetes mellitus, metabolic syndrome, or polycystic ovary syndrome. Individuals with these disorders should be evaluated by a pediatric endocrinologist.

SUGGESTED READINGS

Taïeb A, Boralevi F. Hypermelanoses of the newborn and of the infant. *Dermatol Clin.* 2007;25:327–336.
Weinberg S, Prose NS, Kristal L, eds. *Color Atlas of Pediatric Dermatology.* 4th ed. New York, NY: McGraw Hill; 2007:267–284.
Paller AS, Mancini AJ, eds. *Hurwitz Clinical Pediatric Dermatology: A Textbook of Skin Disorders of Childhood and Adolescence.* 4th ed. Philadelphia, PA: Elsevier Saunders; 2011:20–23.

74

Bullous Rashes

Beth A. Shortridge

Approach to the Problem

Blister-associated rashes in children are divided into two groups: *vesicular* rashes and *bullous* rashes. By definition, vesicles are fluid-filled lesions that are no more than 0.5 cm in diameter and bullae are blistering lesions that are greater than 0.5 cm in diameter. They may be seen in the skin or mucous membranes and may be round or have irregular borders. Compared with adult skin, that of pediatric patients is very prone to blistering. Vesicular rashes are common in the pediatric population, and are discussed elsewhere. Bullous rashes, on the other hand, are a relatively uncommon class of pediatric skin disorders.

Bullae form secondary to fluid accumulation between cells in the epidermis or between the epidermal and dermal (subepidermal) skin layers. Bullous skin disorders can be divided into *congenital* disorders, such as congenital epidermolysis bullosa (EB); *infectious* disorders, such as bullous impetigo and staphylococcal scalded skin syndrome (SSSS), *immunologic* disorders, such as Stevens–Johnson syndrome (SJS), toxic epidermal necrolysis (TEN), chronic bullous dermatosis/disease of childhood, and *toxin-mediated* such as phototoxic or venom reactions.

Key Points in the History

- Systemic symptoms such as fever, fussiness, ill appearance, and diffuse skin involvement are associated with SJS, TEN, and SSSS.

- Congenital blistering diseases, such as EB, are often present at birth or during the newborn period.

- Bullae appearing in the first few days or weeks of life may be secondary to EB, bullous impetigo of the neonate, or SSSS.

- In EB, bullae form at sites of minor skin trauma or friction.

- With the exception of TEN, the more common bullous skin disorders involve only the epidermis and may cause temporary hyperpigmentation and lichenification but do not tend to cause permanent scarring.

- Although many believe SJS and TEN are a continuum of the same disease, one convention is that infectious agents are causally related to SJS, and drugs to TEN.

- Chronic bullous disease of childhood is rare, but it is the most common acquired autoimmune bullous disease in children; it is only rarely present in the neonate.

Key Points in the Physical Examination

- Photosensitivity rashes are seen on exposed parts of the body, primarily the face and extremities.

- Bullous impetigo differs from nonbullous impetigo. Distribution is more truncal with a predilection for intertriginous areas, including the diaper area.

- Nikolsky sign—the ability to use gentle traction with a finger to separate the upper epidermis from the underlying skin in bullous lesions—is commonly seen in systemic bullous disorders, including TEN, SSSS, and EB.

- Mucous membrane involvement is seen in TEN, SJS, and in more severe forms of EB but not in SSSS.

- In bullous impetigo, photosensitivity rashes, EB, and SSSS, bullae are seen on the skin; in SJS/TEN, they are also seen on the mucous membranes of the mouth, nares, conjunctivae, and the anorectal and perineal areas.

- Conjunctivae are involved in SSSS (erythema) and SJS and TEN (mucositis).

- In chronic bullous dermatosis/disease of childhood, the lesions are often annular and appear like a "string of pearls"; lesions initially mimic bullous impetigo, herpetic diseases, or bullous erythema multiforme.

PHOTOGRAPHS OF SELECTED DIAGNOSES

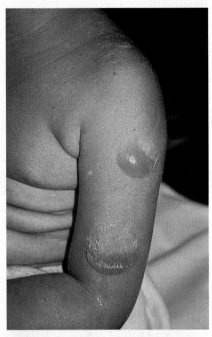

Figure 74-1 Photosensitivity. Large blisters that developed on the second day following prolonged sun exposure. (Courtesy of George A. Datto, III, MD.)

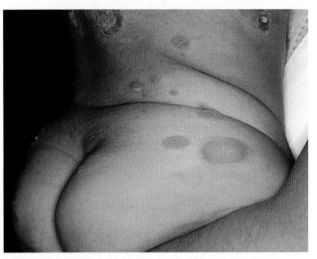

Figure 74-2 Bullous impetigo. (Used with permission from Fleisher GR, Ludwig S, Baskin MN. *Atlas of Pediatric Emergency Medicine.* Philadelphia, PA: Lippincott Williams & Wilkins; 2004:200.)

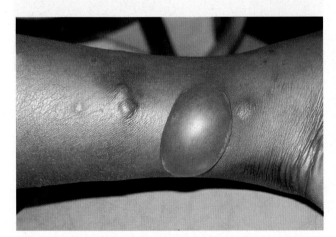

Figure 74-3 Bullous insect bite reaction. (Used with permission from Goodheart HP. *Goodheart's Photoguide to Common Skin Disorders.* 2nd ed. Philadelphia, PA: Lippincott Williams & Wilkins; 2003:3.)

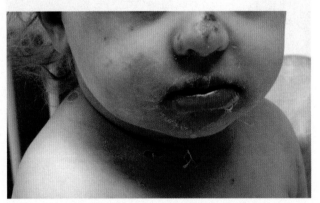

Figure 74-4 Staphylococcal scalded skin syndrome with ruptured bullae. (Courtesy of Gary Marshall, MD.)

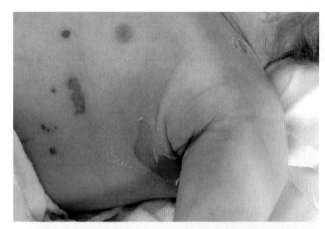

Figure 74-5 Staphylococcal scalded skin syndrome. "Scalded" skin underlying ruptured bulla in SSSS. (Courtesy of Gary Marshall, MD.)

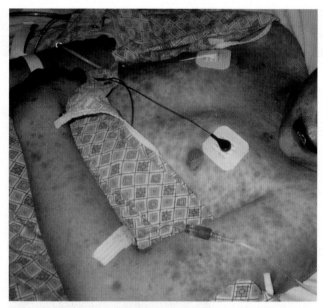

Figure 74-6 Target-like purpuric lesions of Stevens–Johnson syndrome. (Courtesy of Gary Marshall, MD.)

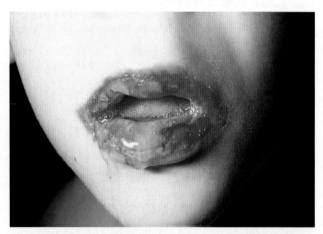

Figure 74-7 Hemorrhagic ulcerative stomatitis in SJS. (Courtesy of Joseph Lopreiato, MD.)

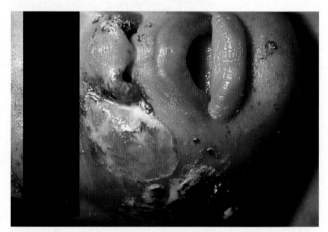

Figure 74-8 Epidermolysis bullosa. Note the ruptured bullous lesion. (Courtesy of Joseph Lopreiato, MD.)

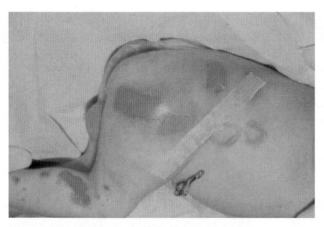

Figure 74-9 Epidermolysis bullosa congenita.
(Used with permission from The Benjamin Barankin
Dermatology Collection.)

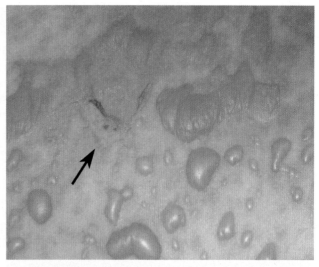

Figure 74-10 Toxic epidermal necrolysis. Nikolski sign
(arrow). (Used with permission from Mulholland MW,
Maier RV, et al. *Greenfield's Surgery: Scientific Principles
and Practice*. 4th ed. Philadelphia, PA: Lippincott Williams &
Wilkins; 2006.)

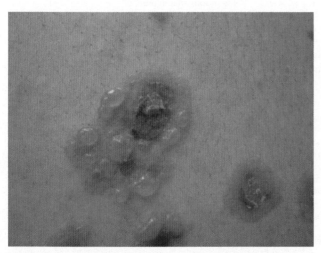

**Figure 74-11 Linear IgA Disease (Chronic Bullous
Disease of Childhood).** Note "pearls on a string" in an
annular pattern. (Used with permission from Dr. Barankin's
Dermatology Collection.)

DIFFERENTIAL DIAGNOSIS

DIAGNOSIS	ICD-10	DISTINGUISHING CHARACTERISTICS	DISTRIBUTION	ONSET/ CHRONICITY
Photosensitivity/ Phototoxic	L56.8 Other specified acute skin changes due to UV radiation	Exaggerated sunburn Occurs in all age groups Vesicles and bullae in severe cases Pruritic Onset after sun exposure: minutes to hours (phototoxic); 48–72 hours (allergic)	Sun-exposed areas of skin Often involves face, upper neck ("V" portion), hands, forearms Covered and shadowed areas of body are spared.	Acute May recur
Bullous Impetigo	L01.03	More common in infants and young children Child does not appear ill. Mucous membranes not involved Bullae leave scaly collarette of peeling skin May have weeping surface under denuded bullae	Warm, moist areas	Acute
Staphylococcal Scalded Skin Syndrome	L00	Onset frequently 3–7 days of life Vast majority, onset <6 years of age Appears as diffuse erythema that blanches Bullae rupture leaving skin "scalded" Conjunctivae, but not other mucous membranes, may be involved. Fluid inside bullae is sterile and clear. May be clinically indistinguishable from TEN	Initial lesions: small pustules in diaper area or lower abdomen or erythema with or without crusting around the mouth, diaper area, or umbilicus Spreads diffusely	Acute
Stevens– Johnson Syndrome	L51.1	Most common in children and young adults Viral-like prodrome, then rapid development of rash and bullae (24 hours) Bullae found on mucous membranes, and in severe cases on skin (SJS–TEN continuum) Target lesions or nonpalpable purpura <10% of BSA involvement in uncomplicated SJS	May be localized to trunk, palms, and soles, or generalized Always involves mucous membranes (mouth, eyes, genitals, perianal, or anorectal area)	Acute following prodrome of 1–2 weeks Duration of oral lesions may last months
Toxic Epidermal Necrolysis	L51.2	More common in adults In children, males more often affected, reverse gender predilection in adults May be clinically indistinguishable from SSSS in neonates Full-thickness loss of epidermis >30% of body surface involvement	Begins with mucous membrane involvement similar to SJS, but progresses to diffuse epidermal involvement with full-thickness loss of epidermis	Acute following prodrome; if drug related, prodrome 1–3 weeks after exposure

ASSOCIATED FINDINGS	COMPLICATIONS	PREDISPOSING FACTORS	TREATMENT GUIDELINES
Pruritus Areas of contact dermatitis Occasional onycholysis	Healing with hyperpigmentation and lichenification May see recurrence even after discontinuation of offending agent Systemic lupus erythematosus may present with photosensitivity.	Drug exposure Skin products Family history	Identification and withdrawal of suspected drug or topical agent Sun avoidance and protection Cool compresses Consider topical corticosteroids.
Outbreaks in close contacts, such as family members Bullae contain *S. aureus* with exfoliative toxin A	Cellulitis from progressive infection (more common in nonbullous impetigo)	*Staphylococcus aureus* producing exfoliative toxin A	Topical vs systemic anti-staphylococcal antibiotics even if systemic symptoms are not present
Fever, fussiness, ill-appearing Positive Nikolsky sign Bullae and underlying skin may be extremely painful. Flaking desquamation after acute phase	Sepsis Cellulitis Loss of hair and nails Osteomyelitis Pneumonia Fungal or bacterial superinfection Fluid and electrolyte disturbances Mortality higher with increasing age	Asymptomatic staphylococcal pustulosis Some consider SSSS in a continuum with bullous impetigo	Multiple cultures from blood and possible sources of infection, but not from bullae, which are considered sterile Systemic anti-staphylococcal antibiotics including anti-MRSA agents if exposure possible Barrier emollients Stabilize patient with fluids and electrolytes Pain management Biopsy in older children to rule out TEN Transfer to burn unit, if indicated Prevention: promote good hygiene practices
Weakness Lethargy Pneumonia Severe eye involvement in most cases: conjunctivitis, ulcerations, uveitis Nephritis Ulcerative/hemorrhagic stomatitis from oral lesions	Severe dehydration Secondary infection Respiratory failure Renal failure Gastric perforation Blindness Mortality: less than 10% Body Surface Area (BSA) involvement <10%; 10%–30% = "SJS/TEN overlap"; >50% SJS/TEN Children have long-term sequelae. Recurs in up to 20% children with SJS/TEN	Infection, including mycoplasma, HSV, and viral upper respiratory tract infections Drug exposure to antiepileptics, sulfonamides, penicillin derivatives HLA-B*1502 genotype in Asians at risk for carbamazepine-induced SJS	Transfer to burn unit if >10% body surface area (BSA) affected with blisters Stabilize and support Identify and remove or treat suspected causative agent(s). Colloidal baths/wet compresses Biological/synthetic or semi-synthetic wraps with or without antimicrobials Histamine-1 blockers Topical analgesics for oral lesions Infection prevention and treatment
See SJS Mucous membrane involvement (eyes, mouth) Positive Nikolsky sign Painful erythematous skin	Fluid and electrolyte imbalance Ocular sequelae in 30% (including blindness) Overwhelming sepsis All organ systems may be involved; gastrointestinal, respiratory, ocular most commonly Mortality up to 30%, but is decreasing with better recognition and improved supportive care	Drug exposure, most commonly analgesics Nonsteroidal anti-inflammatory agents antibacterial, antifungal medications, and antiepileptics Idiopathic etiology more common in children	Same as SJS Transfer to burn unit Pain management Enteral feedings Steroid use is controversial. High-dose early IVIG thought to be efficacious Plasmapheresis—optional

(continued)

SECTION 15 • SKIN

DIFFERENTIAL DIAGNOSIS *(continued)*

DIAGNOSIS	ICD-10	DISTINGUISHING CHARACTERISTICS	DISTRIBUTION	ONSET/ CHRONICITY
Epidermolysis Bullosa	Q81.9 EB, unspecified	Bullae often present at birth Inherited skin disorder Four major subtypes: EB simplex, junctional EB, dystrophic EB and Kindler syndrome; multiple minor subtypes	Most commonly involves hands and feet, but also other areas of minor trauma	Recurrent/Chronic
Chronic Bullous Disease of Childhood	L12.2 Chronic bullous disease of childhood	Linear IgA disease of childhood—autoimmune "string of jewels or pearls" appearance Typically age 6 months to 6 years Tense, not flaccid, bullae Bullae may be hemorrhagic Mucosal lesions less common Mucosal lesions erosions, not vesicular	Widespread More abundant on lower abdomen, thighs, and groin Perioral lesions common in younger children Often annular "targetoid" lesions	Onset insidious Relapsing over months to 4 years

ASSOCIATED FINDINGS	COMPLICATIONS	PREDISPOSING FACTORS	TREATMENT GUIDELINES
Severe types: scarring at previously involved sites Oral involvement Nail dystrophy Palmar and plantar hyperkeratosis; other organ involvement	Hyperpigmentation Superinfection Sepsis In severe types: scarring contractures, ocular, tracheolaryngeal, gastrointestinal complications Skin cancer in adulthood Failure to thrive Fatal cardiomyopathy	Family history Bullae form at sites of minor trauma Diagnosis can be made by prenatal chorionic villous sampling at 10–12 weeks gestation	Avoid mechanical trauma and friction. Padding and cool environment Emollients, hydrocolloid gels Debridement as needed Prevent bacterial infection Treat for bacterial infection as needed Genetic counseling
Constitutional symptoms or prodrome uncommon Pruritus before or with eruption Usually no suspicious drug exposure Several clinical differences from adult disease	Significant morbidity due to extent and duration of lesions Cosmetic and social consequences Adverse events of medications Ocular scarring Mucosal scarring	Clinically nonfamilial Unlikely drug-induced Genetic markers HLA B8, Cw7, and DR3 are implicated in some patients.	Skin biopsy in most cases with immunofluorescence studies Sulfapyridine Dapsone Erythromycin Colchicine Limited use of systemic corticosteroids

Other Diagnoses to Consider

- Pemphigus

- Bullous pemphigoid

- Epidermolytic hyperkeratosis (bullous ichthyosis)

- Toxic shock syndrome

- Bullous scabies

- Insect and arachnid bites

- Thermal trauma

- Bullous varicella

- Juvenile dermatitis herpetiformis

- Erythema multiforme with bullae

When to Consider Further Evaluation or Treatment

- Skin biopsy strongly recommended in atypical SSSS or SJS, all TEN and persistent or refractory disease.

- Patients with suspected SSSS, SJS, and TEN need close monitoring for other organ system involvement and life-threatening complications.

- Complicated SSSS, SJS, and all TEN should be managed in a burn unit.

SUGGESTED READINGS

Cole C, Gazewood J. Diagnosis and treatment of impetigo. *Am Fam Physician.* 2007;75:859–864.
Drucker AM, Rosen CF. Drug-induced photosensitivity culprit drugs, management and prevention. *Drug Saf.* 2011;34(10):821–837.
Fine J-D. Inherited epidermolysis bullosa: recent basic and clinical advances. *Curr Opin Pediatr.* 2010;22:453–458.
Finkelstein Y, Soon G, Acuna P, et al. Recurrence and outcomes of Stevens-Johnson syndrome and toxic epidermal necrolysis in children. *Pediatrics.* 2011;128:723–728.
Gerull R, Nelle M, Schaible T. Toxic epidermal necrolysis and Stevens-Johnson syndrome: a review. *Crit Care Med.* 2011;39:1521–1532.
Mintz EM, Morel KD. Clinical features, diagnosis, and pathogenesis of chronic bullous disease of childhood. *Dermatol Clin.* 2011;29:459–462.

Index

Note: Page numbers followed by "*f*" denote figures.

615